Ultimate Immunity

SUPERCHARGE YOUR BODY'S NATURAL HEALING POWERS

Elson Haas, MD, and Sondra Barrett, PhD

RODALE.

This book is intended as a reference volume only, not as a medical manual.
The information given here is designed to help you make informed decisions about your health.
It is not intended as a substitute for any treatment that may have been prescribed by your doctor.
If you suspect that you have a medical problem, we urge you to seek competent medical help.

Mention of specific companies, organizations, or authorities in this book does not imply
endorsement by the author or publisher, nor does mention of specific companies, organizations,
or authorities imply that they endorse this book, its author, or the publisher.

Internet addresses and telephone numbers given in this book were accurate at the time it went to press.

Printed in the United States of America

Book design by Christina Gaugler

Illustrations by Michael Gellately

ISBN: 978–1–62336–390–1

We inspire and enable people to improve their lives and the world around them.
rodalebooks.com

To all of our students, whose questions guided us to learn more.

*To our children—Sondra's Heather and Ted and Elson's Ishara and Orion,
and Sondra's grandchildren, Ethan, Harper, Micah, and Bennie,
and Elson's yet to come—may you all benefit from the wisdom in this book
and, of course, from the love in our hearts.*

*To our parents, who encouraged us to live life with love
and make a difference for others.*

*To our readers—may your immunity be strong and vital, and keep you well.
And may you enjoy a new, vibrant lifestyle.*

*And lastly to our Mother Earth's immune system—may your waters,
soil, and air be healed, so that the aligned immune systems
of all your children can be healed as well.*

CONTENTS

ACKNOWLEDGMENTS

For both of us, this book has been a labor of love. We hung in there together through all the writing and research—even when we got frustrated, we did our work with great affection, focus, and persistence.

There are so many people to thank for making this book possible. We express our gratitude:

To the thousands of research scientists whose curiosity and persistence showed the way into the vast workings of the immune system and the mind; and to the physicians and patients who helped to expand our understanding.

To Bethany Argisle, our friend and longtime business associate, whose vision and energy led to our collaboration in *Ultimate Immunity*.

To Nancy Fitzgerald, our editor at Rodale, who guided us throughout, improving what we wrote and encouraging us to stretch our limits and make this a valuable book for you, the readers.

To the Rodale Test Kitchen, including JoAnn Brader and Jennifer Kushnier, who lovingly cooked up and tasted our recipes, and to cookbook editor Katie Kackenmeister.

To the Rodale design team, especially Chris Gaugler and Amy King, and to the Rodale production team, including Nancy Bailey, Sara Cox, and Chris Krogermeier, who all worked together to create this beautiful book.

To April Alexandra, who makes Dr. Haas's life easier and more entertaining every day, and who believed in us and nourished us and our immune systems with beautiful meals and garden flowers during our writing and work meetings.

INTRODUCTION

As you enter the pages of this book, we invite you to explore the amazing immune system while discovering more about your own health and learning new strategies for healthier living. *Ultimate Immunity* brings together the science and common sense for creating a balanced immune system and improving your well-being. We'll cover the basics of how your immune system works and what happens when it doesn't operate at its best. Then we'll offer solutions for bringing the many activities of your immune network into harmony by enjoying healthy foods, cooling down inflammation, managing stress, and doing special energy movements. You'll also find simple, practical plans for cleansing and detoxifying your body, calming your mind, and—ultimately—enjoying your life more fully.

We write this book weaving together our two different perspectives yet similar backgrounds that embrace natural, ancient healing methods. Sondra, a medical scientist trained in immunology, is experienced in educating and guiding people with mind-body strategies for healing. Elson is a medical practitioner dedicated to writing and speaking about natural medicine, detoxification, and healing as a personal learning experience. He focuses on helping people get and stay healthy, with an emphasis on preventing disease and supporting healthy aging.

Both of us want to make a difference in your health with simple and effective solutions. In this book, we bring our knowledge and experience together to help anyone who is challenged by an immune condition.

SONDRA: As a laboratory scientist exploring how immune cells fight infections and what makes a normal cell become a cancer cell, I strayed out of the lab and into the lives of people struggling with cancer and autoimmune illnesses. Over the last three decades, I've been bridging biomedical science with the vast array of mind-body strategies—meditation, energy awareness, imagery, shamanism, and expressive arts—that can help people, including myself, manage the stresses of life.

As an educator, I've listened to people's questions about how stress impacts the immune system and what diminishes the damage that stress can make on personal health. I've always been inspired by people's questions and problems—they have spurred me to learn more. And that's why I was so excited to write this book with Elson.

My perspective is unique for a scientist. I have a deep knowledge of biochemistry, immunology, and the workings of the body, along with practical experience in the inner workings of the mind and its impact on our choices and health. My earlier book, *Secrets of Your Cells*, brings together the science, spirituality, and mysteries of our cells. *Ultimate Immunity* permitted me to focus on the amazing immune system, which, in my mind, encompasses the total healing system of the body. This new book is our offering to you.

ELSON: This book is very personal to me. Decades ago, I was able to clear my allergies through using the same principles described in these pages. I also was able to improve my overall health—I believe I prevented many of the illnesses common to my family members. And now, after working with Sondra on this book, I am even more impressed in seeing how much influence our immune system has on our overall health.

Throughout my career, I have always looked for the underlying and deeper causes of disease. To me, our health is the result of our genetic potentials and the actions we choose to take daily. Our behaviors affect the expression of our genes—what we do does influence our genetic proclivities. This is really important to know, that your actions and lifestyle greatly influence whether you get certain diseases or not. There is an exploding new field of research called epigenetics that is beginning to show that how we live life influences which genes are expressed; you'll hear a bit more about this later in the book.

From 40 years of clinical family practice, I often see people get better from embracing natural treatments rather than depending on the usual antibiotics, antiallergy medicines, or steroids. This natural healing approach encompasses shifts in food choices, nutritional and herbal supplements, and the power of the mind.

AN INVITATION

Ultimate Immunity is a guidebook to everything you ever wanted to know about immune health. We build a framework of how the complex immune network functions and then show you what can go wrong, presenting the latest theories and ideas. One thing is certain: Regardless of the cause of any immune illness, inflammation is the underlying factor in almost all of the symptoms, and it's a contributing factor in other illnesses such as heart disease, diabetes, Alzheimer's, and even obesity. So one important focus of the book is how to lessen or "cool down" inflammation.

Because we live in the West and enjoy the benefits of modern medicine, we explain how the typical physician treats immune problems such as frequent infections, allergies, and autoimmune illnesses. Our emphasis, though, is on more natural self-care approaches, and that's how *Ultimate Immunity* becomes your guidebook. You'll learn about the usual medications prescribed for immune problems—but we'll take you beyond the usual and into a variety of alternative and effective approaches. Preventing problems of immune imbalance is much more rewarding than trying to treat them after they emerge. More antibiotic-resistant germs are gaining ground because of the unnecessary use of too many antibiotics. To avoid this, you need to know when and if an antibiotic is truly the answer to your problem, when to consider natural remedies initially to help, and, of course, how to keep your immune system strong and healthy so that it can protect you from dangerous microbes.

First, you'll discover which nutrients and foods are immune superpowers—those that boost immune activities and those that, when deficient, can impair your health. After all, if your cells don't have what they need to function optimally, they'll let you down. Then we'll provide eating programs like the 5-Day Elimination, Healing Plan and the Immune-Power Eating Plan (I-PEP) to make it easier for you to choose those foods that you—and your immune cells—will enjoy and that will empower your health.

> *A healthy outside starts from the inside.*
> —ROBERT URICH

But it's not only food that will keep your immune cells working well. You also need to be active and manage your stress as you enjoy the pleasures of life. You'll have the opportunity to explore different ways to reduce your stress and find the approach that works best for you.

We bring you a broad range of healing strategies, including two complementary approaches—imagery and qigong. Imagery will help you experience relaxation and address a variety of immune problems. Qigong, a moving meditation practice based on ancient Chinese medicine, will help you balance your immune warriors while enhancing your energy.

We've put all these strategies together into a Cool Down Inflammation Prevention Program that we believe will be useful and personally meaningful to you.

> *The environment is everything that isn't me.*
> —ALBERT EINSTEIN

AN ENVIRONMENTAL PERSPECTIVE

You can do all the right things—eat nutritious foods, take helpful supplements, and manage your stress—but if you live near a freeway, stay inside with your eyes glued to a computer screen, or live a lonely life without much social support, you're contributing to potential problems for your immune cells. You are not separate from your environment. The health of your environment affects you at every level. And all of us together affect what's happening on the planet.

> *Humankind has not woven the web of life. We are but one thread*
> *within it. Whatever we do to the web, we do to ourselves.*
> *All things are bound together . . . all things connect.*
> —CHIEF SEATTLE

The health of the Earth is challenged, and many scientists tell us we have little time for healing it. As a result of climate change and agricultural chemicals, the monarch butterflies are disappearing, the moose in Minnesota are nearly extinct, and our oceans and rivers are contaminated with toxic chemicals and metals like mercury. Advances in agriculture, technology, and medicine, which have brought amazing benefits, have also brought some dangerous consequences.

Even if you can't save the world by yourself, you can each do your part. You can make choices to protect yourself and your family from toxicity by using fewer polluting chemicals in your daily life, by purchasing organically grown and nongenetically modified foods, by recycling, by buying fewer packaged products, and so much more.

Each of your choices can help heal climate change and global toxicity. Can you designate 1 day a week for not driving a motor vehicle? Can you lessen your red meat consumption? Can you have a "no screen" day? And since it seems that water may be our most valuable commodity, can you conserve this resource in creative new ways? All of these actions can alter your own health as well as that of the Earth—and help to keep your immune system strong.

IT'S PERSONAL AND IMPORTANT

No matter what symptoms, conditions, or diseases you or your family members may be experiencing, making simple, positive changes in lifestyle behaviors can improve your condition and even your life. From your dietary choices to the ways you handle stress to your efforts to improve your fitness, you have the power to support your immune system and enhance your health.

We are excited to bring you *Ultimate Immunity*. Your immune system provides the foundation for your general well-being and protects you from the bad germs in your environment. When your immune system is strong and balanced, it's less likely to overreact with an allergic response to safe substances in food or the environment, or to trigger an autoimmune condition against your own tissues. It's also less likely to fail when the next flu epidemic arrives. It keeps you well when you maintain balance by taking good care of yourself—your body, your mind, and your spirit. You deserve the best!

> *Take care of your body. It's the only place you have to live.*
> —JIM ROHN

Sondra Barrett, PhD, and Elson M. Haas, MD,
Sonoma County, California

CHAPTER 1

Immunity 101: Getting *to* Know Your Immune Network

You've had a few stressful weeks. There's a deadline looming for a big project you're working on, so you've been eating on the run, grabbing whatever's quick and easy. No time for sitting down to enjoy a meal with your family, and even less time to relax.

Then, from out of the blue, the thing you need the least: You wake up with a hint of a sore throat. By the end of the day, your nose is dripping and you begin coughing. Why now? Maybe your immune system is as stressed out as you are, and you just can't cope with one more assault.

Here's what's probably going on: Worn out with worry and work, you stopped taking good care of yourself and didn't pay attention to what you really needed. So the *cells** that protect you from germs took time out, too, allowing viruses to set up house in your body and ultimately sending you to bed.

But before your head even hits the pillow, you're bombarded with advice. Everybody and their cousin has a favorite home remedy, and ads for cold medicine seem to pop up everywhere. Some of those medicines might weaken the viruses that are knocking you out. But more likely, those little bugs will grab hold and make you feel lousy for a few days.

---

*Italicized terms are defined in the Glossary, starting on page 308.

Are you helpless against everything from the common cold to a bout of pneumonia? Well, not exactly.

What happens when you're exposed to all those microbes that can make you sick is partly up to you. One of our goals for this book is to guide you in knowing how to care for and feed your all-powerful immune healing system. With the right approach, you're less likely to get sick, and if you do become ill, you're more likely to bounce back a bit quicker.

A speedy recovery is thanks to the hard work of your immune system. Your body is constantly exposed to microbes—it's actually home to trillions of *bacteria*. In fact, there are more microbes in your body than your own cells, and yet you avoid getting any kind of infectious illness from these microbes inside you. An amazing collaboration between your cells and the "magic *molecules*" they produce keeps you protected from both what's inside you as well as what can invade from the outside world. How come you don't catch everything that's going around? The short answer: your amazing immune system, the focus of this book.

Sometimes, a vast army of microbes sneaks past your immune defenses and threatens to make you ill with an *infection*—from a simple cold to herpes or measles; from food poisoning to a life-threatening bout of hepatitis. Generally, these infections are self-limited as your body rallies to fight off the invaders; at other times, you need stronger support.

This book provides a treasure trove of information about how the vast immune network works to protect you and how you can nurture it so that potentially harmful microbes—known as pathogens—don't make you sick. You'll learn what the consequences are if and when our immune system is thrown out of balance and becomes misguided. Then you'll need strategies to strengthen it or calm it down. By getting to know and care for your immune system, you can help it deliver better care to you.

MEET YOUR IMMUNE SYSTEM

If it's been a long time since you had high school or college biology, these first two chapters may seem pretty technical and heady. After all, we're providing you with a basic scientific overview of how this very complicated system functions. Don't worry—the rest of the book veers away from hard science. You can read ahead and come back here when you need to understand a specific point.

What exactly is the immune system, and where is it located? Turns out, it's not just parked in one place. It has outposts all over your body. It's really a protection or guardian network, since the immune cells connect with every other system and part of your body. This network encompasses your skin, bone marrow, organs like the *thymus* and spleen, hormones and molecular messengers, as well as your brain, muscles, and even your mind. This network is a master of communications, and it consists of four main parts:

- **Physical barriers,** such as your skin, saliva, tears, and stomach acid
- **White blood cells,** including *phagocytes* and *lymphocytes*
- **Organs** where immune cells are produced (thymus and bone marrow) and where they do most of their work (lymph nodes and spleen)
- **Molecules,** including *antibodies* and *cytokines*

Although the immune system is spread throughout your entire body and has lots of different functions, it features two kinds of immune cells with specific jobs to provide both short-term "inborn" protection and lifelong protection.

PHAGOCYTES are *white blood cells* that engulf and destroy anything they consider to be "foreign." They act fast, yet they'll never remember the foe. They're part of your short-term natural instinctive *immunity*.

LYMPHOCYTES, though, are in the battle for the long haul. They're called in to manufacture specific weapons against their "favorite" microbe. They're smart, trainable cells with additional skills as warriors and managers. In general, their responses take longer to develop than those of the phagocytes, since lymphocytes have to hone their abilities whereas phagocytes are born with their know-how. (One exception: the *natural killer lymphocyte*, or NK cell, which responds quickly after a virus has made its way inside you. The NK cell is part of your *innate immune response*, just like the phagocytes.)

Your immune cells don't operate alone, though; they're influenced by what you think, what you do, and the choices you make every day. Chronic *stress*, depression, poor sleep, or a steady diet of junk food can keep them from working at their best.[1] But there's good news: You can improve and rebalance your immune functions with stress-reduction strategies; healthy, nutritious food; the right supplements; a good night's sleep; and healthy, supportive relationships. And here's a bonus: Laughter and love also strengthen immunity and boost your mood.[2]

Even your attitudes and beliefs contribute to your immune functions. After all, attitudes don't simply stay inside your head. They direct your emotions and your behaviors. Your behaviors and daily choices—whether or not to exercise, smoke, take long walks, or talk to a friend—all affect the health of your immune system and, ultimately, your overall health and well-being.

Although the immune system is viewed as one system, its cells, organs, and chemicals are distributed throughout your body and are in constant communication. Sometimes called a roving sensory network, your immune cells patrol your whole body. When they're working well, you don't even know they're there. But when they're overwhelmed by an invading army of germs or get confused about what's safe and what's not, you may find yourself with infections, *allergies*, or an *autoimmune disease*.

Let's zero in on how this complex network functions and how it protects you from

HOW HEALTHY IS YOUR IMMUNE NETWORK?

To see how the immune network is involved in your health, take a few minutes to reflect on these questions.

1. Do you get frequent colds, more than three a year?   (Y)   N

2. Do you often experience itchy, red skin?   Y   (N)

3. Do you seem to have a runny nose most of the time?   Y   (N)

4. Do you get an upset stomach when you eat certain foods?   Y   (N)

5. Do you put on weight no matter how hard you try to lose it?   (Y)   N

6. Do you often have trouble getting a good night's sleep?   Y   (N)

Score! Tally up your yes and no responses. If you've answered yes to two or more questions, your immune system could use a recharge. The problems you're experiencing could result from a misguided immunity.

a host of problems. Later, in Chapter 2, you'll learn what happens when the network becomes misguided and immune cells destroy your own cells or react to a food or a plant. We call these inappropriate behaviors *hyperactive immune states.*

YOUR BODY'S DEFENSIVE BARRIERS

Every second of every day, you're protected from dangerous microscopic invaders by a powerful, all-encompassing immune network of cells and chemicals that work together to keep the bad guys out, create barriers against physical threats, handle damage control, and even build new tissues.

First of all, there are the physical and chemical barriers. Think of the immune system as a couple of defense teams. The first line of defense, or layer of protection, consists of the physical and chemical barriers at your body's boundaries and entryways. Naturally, your skin and mucous membranes are the first to prevent dangerous microbes from entering your body at its most vulnerable places—those directly exposed to the external environment. Protein molecules in your tears and saliva dissolve microbes that reach these sensitive areas. Other proteins in your saliva prevent microbes from getting beyond your mouth. Your stomach's hydrochloric acid eliminates microbes that make it into your digestive tract.

If potential pathogens get past that first line of defense, there's another lineup waiting for them—the fast-acting phagocyte white blood cells, the first immune cellular team aimed at eliminating bacteria and fungi. These quick-acting scavenger phagocytes are called *neutrophils.* They're first on the scene to kill and eliminate microbes. The neutrophils are short lived, lasting only a few hours. When these first cell responders are done—or even while still in action—the second team of responders, the lymphocytes, enters into protective mode.

All these defense cells—phagocytes and lymphocytes—know to eliminate a bacteria or fungus because they recognize patterns or designs on the microbe's surface, like a scanner recognizes a bar code. These molecular patterns aren't found on your body's own cells or on viruses.

Because viruses don't have molecular designs that neutrophils recognize, another immune cell must step in to detect and eliminate them—and that's the natural killer (NK) lymphocyte. The NK cell is the first responder to a viral invasion, usually

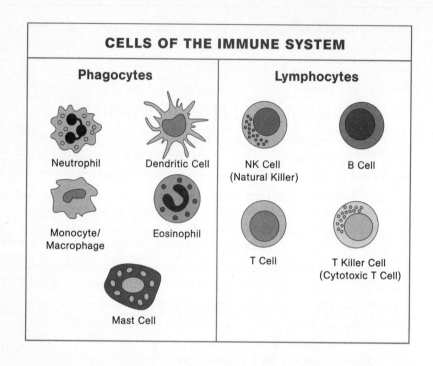

CELLS OF THE IMMUNE SYSTEM

Phagocytes

Neutrophil

Dendritic Cell

Monocyte/
Macrophage

Eosinophil

Mast Cell

Lymphocytes

NK Cell
(Natural Killer)

B Cell

T Cell

T Killer Cell
(Cytotoxic T Cell)

within 4 hours. Then, within 24 hours, other cells come on the scene to broadcast the initial alarm of invasion so that all the immune cells can do their part in protecting you from a viral infection.

First Immune Responders in Action

If an invader penetrates the body's physical boundaries, the phagocytes scan the microbe or particle. Once the invader is recognized as "not self," it's engulfed by the phagocytes, which release a cocktail of chemicals to kill it and break it down. There are two kinds of phagocytes—the quick-acting neutrophils (discussed above) that work in your blood and the more complex, long-lasting *monocytes* that work in your tissues. When monocytes wander out of your bloodstream into your tissues, they get a new name: *macrophages*. Monocytes have more responsibilities than simply acting as a phagocyte: They can also regulate immune responses, not just defend against microbes.

The phagocyte's killing weapons include hydrogen peroxide, *free radicals*, and a variety of proteins. In addition, the macrophages send out signals to the second team of cellular responders, the lymphocytes, to prompt them into action. And this first cellular defense team also initiates the powerful inflammatory response. It's a complex and amazing dance, and some of its most important steps are triggered by the free radicals.

Free Radicals, a Defense and Communication Strategy

Chances are, you've heard of free radicals as bad things that damage your cells and accelerate aging. But they have a good side, too—they help eliminate and destroy microbes. Free radicals (also known as *oxidants*) are highly reactive molecules that are electrically out of balance. That means they carry around just one electron that's always looking for a partner—you may remember from high school biology that electrons like to travel in pairs. To find a mate, those electrons will grab another electron from other molecules or tissues, bringing itself into balance. But that starts a chain reaction, as more and more molecules have their electrons raided and begin stealing from other molecules in turn.

Although free radicals sound like dangerous troublemakers—and sometimes they are—they are also essential for life. Besides helping to kill microbes, they can signal blood vessels to relax and activate other important chemical processes in your body. Where do free radicals come from? Turns out, lots of places. Your phagocytes make them; your body produces them as it breaks down the food you eat; you even manufacture them after an intense workout or when you've been out in the sun for a while. Toxins, like cigarette smoking and air pollution, also create free radicals. Although most of these environmental free radicals aren't so good for you, the ones that your body makes can support your health.

Free radicals can cause trouble through a process called *oxidative stress*. Starved for electrons and pilfering them at will, free radicals can damage your tissues or molecules, and the effects can be serious: *gene mutations*, altered proteins, macular degeneration (an eye disease resulting in loss of vision), skin wrinkles, and many conditions associated with unhealthy aging.

Yet your body can protect you by producing *antioxidants*, molecules that balance the free radicals. And your foods and supplements can supply antioxidants to maintain oxidative balance. Too many free radicals can lead to more *inflammation*, but an antioxidant-rich diet supports your body to stay more in balance. Think carrots, oranges, and lots of green vegetables.

Inflammation Creation

Inflammation is another basic innate immune response. It's initiated by the phagocytes—blood neutrophils and monocytes—and by tissue *mast cells*. What triggers the inflammatory response? One switch that turns on inflammation is when tissues are damaged by burns, cuts, sprains, and other physical traumas. Damaged cells send out the call for inflammation to get into action. Free radicals and chemical signals from the phagocytes also contribute to inflammation. Acute inflammation is a good thing. It protects you from further damage. Chronic *inflammation?* Not so good. It can cause many illnesses, like heart disease, as well as allergy symptoms and chronic pain.

What actually happens during inflammation? Injured tissue cells or a foreign object like a splinter stimulates the damaged cells to release "inflammatory" chemicals. The first chemical released on the scene is *histamine*, which summons blood cells to the area and initiates the entire inflammatory process. Then your brave phagocyte warriors join the battle, engulfing and destroying any toxic agents or microbes that came through the damaged tissues. The *serum*—that's the fluid in your blood—seeps in, flooding the area to dilute any toxins, while *platelets*, cells in your blood, wall off the area to prevent dangerous microbes from moving beyond this region and creating further damage.

THAT'S INFLAMMATION!

- You sprained an ankle and it becomes swollen and painful.

- You burn your wrist taking baked lasagna out of the oven. It hurts for a few hours, then forms a blister, becomes red, and takes several weeks to heal.

- You're allergic to pollens: Your nose gets runny, your eyes itch, and you have a little tickle in your throat.

- After a bug bite, your skin becomes itchy and swollen, and big red bumps appear.

There are four key physical signs of the inflammatory response.

- Swelling
- Redness
- Heat
- Pain

Remember what happened when you got a burn from the oven or a splinter from a piece of wood? The area probably started to blister or bleed as blood rushed to it, and became red, sore, swollen, and probably even hot. If the cells didn't do their job and the area got infected, you started to notice pus—dead white blood cells. These symptoms or signs are all due to the inflammatory cells and chemicals turning on the healing response.

Once this inflammatory process begins, it can take a few days to a few weeks to reclaim the area to its almost-original, pristine state. If you had a cut, new tissue is built, leading to wound healing. It's a great system. But it can be compromised by stress or poor nutrition. In a study at Ohio State University, people stressed by caring for their elderly parents with dementia were given an experimental wound. Researchers measured the time it took for the wound to heal. Those with more stressful situations experienced a longer healing time than those who had a strong support system and help in caring for their parents.[3]

Sometimes the inflammatory process doesn't shut off once it's no longer needed. Such long-lasting chronic inflammation is known as an overzealous hyperactive response. In fact, it's a factor in many conditions not usually considered immune in origin, like heart disease, chronic pain, type 2 diabetes, obesity, and even Alzheimer's disease. Today, scientists and doctors are looking at chronic inflammation as a causative factor of these illnesses, not just a consequence. In the lab, we can measure chemicals in the blood that tell us inflammation is occurring somewhere inside your body.[4] Keeping inflammation toned down through diet, exercise, and stress management[5] helps keep your immune network balanced to prevent many chronic illnesses previously thought to be associated with old age.

Bringing In the Backup Responders

When it comes to immune system strategies, the innate "on call" immune responses of phagocytosis and inflammation may be two of the oldest tricks in the book. Even jellyfish, worms, bugs, and plants use them. But only humans and other vertebrates

I was trimming blackberry vines in my yard when a tiny thorn nicked my thumb, right through my gardening gloves. When a piece got stuck under my skin, I didn't worry at first, since my body usually works out bits that it doesn't want. But this time was different. Soon my thumb became inflamed and painful. By day 5, it was so sensitive that I couldn't hold anything, and I knew that my phagocytes were busy causing the swelling, redness, and pain of inflammation. Even antibiotic ointment and a light wrap didn't seem to help.

I showed my thumb to my nurse practitioner, Judy. After soaking it, Judy used a needle and gently cut the skin to squeeze out the fluids and some blood. Then she rewrapped it and applied a bandage. The next day, the swelling was down and the healing seemed to be in full progress. Within a month, my thumb was all better.

This was an example of a simple immune reaction to a splinter with definite inflammation and increased local activity to wall off any deeper reactions or infection—all without taking oral antibiotics.

(animals with backbones) have evolved to develop the more complex *acquired immunity* made possible by the lymphocytes. Here's how it works.

Following the basic inflammatory process, if there are microbes still present in the damaged tissue, the next layer or team of immune protection is called in. The phagocytes have partners in this next phase called *dendritic cells*, which do their job of pulling apart the microbes into "tasty" morsels called *antigens*. (An antigen is any substance, usually a protein, that stimulates an immune response.) When the dendritic cell parades around with the antigen on its outer surface, a particular lymphocyte will be attracted to and recognize the antigen. In the scheme of immune protection and surveillance, the lymphocytes take over when the phagocytes complete their work. Lymphocytes are primed into action by meeting their one "special" antigen. Because lymphocytes are born with the ability to recognize only one antigen, the lymphocyte response is slower—it takes a while for them to meet—and takes more time than that of the quick-action phagocytes. Some lymphocytes can protect you from future invasions by the same microbe by producing cells that have memory: When you develop an infection or receive a vaccination, memory cells are created to protect you in the future. In contrast, the phagocytes do their job and never remember doing it.

The Decoding Immune Cells: T and B Lymphocytes

In the world of lymphocytes, there are two primary families: the *T lymphocytes* (T cells), born in the bone marrow and educated in the thymus; and the *B lymphocytes* (B cells), both born and schooled in the bone marrow. Each lymphocyte, when it recognizes a specific antigen, initiates the acquired or learned immune response. Now let's look at the different responsibilities of these very capable T and B cells.

THE T LYMPHOCYTES. The T cell is the major cell regulating immune functions. T cells activate an immune response when they discover an antigenic clue—and they can also turn off the immune response when their job of eliminating a particular microbial antigen is finished. There are *T helper (Th)* cells, which manage different aspects of immune reactivity. T helpers are very busy cells. Some of them (*Th1 helpers*) increase the number of infection-fighting T cells, while others (*Th2 helpers*) tell the B cells to get to work. But wait: It gets more complex. Some T cells can become even more specialized *T regulator (Treg)* cells, which slow down, turn off, or accelerate a variety of immune processes. Then there are also the T cells that kill infected cells; these are called *cytotoxic* or *T killer cells*.

THE B LYMPHOCYTES. Since the T cells are the regulators of immune activity, they also trigger into action the B lymphocytes to produce protective antibody molecules. Antibodies, also known as *immunoglobulins*, are proteins that pair with a specific antigen and help remove it from the body. (See "Antibodies to the Rescue!" on page 15.)

THE IMMUNE DANCE

As we've seen, a lymphocyte is born with the ability to recognize only one specific antigen. In the scheme of immune protection, this means the lymphocytes travel throughout your body looking for the antigen they recognize carried on the surface of a dendritic cell. Once the T cell finds its "chosen" antigen, it tells your body to produce more T cells that identify this one antigen. The T cells can expand their abilities by becoming T helpers, which produce chemical signals to turn on another

SMART CELLS IN A NUTSHELL

Here's a quick guide to how your immune system works.

Recognizing and dismantling the invader. (1) The cells that begin the immune dance are the phagocytes and the *antigen-presenting cells (APCs)*. The APCs process antigens from the invaders and include the dendritic cells. The offending organism, recognized as dangerous, is taken apart into pieces called antigens. These antigens stimulate immune recognition and specific immune reactions. Once the immune cells recognize the invader, an almost magical dance is choreographed.

Carrying the marks of an invader. (2) The antigen-presenting cell now carries the antigen on its outer surface, like a flag (or like the lightning bolt on Harry Potter's forehead!). Then it travels around the body until it meets T helper cells that recognize this particular antigen. (3)

Messaging with molecules. Communication? Invasion! Once the appropriate T helper cell recognizes its specific antigen, that signals it to make more T cells that recognize that antigen. (4) The signaling molecules that tell the immune cells what to do are called cytokines.

Looking for partner B cells. (5) The expanded army of T cells with the antigen flag of the invader on its surface goes on the prowl to find a B lymphocyte that recognizes the same antigen. The T cell activates the B cell to make more B cells capable of recognizing that antigen.

Expanding B cells and producing antibodies. (6, 7) This population of educated B cells expands and matures into *plasma cells* that produce antigen-neutralizing protein antibodies.

Halting the action. (8) Once the immune defenders have duly eradicated the invader, another set of molecular signals trigger the balance switch: The Treg cells send out their brand of cytokines to turn off the actions.

round of protectors, the B cells, which produce antibodies—proteins that recognize and help remove specific antigens. T helpers (Th) may develop into T regulators (Treg), which can turn the immune response on or off. T helpers also activate another family of T lymphocytes, the T killer cells, which eliminate infected cells and produce more toxic chemicals.

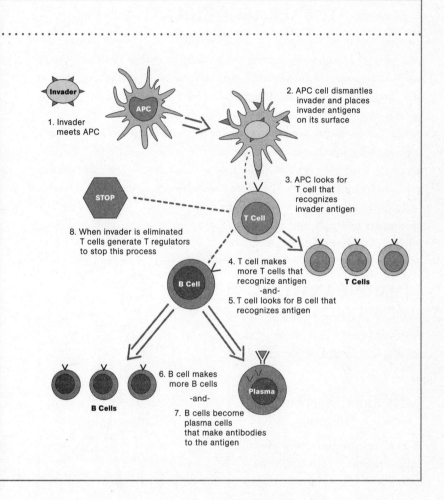

1. Invader meets APC

2. APC cell dismantles invader and places invader antigens on its surface

3. APC looks for T cell that recognizes invader antigen

8. When invader is eliminated T cells generate T regulators to stop this process

4. T cell makes more T cells that recognize antigen
-and-
5. T cell looks for B cell that recognizes antigen

6. B cell makes more B cells

-and-

7. B cells become plasma cells that make antibodies to the antigen

Think of the immune cells doing a do-si-do dance—meeting new partners, handing off antigens to another, and completing the dance by delivering what's special from each of the immune cells. Cells have a unique messaging system of hundreds of different chemicals called cytokines. The word "cytokine" means traveling ("kine") between cells ("cyto").

IT'S ALL ABOUT IDENTITY

An important feature of immune cells is their ability to discriminate between "me" and "not me." Immune cells carrying invader antigens on their surface membrane need to show a sign of "self" so that other immune cells won't attack them. Think of the immune cell as a two-handed creature: One hand feels or recognizes the invader antigen while the other hand shakes hands with its self-markings.

Early in the development of your immune cells, even before you're born, T cells learn to distinguish self-markings. Those that can't recognize "self" from "other" are destroyed. It's as if there's a bar code on your cells that says SELF. Immune cells that can't read the bar code must be eliminated since by being there, they could later in life attack your own. As you'll learn in Chapter 2, some normal immune cells may lose their ability to decipher self-markings. That can lead to an autoimmune disease, which means your body attacks itself.

IMMUNE ANATOMY

Where do all these immune cells come from, and where do they perform their amazing jobs of protection? Let's find out.

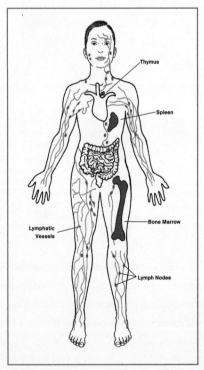

The Bone Marrow and Thymus

As mentioned earlier, most immune cells—lymphocytes and phagocytes— originate in the bone marrow, which is considered a primary immune organ; the thymus is the other primary immune organ. In fact, all blood cells, including red blood cells, white blood cells, and platelets, are created in the bone marrow from stem cells. The lymphocytes, which start out in these localized regions, travel

ANTIBODIES TO THE RESCUE!

Antibodies are protective proteins your body manufactures to help remove specific antigens. Antibodies are also known as immunoglobulins (Ig) that neutralize or coat an invader, rendering it harmless. Typically, their names are written as Immunoglobulin G, or IgG. All antibodies are produced by B cells that have matured into immunoglobulin-producing machines called plasma cells. Immunoglobulins are primarily effective against microbes and antigens that travel in the fluids of the body but not if the antigen is inside a cell. The primary types of antibodies include IgG, IgM, IgA, and IgE, each active in a different part of the body or stage of immune protection.

IgG is the most predominant antibody molecule in the body and can neutralize bacterial toxins and coat microbes to make them more "tasty" and enticing to the phagocytes. (*Note:* A pregnant woman passes her IgG across the placenta to her baby, thereby providing passive immunity to the newborn. "Passive immunity" means the baby is protected by the mom's immunity, not by any immune response made by the baby.) IgGs are the memory antibodies that stay with you for future recognizance of any microbes they have fought during your life.

IgM is the first antibody your cells make following exposure to an antigen during an infection or after an immunization. They are active early in the elimination of microbes.

IgA plays an essential role in gut or *mucosal* immunity, so it's not surprising that most IgA is made by immune cells in the intestinal lining. It is the primary antibody in your body's secretions (saliva, mucus, tears, and colostrum) and is considered a first line of defense against upper respiratory and gastrointestinal infections. *Salivary IgA* is often lowered by stress and can be elevated by laughter, music, a sense of community, and stress reduction.

IgE is normally very low in the blood but elevated in situations of allergies and parasitic infections, where it plays a significant role in allergic and inflammatory responses.

throughout your body via the bloodstream and the lymphatic vessels. Some lymphocytes stay in the bone marrow to get further educated; they become the bone marrow–derived cells, or B cells. Lymphocytes that travel to the thymus to mature and get their education become thymus-derived cells, or T cells. The thymus, located above the heart, is considered a major regulator of immune functions. Stress and aging are two factors that can shrink the thymus. One way to keep your thymus happy is to gently tap high on your chest and hum. This is a natural health-enhancing practice called the Thymus Pat and Hum; see page 186 for details.

The thymus is largest when we're babies and tends to shrink with age. Only 50 years ago, when scientists didn't know the role of the thymus, it was thought that a large thymus contributed to crib death (now known as sudden infant death syndrome), and it was treated with radiation to shrink it.[6] Decades later, those who received that incorrect treatment as babies have a greater incidence of thyroid *cancer* and breast cancer.[7]

The Lymphatic System: Lymph Nodes and Spleen

The lymphocytes, regardless of where they went to school, travel to the lymph nodes and spleen (the secondary immune organs) to finish developing their specific repertoire, like mastering antibody production. The tissues that make up the lymph system additionally function as filtering centers, catching stray microbes that have reached them through the blood or lymph vessels.

LYMPH NODES are small bean-shaped tissues clustered in your neck and armpits, in your abdomen around your digestive organs, in your groin, in areas near your heart, and along your spine. They are powerful defense outposts stationed along the lymphatic vessels, filtering out and trapping wayward microbes.

Have you ever experienced swollen and achy glands in your neck, throat, and even armpits when you had a sore throat? That's because when there's an infection, nearby lymph nodes, also known as lymph glands, become inflamed and enlarged due to the poisonous microbes and the increasing numbers of immune cells to eliminate them. And when it comes to your lymph nodes, stress—not just infection—is another culprit. During times of stress, young lymphocytes in your nodes and thymus are often destroyed. When you're chronically stressed (as you'll learn more about in Chapter 5), the developing T cells are often thwarted and eliminated, perhaps to conserve energy.

THE SPLEEN performs similar jobs to your lymph nodes.[8] About the size of your fist, your spleen is located on your left side under your rib cage and behind your stomach. It filters out unwanted material from the blood, including old red blood cells and microorganisms. It also stores blood and is home to antibody-producing immune cells. If your spleen is removed due to trauma or disease, you have a higher risk of certain bacterial infections. People who've had their spleen removed are advised to receive specific *vaccines* to protect against bacteria usually defended by antibodies made in the spleen. They also need to be vigilant at any sign of an infection. Vaccines recommended include those for pneumococcus, meningococcus, and *Haemophilus influenzae* type B.

OTHER LYMPHOID TISSUES include the tonsils, adenoids, and the appendix. Since we can live without them, they're not essential to immune health, although they are certainly helpful. Just a few decades ago, it was routine to surgically remove the tonsils and adenoids of children who suffered frequent sore throats, but that practice is rare now. The appendix is another example of lymphoid tissue with uncertain immune activity. Appendicitis (inflammation of the appendix) does require immediate surgical removal to prevent life-threatening infection of the whole abdominal cavity.

The Lymphatic Transportation Highway

Your thymus, spleen, and lymph nodes connect to each other through tubes or channels of both blood vessels and lymphatic vessels that make it easy for the immune cells to travel through the body searching for invaders.

The lymph nodes, lymphatic vessels, and lymph fluid are all part of the vast *lymphatic system*, a filtration network of tiny vessels that drain *lymph*—a clear fluid containing water, proteins, and other substances—throughout your body via the lymphatic vessels and the bloodstream.

Since water, proteins, and other substances continuously leak out of tiny blood capillaries into the surrounding tissues, they must be recycled back into the blood to prevent tissue damage. The lymphatic system comes to the rescue, returning the leaked materials to the bloodstream. Wherever there are blood vessels, there are lymph vessels close by—the two systems work together. If the excess fluid couldn't be returned to the blood, our tissues would become swollen and we'd get really sick.

Since only a few lymphocytes can respond to any specific antigen, the T lymphocytes continuously circulate throughout the body, increasing the likelihood of the right cells finding the right antigen. They patrol your body, searching for invaders, by circulating in the blood vessels and the lymphatic vessels. Then, from the bloodstream, they crawl into the tissues and may stay there or make their way back into the lymphatic circulation.

"Naïve" T cells, those that have not yet detected their antigen, enter the lymph nodes from the blood to "sample" the node for foreign antigens that have come from lymph vessels. In contrast, memory T cells, those that have already met and responded to their "chosen" antigen, preferentially migrate to the sites where they first came in contact with that antigen—kind of like salmon swimming back to their place of birth. In summary, here's a look at the important work your lymphatic system performs:

IT BALANCES THE FLUIDS AND PROTEINS IN YOUR BODY. About a quart of the blood fluid with its proteins leaks out of the cells into the space between the cells and tissues every day, which could be life threatening. But the lymphatic system drains fluid from the tissues back into the bloodstream.

IT FILTERS YOUR BLOOD TO TRACK DOWN DANGEROUS MICROBES AND TOXINS. The lymphatic system acts as a highway, transporting white blood cells to and from the lymph nodes and antigen-presenting cells (APCs) to the lymph nodes. The APCs reveal the toxic or microbial antigen so that the lymphocytes can recognize it, react, and help in its removal.

IT AIDS IN YOUR NUTRITION by absorbing fats from your food and transporting fatty acids from the small intestine to the liver to be metabolized.

Keeping It Moving

Your blood circulates up and down from your pumping heart, but the lymph fluid in your lymphatic vessels moves in only one direction—*up* from the lower part of your body or *down* from your head and neck. Most of it empties into the venous system near the left shoulder. But unlike your system for circulating blood, there's no pump for your lymphatic system. Instead, your lymphatic vessels are squeezed by muscle contractions in a slow process that moves the fluid within them at a rate of about 4 ounces an hour. But you can speed up the efficiency of your lymphatic circulation all by yourself, by exercising, doing deep abdominal breathing, or getting a massage. Exercise—walking, swimming, pumping iron—makes the muscles contract more strongly, squeezing the lymph vessels, which increases the flow of lymph to about 60 ounces an hour.

Just like you, your lymphatic vessels like a good massage. Large muscles surrounding the lymphatics need massage and movement to get the lymph moving, which helps remove waste, toxins, and excess fluid. Self-massage (see Chapter 6) stimulates movement of the lymph and is especially beneficial when you feel a cold coming on or during times of severe antigenic stimulation, such as during allergy season or being outdoors in polluted cities.

Clogging the Circulation

Do you ever have swollen ankles? This may be both your circulatory and lymphatic systems telling you something is off. Standing or sitting for a long time can result in swollen feet and legs because your blood and lymph fluid pool in a process called *edema*. That happens when fluid rapidly flows out of tissues and not enough gets back into circulation. The condition called *lymphedema* refers to swelling in an arm or leg due to a blockage in the lymphatic system, usually because of the removal of lymph nodes as part of cancer treatment. You might look at this as a block in a gas line: Gas builds up in one place and can't get through the whole system. The range of swelling goes from barely noticeable to extreme. Following cancer treatment, lymphedema may not appear for years, especially post–breast cancer, but it can be alleviated by lymphatic massage or pressure dressings.

Your Gastrointestinal Tract: The Main Immune Area

Most of what's in your gastrointestinal tract isn't actually *you*. You provide a home to trillions of microorganisms that live all over your body—on your skin, in your mouth and nose, and, most of all, in your belly. The average human body has 10 times as many microbes as its own cells. This collection of microbes that normally occupy you is called your *microbiome*, and it's as unique to you as your fingerprints. The connection between the microbes in your gut and the health of your body is an exciting and vast new area of research. What is most amazing about our intestinal bacteria is that, for the most part, we live together peacefully. The bacteria aid in digesting food, make some of your vitamins, and prevent disease-causing microbes from causing damage. They even help your immune cells develop and mature.[9] They can influence your weight[10] and the way you metabolize medications. Experience a round of antibiotics and you may discover you're now hosting a virulent set of intestinal microbes that had been held in check by your peace-keeping microbes. Persistent diarrhea is a potential consequence of the imbalance caused by antibiotics wiping out the protective microbes.

Those microbes that live in cooperation with us have induced a tolerance by the immune cells that live with them in the gut. That means the cells "tolerate" the germs and don't launch an attack on them, even though they're not "self." Oral tolerance is the ability of the immune system to recognize substances taken in orally and suppress or weaken any immune response to the substance. This may account for the balance we enjoy when we do not react to most foods we eat.

The immune cells in the gut are known by two different names—gut-associated lymphoid tissue (GALT) and *mucosal-associated lymphoid tissue (MALT)*. The gut or mucosal immune tissues are where we are first exposed to most of the potentially dangerous invaders. So it's essential that the immune cells can distinguish those that are a danger to us from those that are friendly. Once again, the immune cells' ability to recognize patterns is what helps them determine safe from dangerous bacteria in our gut. This gut region produces an almost endless supply of mucus, which ensnares bacteria and keeps them from moving to a more vulnerable part of your body. Plus, your cells in the region supply chemical signals that activate immune responses and inflammation when needed. Your intestines contain the most lymphoid tissue in your entire body, and the center of all the action is your small intestine.

The Immune Communications System

Because your immune cells are stationed all over your body, they need ways to communicate with each other. They do this through an amazing system of molecular signals. The two primary kinds of molecules that make up the magical immune communications repertoire are:

- **Cytokines.** These proteins communicate between cells, helping to manage and regulate your body's immune responses. There are at least 100 different cytokines.
- **Leukotrienes and prostaglandins.** Your body makes these molecules in response to inflammation. *Leukotrienes* and *prostaglandins* can activate, prolong, or turn off inflammatory responses.

Cytokines

Cytokines are the bossy molecules. Think of them as signals telling other cells on the immune team what to do. Some are chemoattractants, giving the "come hither" message. Cytokines are protein molecules that send chemical signals to direct a cell to engage in a specific kind of activity. They express a molecular language that immune cells can listen to and interpret. The result? Immune functions are activated and regulated. There are hundreds of different cytokines, and they do lots of different jobs. They signal the growth and development of immune cells, wound healing, inflammation, and proliferation of blood cells. Other cytokines attract cells to come to a site of injury or infection—they play an important role in inflammation.

We used to think cytokines affected only immune cells. However, recent research has revealed that the brain and immune cells "talk" to each other. In fact, some cytokines (*interleukins*—IL-1 and IL-6) are responsible for causing fever when we have an infection.[11] To do that, the cytokine travels from your immune cells up to your brain and changes the thermostat. Your immune network is really smart! Though a fever may make you uncomfortable, many microbes cannot survive if the body temperature is raised even a few degrees, so your fever actually helps to zap the offending bugs. Plus, those higher temperatures accelerate most immune processes. And IL-1 enhances the deep, slow wave, restful kind of sleep that promotes healing.

As scientists learn more about the intricacies of all the immune cells and especially the cytokines, they'll be able to devise better treatment and prevention strategies for many immune illnesses. Sometimes just one little molecule can make a difference in a health outcome. (Ever hear of interferon? That's a cytokine made by our cells in response to a viral infection and has been used as a drug in the treatment of hepatitis and even some cancers. And a form of interferon is being used in the treatment of multiple sclerosis.)

HOW CYTOKINES WORK

A cell has a docking or receiving site called a *receptor* on its outer surface. This receiving site can detect and recognize a particular cytokine. The cytokine can then land on the cell surface and trigger or tickle a specific response inside the cell. Only cells with a receptor for the cytokine can respond to it. This receptor docking site is a standard way many cellular communication systems work. For instance, the stress hormone adrenaline can land on cells that have docking sites for it and initiate a response, like heart cells being made to beat faster.

Leukotrienes and Prostaglandins

The second set of chemical communication potions are also produced by your white blood cells: Leukotrienes and prostaglandins help manage your inflammatory responses. When your cell membranes are damaged or stimulated, they release these fatty molecules. Cell membranes are composed of a variety of fat molecules that are influenced by what you eat. If you eat a lot of red meat, the molecules released will carry more inflammatory prostaglandins and leukotrienes. A diet that favors wonderful omega-3 fatty acids, such as those from salmon, will cause fewer inflammatory messages to be released.

THE INVADERS: DISEASE-CAUSING MICROBES

Now that you've learned how your complex immune network works, let's look at what it's defending against: the dangerous microbes that can make you sick. Each kind of infecting agent—bacteria, virus, fungus, and *parasite*—uses a different ploy to infect a person and cause disease. Of course, your intelligent immune system has evolved a slew of ways to counter each type of attack. The general plan: Pathogens are first removed by scavenger phagocytes, followed by the lymphocytes doing their specific activities. Now to the specific differences.

BACTERIA. The most common bacterial infections are strep throat, staph skin infections like boils, bacterial bronchitis, and urinary tract infections (mostly caused by E. coli). Since most bacteria move in the fluids of your body, not inside your cells, the phagocytes can engulf and eliminate them. This happens even faster if the lymphocytes have already made antibodies against that microbe.

VIRUSES. These much smaller creatures cause a wide variety of infections that can't be treated by antibiotics. Since viruses take over the cells of their host—you—zapping them also kills the human cells they've hijacked. Viruses must enter your cells to grow, and when they do, they leave clues on the outside of the infected cell showing that an invader is inside. That makes it easier for the T killer cells to recognize and eliminate the infected cell. Common viral infections include the cold, influenza, oral and genital herpes, hepatitis, and HIV.

YEASTS (FUNGI). Some of the most popular foods we enjoy—mushrooms, blue cheese, bread, and beer or wine—are all made by or with *fungi* and yeast. But some yeast can deliver diseases, like *Candida albicans*, a common cause of vaginitis and intestinal

YOU'RE NOT SICK: IT'S EVIDENCE OF YOUR IMMUNE CELLS AT WORK

When you have an infection, you often feel crummy, you come down with a fever, and you may be achy or sleepy. The same thing can happen following an immunization. In fact, one of the main complaints with immunizations is that people may develop symptoms, like a mini flu, for a few days—feeling achy, feverish, and tired. These symptoms or side effects are actually signals of an activated immune system. In a study of experimentally induced influenza (flu) infection, participants who took aspirin to prevent these symptoms actually prolonged their illness compared to the people who took acetaminophen (Tylenol).[13]

overgrowth. This can lead to inflammation of the gut lining. It can even ferment your foods, especially carbohydrates, and that leads to gas and bloating. Athlete's foot and other skin infections are caused by fungi, too. (Fungi can be especially dangerous in people whose immune systems are already not working at their best.) Fungal invasions are countered by a complex collaboration between the macrophages and dendritic cells, which then enjoy close encounters with T cells to eliminate the fungi. However, a potent inflammatory response also plays an important role in getting rid of these invaders.

PARASITES. Parasitic infections are caused by organisms called protozoa—one example is giardia—or by worms. These are very different from other infectious microbes: They have complex life cycle stages, can live a long time in the human body, and can change themselves to avoid being zapped by your immune system. Parasite infestation may be more common than many physicians and patients realize, and it can cause chronic digestive upset, gas and bloating, loose *bowels*, and occasional abdominal pain, as well as fatigue and headaches. People don't necessarily have to be immune deficient to become infected or infested with parasitic bugs; it may have more to do with the level of exposure. Parasites are the most complex group of invaders to eradicate. They can live inside or outside of cells, and they require a variety of immune strategies for effective removal. Often they trigger an inflammatory response that releases toxic chemicals to destroy these invaders. Antibodies help eliminate parasites, too. There are new and innovative tests that are better able to find and diagnose parasites. Ask your doctor about special stool testing if you suspect you may have parasites.

Let's take a look at how vaccines or *immunizations* work, since they're so common and play such an important role in public health.

Vaccines prevent deadly or crippling diseases like smallpox and polio. In general, a vaccine contains antigenic material from a specific organism. There are two main types of vaccines: those made from whole cells and those containing only antigens, not cells, from the pathogen (usually part of the cell wall). Whole-cell vaccines use a weakened or killed microbe.

Vaccines help prevent outbreaks of infectious diseases and save lives.

They've contributed to the near elimination of some diseases such as smallpox worldwide and polio in the United States. Some people, though, choose not to have their children vaccinated. Yet when 85 to 90 percent of the population is vaccinated against a contagious disease, most everyone is protected—even those not immunized—in what is known as "herd immunity."[12] Some people, such as pregnant women or those whose immune system isn't strong enough, can't receive certain vaccines. That's why it's important that people around them should.

THE TAKEAWAY

Scientists are constantly learning more about your immune system, and new information is always changing and enhancing what we know. The exciting thing about the evolving science of immunity is that it helps us better understand how to keep your cells and your self healthy.

Throughout your life, the immune system undergoes many changes. It's just developing when you're born, probably reaches its peak when you're a young adult, and slows down as you age. Yet at each season of life, you can find ways to maintain and improve your immune health.

In this chapter, we've looked at how the amazing immune system does its incredible jobs.[14] Next, let's see what happens when things don't function as they should. What goes wrong in your body? You can get sick with infections, or you develop allergies or autoimmune problems. But don't worry. In the chapters that follow, you'll learn solutions for taking care of yourself and preventing illness. Read on!

CHAPTER 2

The Out-of-Balance Immune System

We've explored the amazing ways your immune system works to keep you healthy and protect you from dangerous infections. But what about when things go wrong? In this chapter, we'll look at what happens when your immune system gets out of balance. And these days, a malfunctioning immune system is more likely to be working too hard than loafing on the job. So instead of resulting in a slew of infections, that hyperactive immune system serves up a number of common conditions, from allergies, asthma, and autoimmune disease to chronic inflammation.

You know: those constant sniffles and sneezes in the spring that have you wondering if they are from a cold or an allergy. What about those early-morning aches and pains—are they just unwelcome signs of age and inactivity, or are they the result of an overactive immune system causing inflammation? And when your doctor tells you you're at risk for heart disease, even though your cholesterol numbers are normal, could the problem really be your immune system? Let's zoom in on all these bothersome hyperactive immune conditions and see what's up.

ALLERGIES. When your immune system goofs, making an inappropriate response to something that's perfectly safe to most people—like a flower, a peanut, or a dusty attic—an allergy is what develops. With an allergy, your body launches an unwelcome *immune response* to something coming in from the outside: inhaled pollen, ingested wheat, or even the touch of latex or detergent. You know the drill: runny nose, itchy eyes, skin rash, or even an upset tummy.

ASTHMA. Caused by an allergy, an irritant, or both, asthma is a chronic inflammatory disease of the respiratory tract. It can lead to difficult breathing, wheezing, feeling tired, and being short of breath. Sometimes, you even feel like you can't get enough oxygen.

AUTOIMMUNE DISEASE. Autoimmune illness is another case of mistaken identity, but this time it's a misguided attack on something inside you rather than something from outside. It happens when your immune system doesn't recognize your own tissues or body proteins as "you." Remember, your healthy immune system knows the difference between what's safe or "self" and what's a threat or "not self." But when your immune system goes into overdrive or is misguided toward a mistaken identity, it can turn on you. In this hyperactive condition, it loses its ability to discriminate between what to react to and what to leave alone, such as your own cells or proteins.

CHRONIC INFLAMMATION. This occurs when a tissue is damaged and the normal immune reactivity persists long after it's needed. It's different from acute inflammation, which happens when you get a splinter or a paper cut: Your finger bleeds, gets red and swollen, hurts a bit, and gets better in a few days or a week, when the tissue is cleaned up and repaired. Yet sometimes, this very essential immune response forgets to stop when the danger is over. If it continues too long, it damages your body instead of repairing it. Chronic inflammation is one more example of hyperimmune activity, in which the response keeps going after its job is done.

Hyperactive immune states can lead to irritation, organ damage, tissue destruction, and chronic illness. Prolonged symptoms like aches and pain, joint swelling, itchy skin, and other reactions are good clues that your immune response may have gone into hyperdrive. Like a hyperactive toddler, it's just plain out of control.

HOW DOES YOUR IMMUNE SYSTEM GET UNBALANCED?

As usual, there are lots of explanations. Both biological factors and lifestyle choices—including your genes, stress levels, dietary choices, and even feelings of loneliness or anger—can impact the workings of your immune system. And your gender can make a difference, too. If you're a woman, you're likely to have a more vigilant and vigorous immune system than most men. There are other factors as well. If you're clinically depressed, your immune response is likely to be depressed or underachieving.[1] If you don't get enough protein in your diet—you guessed it—your immune system suffers. Did you live in a too-clean environment as a tot? Even that can undermine your

IMMUNE IMBALANCE CAN BE CAUSED BY . . .

Genes. These provide clues to your ancestors' health issues and your propensity toward certain diseases. Yet these are not carved in stone: Your lifestyle behaviors—diet, exercise, stress—can influence the way your genes express themselves. (See the discussion of epigenetics on page 45.)

Stress. Both physical and mental/emotional stress—including insomnia, anxiety, depression, relationship problems, daily hassles, and life in general—play a role.

Illness, infections, and trauma. These issues activate immune responses and can stress or weaken them. Infections influence other factors here, including digestion and microbial balance.

Poor diet. Eating an unhealthy diet can lead to toxicity, weakness, and depletion of nutrients such as zinc, vitamin A, or protein, all of which are needed for normal immune function.

Weakened digestion. Poor digestion can lead to a leaky gut or abnormal microbes.

Medications. Some medicines—such as steroids, antibiotics, hormones, or chemotherapy agents—are factors.

Environmental toxins and free radicals. These include chemicals from air, water, and food at home, at work, and out in the world around you.

Overcleanliness. Too clean an environment during infancy and early childhood is a surprising factor affecting you later in life.

---

immune health. Some of these factors you can't change. You can't, for instance, travel back in time and relive your childhood in a dirtier home. But you've got lots of control over many factors. It's a good idea to focus on those things that you can readily change, because you can make a positive difference in your overall health.

Let's delve into some of the most common factors that contribute to throwing your immune system out of balance.

Your Genes

You inherit your genes from your parents and grandparents and ancestors going back dozens of generations. Those genes provide the information for how robust your immune cells can be. Your immune genes may even be linked to your sexual attraction—that certain something that captures the interest of a significant other. Here's how it works: Your immune cells are covered on their surface by chemical clues of self-identity—kind of like bar codes—called *human leukocyte antigens (HLAs)*. These self-markings are shed into your sweat and saliva, giving you your own unique smell. That's how a dog finds a lost child in the woods: by recognizing the child's scent on a piece of clothing.

And that's the basis for a pioneering study out of Switzerland.[2] Sweaty T-shirts from college men were placed into boxes, and women were asked to sniff the shirts and decide if they'd be attracted to the owners based on the smell alone. The results: Women had very different immune markers than the men whose shirts they selected as coming from someone they'd be attracted to. How come? What's the biology underlying this strange experiment? The women were attracted to someone immunologically different. Two people with similar immune markers (indicating similar immune responsiveness) would likely produce offspring with more limited immune abilities, while those with different immune markers (and different scents) would have children with more diverse immune capabilities and better chances of survival. So your cells and your scent carry clues to your immune abilities, yet your natural scent is typically covered over with perfumes or aftershave and even changed by hormones, meaning we may not be using this hidden biological feature of our immune identities in picking a partner.

Those markers of identity and your unique smell are biological clues to how robust your immune responses will be. The inherited tendencies toward underactive or overactive immune responses are just that—tendencies, not destiny.

An occasional infection, for example, doesn't mean you've got underachieving immune cells. Many of us, however, have inherited the opposite problem—a tendency toward hyperactive immune states of allergies, asthma, or autoimmune illnesses. If one of your parents has allergies, there's a 25 to 50 percent chance that you'll have allergies, too. If both parents have allergies, your chances go as high as 75 percent. Any kind of hyperactive immune state in the parents increases that possibility in their children, even though they're likely to get a different immune illness or condition—allergies or autoimmune illness. One family member may have type 1 diabetes, while another develops rheumatoid arthritis. Your genes play a big part, but not the only part, in your immune health.

Balancing your immune system is a complex dance. Your cells can activate one immune response while preventing or reducing another immune response. A cell may produce molecules that can both turn on and turn off inflammation. That makes the specific biochemical cause and effect difficult to determine; sorting out and understanding what issues underlie any disease diagnosis is often simply speculation. Even so, there are many strategies to help balance a wayward immune system, and knowing what throws off the balance is a good first step.

Your Stress Levels

Life is loaded with stress, from minor disappointments to the loss of a loved one; from lack of sleep to anxiety, depression, or loneliness; from an argument to a vacation. As you'll learn in Chapter 5, your mental state plays a big part in what feels like stress to you.

But first, what exactly *is* stress? In simple terms, it's your body's response to anything threatening, whether real or imagined. The stress response prepares your body to fight or flee, ramping up everything it needs for immediate survival, like energy production for your muscles to get you moving. Whether the stress response is acute and immediate or chronic and long lasting affects your immune balance. For example, with acute stress, if you're in a fight, your immune cells are activated to protect you from an infection in case you get thrashed. Sometimes, though, stress can go on for a long time. Chronic stress may put you at risk for more infections because stress hormones, like *cortisol*, slow down your immune response. Unlike that of your long-ago ancestors, your stress may not result from run-ins with wild animals. It's more likely to be self-created as you worry over past problems and anxieties and your body responds as if the problem were still an assault. A near accident, a difficult marriage, fear of losing a job—your body reacts to all these as real dangers. Yet if stress dampens your immune response, you might expect that the symptoms of hyperactive immune states would disappear. Not so. Paradoxically, symptoms of autoimmune disorders, allergies, and asthma often get worse when you're stressed out. Chronic stress throws your immune system even further out of balance.

Many factors can dislodge the balance of your system through the molecular "cocktails," the combination of biochemicals your body releases. Stress can both stimulate and suppress your immune responses. There are hundreds of biochemical communications managing the vast number of immunological reactions happening inside your body. Simply knowing that ongoing stress plays a role is reason enough to find good ways to manage it. One idea: Turn off the television news for a week—you'll be amazed at how much calmer you feel. (See more ideas in Chapter 5.)

Your Illnesses, Infections, and Traumas

Illness can deplete the cellular resources and molecular energy needed for healing. When your cells and molecules are busy repairing a broken bone, for instance, they may not be as available for restoring immune activities. You can become more vulnerable to infections when you're recovering from other health problems. That's why it's important, while healing from an illness, to get plenty of rest, eat nutritious foods, and graciously accept help from your family and friends.

Infections themselves alter your immune balance in various ways. For some people with genetic susceptibility, an infection can even bring about new immune problems, like allergies or autoimmune illness.

Your Diet and Your Digestion

Your body needs loads of important nutrients to maintain a healthy immune system. When even one nutrient is in short supply, things can go wrong. So eating a well-balanced diet will help keep your immune system more balanced. We'll delve into nutrition and immunity in more detail in Chapter 4; for now, let's take a quick look at the basics.

Two important points: First, healthy digestion begins with chewing every mouthful of food to liquefy it and make it easier for your body to use the nutrients. Second, consuming "beneficial" bacteria, called *probiotics*, is vital. These "good bugs" live in your intestinal tract, where they play a part in digestion, regulating immune cells, protecting you against the "bad" microbes, and providing you with many essential vitamins and minerals. If you lack some of these beneficial bacteria, you may be able to add more by eating yogurt with live probiotics or taking a probiotic supplement to help restore the healthy bacteria and improve your immune balance.

Your Medications

The pharmaceuticals you take can alter your immune activity. Those antibiotics your doctor prescribes for an infection? Along with getting rid of illness-causing bacteria (they do not rid your body of viruses), they may diminish the beneficial microbes in your gut. Your good-guy gut microbes prevent the bad-guy microbes from staging a hostile takeover, and if the beneficial microbes are eliminated by the antibiotics, this can lead to uncontrollable diarrhea and the need for even more drugs in an unending cycle. Many physicians actually recommend that their patients on antibiotics also take probiotics. Other pharmaceutical culprits that can throw your immune system out of whack include steroids, sex hormones, and chemotherapy agents. Your doctor has prescribed these drugs because he or she believes you need them, so follow instructions carefully. Once these medications are stopped, your immune health should slowly return to normal.

Your Environment: Toxins and Free Radicals

Remember those toxins and free radicals from Chapter 1? These chemicals can damage your immune cells and protective proteins, thus altering your immune balance. Make an effort to avoid these whenever possible by using fewer or no synthetic or toxic chemicals in household cleaning products, garden supplies, and cosmetics and by not smoking. Your cells can get rid of free radicals if they maintain a good supply of free radical quenchers called antioxidants. A diet rich in fresh fruits and vegetables works to keep your chemical oxidant stressors in balance.

Your Hyperclean Childhood

One theory about the cause of allergies and autoimmune illnesses is that as babies, we're not exposed to enough microbes.[3] In North America, we're just too clean. And what we're fed as infants—breast or bottle—helps set the immune system balance point. Children who are breast-fed for 3 to 6 months have fewer allergies than children who are not.[4]

Understanding the many factors that throw off immune balance—from what we eat

ULTIMATE IMMUNITY

Bill Patterson, 60

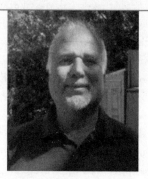

Bill Patterson was doing all the right things— or so he thought. He stayed away from processed foods, ate lots of fruits and veggies, and went hiking nearly every day. So when he went to see Dr. Haas for a checkup 7 years ago, he was blown away by what he learned. His cholesterol count was way above 200, and his weight wasn't much lower than 200. He had lots of allergies, and he always seemed to catch whatever cold was going around.

Dr. Haas took a look at Bill's food diary, scanned his blood test report, and announced that it was time for some changes. The problem: immune conditions. Turns out that Bill was allergic to a wide range of foods, including wheat and dairy, which caused immune reactions like bloating, sleep troubles, and weight gain. The solution: the healing power of the Immune-Power Eating Plan (I-PEP) and the Cool Down Inflammation Prevention Program.

Bill started out on the elimination diet, adding in supplements like magnesium, red yeast rice (for lowering cholesterol), fish oil, and niacin. Within 5 weeks, he'd lost 25 pounds. When he switched over to the I-PEP program and added weekly qigong classes to his hiking routine, the weight loss continued and he began sleeping better than he had in decades. "It was a wonderful, deep sleep that left me waking up feeling refreshed," he says. The most amazing result, though, was Bill's new cholesterol levels, which dropped almost 100 points.

Now, 7 years later, Bill has maintained his fit 160-pound weight and hasn't had a single cold or flu or missed a day of work. He's still hiking, and his routine now includes occasional 3- or 4-hour treks to the local hilltops with friends; when the weather is good, he adds an occasional swim. His new way of eating has inspired a new passion for food—he's taken a culinary class at a local college and has become a regular at the farmers' market.

"Dr. Haas's eating plan really showed me the light," Bill says. "The results have been amazing."

as babies to how we live as adults—can assist you in finding ways to prevent or manage conditions that could result from your immune responses being either too much or too little. In the developed world, it's the "too much" variety of immune reactivity that's on the rise, so let's look next at problems associated with a hyperactive immune system.

HYPERACTIVE IMMUNE STATES

A hyperactive immune state means that your immune system hasn't heard the closing bell to stop work. It keeps on the attack even when the danger has long passed. It also could mean that those immune cells forgot how to distinguish friend from foe, perceiving perfectly safe peanuts—or even your own tissues—as dangerous invaders. The air itself may create havoc in your body. A hyperactive immune state encompasses four health conditions or problems: allergies, asthma, autoimmune diseases, and chronic inflamation.

Allergies

You know what to expect: You sneeze every time you walk into the house of your cat-owner friend. Your eyes get itchy after you try new eye makeup. Your stomach gets queasy and your skin breaks out in itchy red blotches when you eat the first strawberries of the season. What's going on?

One of every five Americans has allergies, with symptoms like itchy eyes or skin,

---

The Immune Diaries   **Sondra**

When I was a preteen, every spring and fall, like clockwork, I suffered from a chocolate allergy. I'd get hives—big, itchy red spots—whenever I had a candy bar or a cup of hot chocolate. By the time I went to college, I was happy that my reactions to chocolate disappeared. To this day, I'm grateful to be free of that allergy! My father had allergies, and so does my son—but not to chocolate. It turns out that when your body reacts to an allergen with hives, the allergy may be outgrown. Many children outgrow their food allergies by the time they reach their 4th birthday,[5] though some, like me, have to suffer all the way through their teens.

COMMON ALLERGENS

Allergens can be anything, and they're found everywhere—in the air, in our foods and drinks, on the things we touch. The most common ones:

- Pollens from trees, flowers, and shrubs
- Dust mites
- Mold
- Animal dander, especially from cats and dogs
- Insect stings
- Latex
- Medications, including penicillin and other antibiotics, sulfa drugs, insulin, and anticonvulsants (note that side effects are different from allergic responses.)
- Foods, especially cow's milk, eggs, seafood, peanuts, tree nuts, soy, and wheat

runny nose, difficulty breathing, digestive upset, or even confused thinking. Almost anything can trigger an allergy in any part of the body. Some allergies last a lifetime, others are only seasonal, and some you may outgrow.

You can develop allergies at any age—some allergies may not begin until your thirties or forties. Some may last a lifetime, while others may disappear as the years go by. The more severe the reaction, the more likely the allergy will last a lifetime. Nobody is really sure why a particular substance triggers an allergy or why one reaction is more severe than another. So for now, we'll stick with some of the scientific theories as well as our own ideas.

Besides a genetic predisposition, an allergic response may be linked to how many other "assaults" your body and mind are dealing with, how well your digestive system functions, and even the integrity of your important microbiome. Your microbiome, or *biome*, is made up of the microbes that live peacefully in your gut. It's said that between 400 and 500 different species of bacteria live with you. As we learn more about these important bugs in the belly, we'll learn about how they impact health, from preventing weight gain to providing nutrients to educating immune cells. In addition, environmental assaults, such as being around cigarette smoke or air pollution, as well as lifestyle habits like poor nutrition and stress, can increase the likelihood of an allergic response.

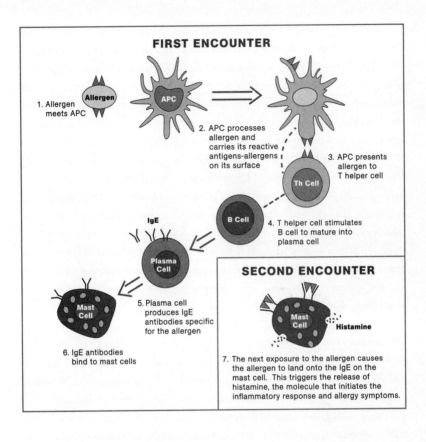

FIRST ENCOUNTER

1. Allergen meets APC

Allergen

APC

2. APC processes allergen and carries its reactive antigens-allergens on its surface

3. APC presents allergen to T helper cell

Th Cell

B Cell

4. T helper cell stimulates B cell to mature into plasma cell

IgE

Plasma Cell

5. Plasma cell produces IgE antibodies specific for the allergen

Mast Cell

6. IgE antibodies bind to mast cells

SECOND ENCOUNTER

Mast Cell

Histamine

7. The next exposure to the allergen causes the allergen to land onto the IgE on the mast cell. This triggers the release of histamine, the molecule that initiates the inflammatory response and allergy symptoms.

STEPS IN TRIGGERING AN ALLERGY

1. Initial exposure to an allergen occurs.

2. Immune cells produce IgE antibodies.

3. IgE attaches to mast cells.

4. The subsequent exposure to the allergen occurs.

5. IgE antibodies on mast cells recognize the allergen and attach.

6. IgE-allergen on mast cells triggers the release of histamine that initiates inflammation and allergic symptoms.

An allergic response starts first with exposure. You can't respond to a substance you've never encountered. Substances that trigger allergic responses are called allergens. The allergic process you suffer starts when you inhale, touch, or eat the allergen. And what becomes an allergen to you can develop at any time and without warning. You may have smelled those flowers, eaten those strawberries, or petted your friend's cat a hundred times with no unpleasant reactions. Yet your immune system can change at any moment and begin recognizing the substance as dangerous.

How come? We don't know exactly *why* this happens, only *what* happens at the cellular level: the development of IgE antibodies. The IgE molecule is specific for a particular allergen—let's say it's peanuts. The first step is exposure. After exposure to an allergen, the next step is the production of IgE antibodies that attach to certain cells in your body called mast cells, whose job is to detect allergens and irritants. The third step occurs the *next* time you come into contact with peanuts. Your mast cells, armed now with both IgE to the peanut and the peanut allergen that you've just eaten, kick the inflammatory response into action by releasing its histamine, thus causing your allergic symptoms.

Let's look a little more closely at how this plays out. When the IgE on your mast cells connects to a piece of the peanut, it unlocks its release of histamine, the major chemical of inflammation. Think of the IgE on the mast cell as the lock and the peanut allergen as the key. When they're connected, it's "open sesame," and histamine floods the area. Histamine quickly finds docking sites on cells (remember the receptor sites we talked about in Chapter 1?) in your nose or throat, skin or digestive tract, triggering allergy symptoms in those tissues and setting off the rest of the inflammatory response. If you have allergies, you may take antihistamines to prevent or at least reduce this reaction from occurring, because they block the histamine receptor sites.

Severe Allergic Reactions

Not all allergic reactions are created equal. IgE is responsible for immediate allergic responses that can range from very mild to life-threatening *anaphylaxis*—a severe and rapid whole-body reaction that can occur at any time, even if you've had only a mild reaction to the same allergen in the past. Although any allergen may trigger this extreme response, more typically, it's triggered by an allergy to a drug, shellfish, peanuts, or an insect bite. An anaphylactic response requires immediate medical

YOU KNOW YOU'VE GOT AN ALLERGY WHEN . . .

INHALED OR SKIN ALLERGENS

Itchy, runny nose

Sneezing

Itchy, watery eyes

Nasal congestion

Hives (raised, red itchy bumps on the skin)

Generalized rash or eczema

FOOD ALLERGENS

Stomach upset or cramps

Nausea or vomiting

Dizziness or fainting

Hives or flushing of the skin

Headaches

Brain fog and fuzzy thinking

Fatigue

Swelling of lips, tongue, or face

DRUGS

Hives or general skin rash

Itchy eyes

Swelling of lips, tongue, or face

Gastrointestinal symptoms

Wheezing

attention since symptoms can progress rapidly to extreme difficulty breathing, dizziness, swelling or tightness of the throat, and a rapid drop in blood pressure. Other symptoms may include swelling and itchiness all over your body, redness, tingling of the extremities, nausea, and fatigue. People who tend to have severe allergic reactions usually bring oral antihistamines and an EpiPen (injectable epinephrine in a special syringe) wherever they go to slow down and prevent these life-threatening responses should they occur.

Testing for Allergies

How do you know whether your rash or upset stomach is caused by an allergy, an infection, or some other irritant? It's not always easy to sort out in the moment, but two common medical procedures can help: skin tests (on the body) and in vitro (outside the body, in the test tube) blood tests. These aren't always conclusive, though, and may not provide useful diagnostic information, at least immediately. You may test positive for a particular allergen yet never have any apparent symptoms from it, or you may have a negative blood test yet still have some reaction. This is especially true for food allergies. Of course, the benefits of a positive allergy test are important—it can tell you which substances to avoid. Skin testing can be time consuming, costly, and even potentially dangerous if you're acutely sensitive, but when testing for only a few suspected allergens, the method is relatively inexpensive and quick to provide answers and confirm suspicions.

There are two kinds of skin tests—scratch and intradermal. With skin "scratch" tests, your skin is gently scratched and the individual potential allergen extracts are applied to the skin surface. For an intradermal test, the allergen is injected under your skin. If you're sensitive to a specific allergen, a reddened area called a wheal and flare (like a hive) appears within 5 to 15 minutes. Skin reactions can range from mild redness to swelling at the site. A word of caution: If you're extremely sensitive, skin testing could lead to a severe or even anaphylactic reaction (though rare). Plus, skin reactions are affected by medications you might be taking, especially steroids and antihistamines, which may prevent and mask allergic reactions and therefore not provide accurate results.

On the other hand, in vitro allergy blood tests are much more objective, with no personal risk of dangerous reactions. However, results may be less accurate. Here, too, the results can be affected by medication, especially steroid drugs that lower immune reactions.

Seasonal Allergies

Did you know that the "ugliest" plants are said to be responsible for most seasonal allergies? It turns out that there's a relationship between how pretty a plant is and its allergy-inducing pollens. According to allergist Robert Valet[6] at Vanderbilt University Medical Center, flowers that smell or look attractive capture the attention of insect pollinators so that their pollen doesn't generally float in the air—instead, insects capture it from the plant. Because plants like ragweed or mugwort aren't very colorful or pretty, insects aren't attracted to them, and the free-floating pollens from these plants contribute to many seasonal allergies. Seasonal allergies are due to the pollens in the air. If the pollens don't get airborne, there's less likelihood that they'll be the culprits.

If you have a runny nose or sneeze a lot in the summer, you may think it's a cold, but it could be an allergy caused by grass pollens or weeds. It's easy to confuse the possible causes for what you're feeling.

IS IT A COLD OR AN ALLERGY?

SYMPTOMS	IT'S A COLD	IT'S AN ALLERGY
How long do symptoms last?	Usually less than 2 weeks	Often more than 2 weeks
Do symptoms get worse?	Yes	Not usually
Is it itchy or does it cause wheezing?	Not typically	Yes, you've got itchy eyes, sneezing, and sometimes wheezing

The Allergy Paradox

Few childhood infections? More allergies! Scientists say that infections early in life train the T cells to favor those that fight infection rather than develop the T cells responsible for allergies. Two types of T helper cells are necessary for immune protection: Th1 and Th2. Th1 cells drive the cellular immune response to fight infections against viruses and microbes hidden inside our cells. Th2 cells drive the antibody (and allergic) response. So when kids don't get a lot of childhood infections, the Th1 cells have weakened abilities, while the Th2 cells, unrestrained, generate lots of antibodies that can propel an increase in allergies and autoimmune illness.[7] Think of Th1 and Th2 as cells on a seesaw. When one type of T cell goes up, the other goes down. An infection requires lots of Th1 cells to fight it off. Allergies, on the other hand, require an abundance of Th2 cells.

Another reason allergies are more common in affluent, developed countries compared to poor countries with less sanitary conditions is that North Americans are just too clean: We're not exposed to enough germs while we're growing up. This theory is called the hygiene hypothesis.[8] We use germicidal bath soap and put hand sanitizers in our kids' schoolbags—in fact, antiseptics are required in many schools. With all the vaccines children get, they don't get deadly infections—a good thing— but they also don't develop as much natural immune responsiveness to pathogens in the environment.

Yet in developing countries, where people have to fend off numerous parasitic or worm infections, allergies are rare. How come? One reason scientists have offered is that their immune cells are so busy fighting off infections that the immune cells that would contribute to allergies are outnumbered. Remember the Th1/Th2 balancing act.

People with long-term worm infections don't have allergies, and they produce a lot of *anti-inflammatory* cytokines, which regulate the balance. A few physicians are even attempting short-term infection with helminth worms in their severely allergic patients. Early evidence suggests this strange approach may be useful but requires much more research.[9] In a related study, in a slum in Caracas, Venezuela, children naturally infected with worms showed no allergies to dust, mold, and other airborne allergens. Then half the kids were given medication for 22 months to eliminate the worms; those who lost their intestinal parasites developed allergies.[10]

Another theory for why infections, such as those from intestinal parasitic worms, prevent allergies is related to the microbiome. Children raised on farms or under less sanitary conditions have a more diverse population of microbes in their gut, which is thought to keep the immune system in balance.[11]

Food Allergies and Sensitivities

Over the last decade, food allergies have increased, affecting more than six million people in the United States. Why have peanut allergies[12] reached such epidemic proportions that these snacks have been banned from many airplanes and schools? While eight foods account for 90 percent of food allergy reactions, peanuts have received the most attention, no doubt because the reactions can be so severe, even deadly. You probably know someone who doesn't tolerate wheat, which can produce a wide range of reactions from wheat allergy or gluten sensitivity or intolerance to autoimmune celiac disease. (Look later in this chapter for more about immune problems with wheat.)

You may think you're allergic to a food when, in fact, it's acting as an irritant to

---

THE TOP EIGHT FOOD ALLERGY CULPRITS

1. Cow's milk
2. Eggs
3. Corn
4. Peanuts
5. Shellfish (such as crab or shrimp)
6. Soy
7. Wheat/gluten
8. Tree nuts (such as almonds and walnuts)

---

your system, not as a true allergen. The symptoms may be similar—they both trigger inflammation—but what's triggering the inflammation is different. An allergen provokes an immune antibody response whereas an irritant doesn't involve antibodies; you can look at the latter as a chemical irritant.

Eliminating troublesome foods or environmental irritants may prevent your body's unpleasant responses. You may improve your digestion, breathing, energy, and even your sleep by staying away from foods that aggravate your body. This process, known as the elimination diet, can be empowering. It's an important part of improving your health and de-stressing your immune system. Learn more about it in Chapter 4.

Asthma

Asthma is a chronic inflammatory disease that affects the lungs and airways. When these tissues become constricted and partially blocked because of inflammation, you don't get enough air—and that can be terrifying and even life threatening. Chances are, you know somebody who has asthma. It may be yourself.

There are two kinds of asthma: First, there's allergic asthma, which is triggered by exposure to allergens such as pollen, mold, or cat dander. The other, less common form is mostly nonallergic, triggered by irritants such as tobacco smoke or air pollution. But whatever the underlying biology, irritants can worsen any kind of asthmatic attacks. A person prone to asthma can react to both irritants and allergens. Cold air, strong chemical odors, perfumes, scented products, vigorous exercise, and even intense emotions can bring on an asthmatic attack.[13]

My dad was a lifelong hay fever sufferer—he had numerous allergies to pollens as well as asthma. Sometimes his sneezing and coughing symptoms got so bad that they escalated to awful asthmatic attacks. He even had an oxygen tank to help him breathe at times. His asthma attacks were also affected by strong emotions, positive or negative. In fact, the day he saw his first grandchild, his breathing became so constricted that he had to be rushed to the hospital. His allergies and emotions multiplied the severity of the reactions in his lungs. According to a recent study, most people who have asthma also have allergies. Whether it was an allergy or irritant that caused my dad's asthma attacks, they were almost always life threatening.[14]

Though fewer than 10 percent of Americans suffer from potentially deadly asthma, the incidence appears to be increasing. We don't know exactly why, but some theories suggest possible culprits as more environmental toxins, pollutants, or gut and digestive problems, and even excess vaccine stimulation. Interestingly, there are more allergies in developed countries like the United States than in developing countries like those in central Africa, for example.

Wheat Allergy, Wheat Sensitivity, and Celiac Disease

You get a bloated belly or a bellyache when you eat bread—but you love it and don't want to give it up. Your child has temper tantrums and constipation after eating a dish of pasta. Your Aunt Sue has splitting headaches after her morning sweet roll. And your younger brother can't eat wheat at all. What's going on in your family?

There's a broad spectrum of reactions to wheat products from allergies and sensitivities to inflammation. Reactions to wheat can cause *celiac disease*, which is an autoimmune condition—that's why we discuss it here, between allergies and autoimmunity. Wheat and its inherent proteins—*gluten*, gliadin, and perhaps others—are the culprits that contribute to a slew of immune problems. These proteins are found in flour products and baked goods that use wheat, rye, or barley, although wheat products contain higher amounts of these reactive proteins. Even soy sauce can be a source of gluten, since it often contains wheat. (Be sure to read labels carefully!)

It's not always easy to tell if you've got a true wheat allergy or just a sensitivity. In a true wheat allergy, your immune cells produce IgE antibodies against wheat proteins, which then trigger a typical allergic response. Gluten sensitivity/reactivity, in comparison, is an issue of irritation and inflammation with either no antibodies against the proteins or—more commonly—IgG antibodies to the gluten and wheat, leading to a delayed reaction.[15] (Remember, for something to be an allergy, IgE antibodies must be produced by the immune cells. IgG reactions are more common and are deemed a hypersensitivity reaction, not an allergy.)

Some people may have a sensitivity, rather than an allergy, to wheat. In that case, the symptoms may not only involve the digestive tract but also manifest as other reactions, like headaches, nasal and sinus congestion, mood changes, and fatigue. Sensitivity may come from overeating gluten products, a change in microbial balance, intestinal inflammation, or repeated courses of antibiotic or anti-inflammatory medicines. In other words, being hypersensitive to wheat proteins is an inflammatory response, while an actual allergy to gluten is a result of an immune antibody response by your lymphocytes.

Then there's celiac disease, an autoimmune condition in which you can't tolerate even small amounts of gluten. Your body produces *autoantibodies* against one of the proteins in your intestines, and that leads to intestinal inflammation and damage. The immune attack is on your gut lining, and it's made worse by eating gluten, which interferes with nutrient absorption, causes major digestive upsets, and, in rare instances, results in death. Sometimes, celiac disease is sparked by a viral infection that initially damages the lining of your GI tract, and it's worsened by eating anything containing gluten. The diagnosis of celiac is made by a biopsy of the intestinal lining. People with celiac often have other autoimmune illnesses as well, such as type 1 diabetes. Compared to wheat allergies and general reactivity, celiac disease is rare—but it can be debilitating. Symptoms of celiac disease can include:

- Abdominal bloating, gas, and pain
- Diarrhea or constipation
- Weight loss or weight gain
- Fatigue
- Itchy skin rash
- Missed menstrual periods
- Infertility or miscarriages[16]

The growing market of gluten-free products topped more than $2 billion in sales in 2012 as the awareness and incidence of gluten reactions increased worldwide. Celiac disease is on the rise.[17] It's estimated that 1 percent of people in the United States, or about 1.8 million, have celiac disease, four times the number of people diagnosed with it 50 years ago.[18] Before these people were diagnosed, they probably suffered a lot of abdominal pain and endured malnourishment. That's because with celiac disease, you can't absorb your food properly. It can affect people of any age, including those over 50 who've enjoyed bread all their life.[19]

THE RANGE OF GLUTEN/WHEAT REACTIONS

Is your tummy fighting a war from within? Diagnosis is sometimes difficult, but here's a quick guide to symptoms.[20]

	GLUTEN SENSITIVITY	WHEAT ALLERGY	CELIAC DISEASE
Symptoms	Stomach issues, bloating, headaches, memory issues, balance problems, fatigue, depression	Hives, nasal congestion, nausea, and even anaphylaxis, although rare	Bloating, diarrhea, malnutrition, osteoporosis
Immune biology	Inflammation and sometimes IgG delayed antibody reactions	IgE antibodies to wheat proteins causing immediate reactions	Autoantibodies to tissue proteins like the intestinal membranes
Intestinal damage	Not usually	Limited yet some inflammation	Leaky damaged intestines, increased permeability
Triggers	Gluten, amount unknown, but worsened with regular intake	Wheat proteins and may react with other grains, rye, and barley	Tiny amounts of gluten
Treatment	Gluten-free diet; small amounts may be tolerated	Avoiding wheat products	Strict gluten-free diet

Some scientists think the growing problems with wheat sensitivity and celiac disease are linked to newly developed wheat strains that produce a lot more different proteins. The solution to any of these conditions, however, is simple but not necessarily easy: Take gluten products out of your diet. You may never get a clear diagnosis, but your health may improve significantly when gluten is gone.[21] As with any reaction, you can cautiously retest yourself by first eating small amounts after a few weeks' break. If you are reactive in any way, your body will let you know.

You may discover that whether your reactions to a food are due to an allergy or intolerance or are autoimmune in origin, the best solution is simply to avoid the food.

But with autoimmune diseases, avoidance isn't always the entire answer—the damage has already been done and other treatments may be necessary.

AUTOIMMUNE DISEASES

Maybe this story sounds familiar: Back in high school, you complained of aching joints. Your mom thought you just wanted to get out of swim practice, your grandma said it was growing pains, and your doctor said it was inflamed tendons. Fast-forward: In your early twenties, while busy launching your career and your social life, your joints began to bother you again. Too much exercise, you figured, so you slowed down a little. When that didn't help, you went back to the doctor, who ruled out arthritis. The diagnosis: inflamed joints. A few years later, after a vacation in the sunshine, you come home with aches and pains, hurting joints, and sun sensitivity, with a red rash on your face and neck. Back to the doctor once more for a final diagnosis—a very scary one. It's lupus (SLE, or systemic lupus erythromytosis), the doc says, a serious autoimmune illness with no known cure yet manageable with medications and lifestyle.

Nearly 25 million Americans, and most of them are women, have an autoimmune illness. We know of about 100 different autoimmune illnesses, and there seems to be a new one discovered every year. What exactly is autoimmune disease? Like an allergy, it's the result of an inappropriate hyperactive—and misguided—immune response to substances that shouldn't be dangerous. But this time, the immune cells attack your own tissues or proteins instead of attacking ordinarily harmless materials

---

EPIGENETICS

Epigenetics refers to changes in the way our genes are expressed—not to changes in the genetic code itself. How does this happen? Environmental influences may turn a gene on and off, regulating the way it works. Some environmental factors[22] shown to have epigenetic influence are diet, the gut microbiome, stress, pollutants, exercise, medicines, smoking, alcohol, and even emotions and beliefs. Epigenetic influences can occur anytime—before a baby is even born and all the way through adulthood.[23]

---

from outside your body. With an autoimmune disease, your own body, your "self stuff," is mistakenly identified as the enemy. So your immune cells launch an attack against *you*, mistakenly destroying your cells or molecules.

Are You at Risk for Autoimmune (AI) Disease?

How do you get an autoimmune disease? Four primary factors put you at risk:

- **Genetics and family history.** Does someone in your family have an autoimmune illness? Genes play a big part in your vulnerability.
- **Environmental triggers.** Have you been exposed to airborne chemicals, a lot of sun, or heavy metals like lead and mercury?
- **Infections.** Have you had any recent infections? These might alter your immune balance and cell identities.
- **Gender.** If you're a woman, you're at greater risk than a man.

Let's look at these factors in more detail.

GENETICS. Just as with allergies, you can have a genetic predisposition to autoimmune disease. In fact, research in animals has shown that allergies and autoimmune illnesses are linked to the same genes.[24] With autoimmune illnesses, there's often clustering in families—if one member of the family has an autoimmune illness, it's likely that others in the family may suffer from either the same or a different AI. President John F. Kennedy had Addison's disease, an autoimmune disease that attacks the adrenal gland, as did his younger sister Eunice. His son John F. Kennedy Jr. had Graves' disease, an autoimmune illness involving the thyroid gland. These family clusters are related to the kind of immune reactivity they inherited, which can be determined by detectable markers, like bar codes, on the surface of their immune cells.[25]

ENVIRONMENTAL RISKS for autoimmune disease include exposure to certain toxins, heavy metals, free radicals, or chemicals that are in the air, in the ground, or in the food we eat. Environmental assaults also include sunlight and infectious microorganisms. When we look at the triggering or causative factors for autoimmune illnesses, after a genetic predisposition, everything in the environment can be a factor.

INFECTIONS may be the most common factor that trigger an autoimmune illness.[26] Scientists have some ideas about why this is so. One theory is called molecular mimicry:

It holds that infectious microbes can make your immune system lose its ability to recognize its own healthy tissues.[27] How? If the antigens of a microbe that has infected you closely resemble an antigen on your cells or proteins, your immune cells begin attacking tissues that look like that microbe. The microbe's molecules mimic or imitate your own, and your immune cells no longer can distinguish the difference.

Microbes can be a factor in AI in other ways as well. They may alter the expression or identity of your own cells or proteins so that they're no longer recognized as "self." Microbes contain *enzymes* that can chew proteins into smaller pieces; if those proteins are part of your cells, they would no longer be a molecular marking of self. It's as if a microbe could remove or change the last number of a ZIP code; the changed number will now represent a different place.

Another theory: An infectious agent can initiate an autoimmune response by unmasking antigens on the cells that had been hidden. Think of it this way: Suppose the cell "self" markers cover up another set of antigenic markings on the cell. The infectious agent could strip off the protective coverings and now make visible previously hidden antigens. Your immune cells haven't seen these before, so they decide that these are new and unfamiliar antigens—and launch an attack. Get out of town!

Finally, some scientists suggest that autoimmune diseases, just like allergies, may also be linked to the hygiene hypothesis—we're just too clean! In the end, the causes of the vast range of autoimmune diseases are still a mystery.[28]

GENDER. Eighty percent of AI diseases occur in women, especially those in their childbearing years. So sex hormones must play a role. In general, women tend to produce higher antibody levels and experience more vigorous immune responses after immunizations or infections than men do. And women are often more resistant to certain infectious agents than men. This tells us that women in general show a stronger and more hyperactive immune response and that immune warriors must abound in women.[29]

Autoimmune illnesses typically affect adolescent girls and young women. Levels of female sex hormones are elevated during puberty and through the childbearing years. Although no definitive cause-and-effect relationship between autoimmune illness and sex hormones has been proven, certain observations suggest that sex hormones are involved, even though the mechanisms aren't fully understood. For instance, *estrogen* stimulates B cells, antibody production, and cytokines that increase susceptibility to autoimmune disease.[30] Women with multiple sclerosis often show reduced symptoms when they're pregnant, perhaps because of lower levels of estrogen, which stimulates the immune system, and higher levels of progesterone, which suppresses it. Plus, women's higher levels of prolactin and growth hormone may also increase autoimmunity.[31]

While sex hormones don't cause AI, abnormal or higher sex hormones, especially estrogen, may enhance the effect of other factors that contribute to AI, such as genetics, infections, and toxins. And women with existing AI can experience anything from a worsening or even disappearance of symptoms of their illness during pregnancy or different phases of their menstrual cycle.

All sex hormones—estrogen, progesterone, and testosterone (an androgen)—are steroid hormones that do alter immune balance. Estrogens tend to enhance immune responses, especially antibody production, while androgens and progesterone are immune suppressors. That's why pregnant women often experience improvement in their AI symptoms. This dimming of the mom's immune response makes her more vulnerable to infections even as it ensures that her immune cells recognize the fetus as "self," not as something foreign.

Estrogens, when activating immune responses, can also be proinflammatory hormones. In both men and women with rheumatoid arthritis, estrogens are elevated in the synovial fluid in their joints and in their blood.[32]

Like progesterone, testosterone has been shown to suppress immune responses and affect brain development. It turns out that the left hemisphere of the brain is involved in both immune regulation and processing of language. As baby boy embryos develop, the increasing levels of testosterone affect their brain and their immune responses. And what do we see more of in boys than girls? Learning disabilities, particularly with language. We also see more allergies in boys than girls. Is this a testosterone effect? Scientists aren't sure. Childhood asthma is also more prevalent in boys, although by age 20, adult-onset asthma is the same in men and women; by age 40, more women than men have the condition. Recent pioneering studies at Stanford University showed that men with high testosterone levels have lower responses to the influenza vaccine than women or men with low testosterone. The mechanism for this lowered immune response was the effect of testosterone on genetic expression.[33] Only more research will give us the answers to these intriguing differences between men and women.

One thing we know for sure: Autoimmune conditions result from a misguided hyperactive immune system that produces autoantibodies (antibodies against "self") or autoreactive T cells (T cells that mistakenly attack the "self"). Before you're born, most of the T cells that can attack you are eliminated, although a few remain. And infections, toxins, or environmental factors may trigger them into action.

An Inside Look at Common Autoimmune Conditions

There are two primary kinds of autoimmune diseases: those affecting specific organs or selective proteins, such as Hashimoto's thyroiditis (thyroid), diabetes mellitus type 1 (pancreas), and multiple sclerosis (nervous system); and those involving the whole body (systemic), such as rheumatoid arthritis, SLE (lupus), and scleroderma. There are many more AI issues that we don't address in this book, including autoimmune hepatitis, alopecia (hair loss), Guillain-Barré syndrome (nerves), hemolytic anemia, myasthenia gravis, and pernicious anemia.

GRAVES' AND HASHIMOTO'S DISEASES. Among the most common autoimmune illnesses in the United States are those affecting the thyroid. Graves' and Hashimoto's affect the thyroid cells and function, and both are due to misguided antibodies to thyroid tissue. Although Graves' tends to cause an excessive thyroid response and Hashimoto's leads to low thyroid function, this is not always the case. Many people (with either disease or no disease) may have antibodies to thyroid proteins yet experience relatively normal thyroid function; others may benefit from some thyroid hormone replacement to turn down the thyroid gland hormone production.

INFLAMMATORY BOWEL DISEASE (IBD) includes Crohn's disease and ulcerative colitis. They both cause bothersome symptoms from pain to bloody diarrhea. While Crohn's disease has long been known to be autoimmune, ulcerative colitis has only more recently been considered autoimmune. Crohn's affects the end of the small intestine (the ileum) and is associated with more pain, while colitis affects the large intestine and tends to cause more bloody diarrhea. The two conditions seem to cross over, and an accurate diagnosis is often difficult. The treatment can involve oral sulfa antibiotics as well as steroids and immunosuppressive drugs. Surgery may be employed for serious cases that do not respond well to drugs.

PSORIASIS has recently been found to have autoimmune aspects[34] and manifests as red, shiny, raised well-defined patches on the skin. These patches occur more frequently on the arms and legs, though they can appear anywhere, including the scalp. They can itch or be painful, yet that's not typical. Psoriasis tendencies can cause nail

COMMON AUTOIMMUNE DISEASES

THE DISEASE	THE ORGAN OR TISSUE ATTACKED	THE STORY: WHAT HAPPENS WHEN DAMAGED?
Graves' disease	Thyroid—autoantibodies to thyroid stimulating hormone (TSH)	Thyroid function usually is elevated, as cells make too much thyroid hormone.
Hashimoto's thyroiditis	Thyroid—autoantibodies made to a part of the thyroid cell, called thyroid microsomal antibody or, its newer name, thyroid peroxidase (TPO) antibody	Thyroid can be inflamed and cells eventually do not make enough thyroid hormone, yet the thyroid can function normally for many years.
Rheumatoid arthritis	Joints, the tissues (synovium and cartilage) lining the joints throughout the body—antibodies, T cells, and phagocytes cause inflammation and breakdown of the joints	Lining of the joints becomes inflamed, painful, swollen, stiff, and, often, deformed.
Vitiligo	Pigmented skin cells—antibodies to the pigment cells, called *melanocytes*	Cells that provide pigment to the skin can't do so, which results in white blotches of skin and hair that turns gray early.
Diabetes, type 1	Pancreas—antibodies damage the insulin-making cells	Elevated sugar in the blood can damage tissues, kidneys, eyes, heart, etc.
Irritable bowel disease (IBD), includes Crohn's and ulcerative colitis	Digestive tract lining and membranes—acute and chronic inflammation	Can result in abdominal pain, ulcers and intestinal bleeding, and diarrhea, along with nutritional deficiencies from poor digestion and assimilation.
Multiple sclerosis (MS)	Myelin sheath protein that surrounds and protects the nerves—affects nerve conduction	Nerve, brain, and spinal cord damage ultimately results in inability to walk, speak, control bladder and bowel, or breathe.

ridges and marks under the nails. The worst scenario may be serious arthritis, called psoriatic arthritis, with painful joint swelling. Stress seems to worsen outbreaks, which is the case for most, if not all, autoimmune illnesses.

RHEUMATOID ARTHRITIS, OSTEOARTHRITIS, AND PSORIATIC ARTHRITIS can all be debilitating diseases caused by T cell and antibody immune reactions that enhance inflammation and damage the joints. Inflamed tissues in the joints cause heat, swelling, pain, and, eventually, destruction of the bones and joint. To manage any form of arthritis, reducing inflammation and the contributing immune reactions is key. Osteoarthritis has always been thought to be a "wear-and-tear" joint breakdown

THE DISEASE	THE ORGAN OR TISSUE ATTACKED	THE STORY: WHAT HAPPENS WHEN DAMAGED?
Psoriasis	Skin—T cells attack the skin, causing inflammation and rashes and, in some cases, joint inflammation	Patches of thick, red, scaly, inflamed, irritated skin develop. Some people with psoriasis have a form of arthritis that affects joints, back, and tips of the fingers and toes.
Lupus (SLE)	Connective tissue—proteins that are part of the gene structures with antibodies to the cell DNA and within all tissues of the body	Nuclear proteins in any tissues could be affected, although most commonly includes the joints, skin, and blood vessels, causing rashes, joint pains, and many other pains.
Sjögren's syndrome	Glands that make moisture saliva and tears, as well as joints and other areas	The moisture needed but not produced results in dry eyes, dry mouth (with trouble swallowing and loss of taste), and dryness in other places that need moisture for proper functioning.
Scleroderma	Connective tissue in skin and blood vessels—abnormal growth	Leads to thickened skin, pain, stiffness of joints, and trouble swallowing.
Celiac disease	Intestinal lining—a protein in the intestinal lining is attacked	When wheat/gluten is eaten, the immune system damages the lining of the small intestines, causing digestive upset and other symptoms.

due to inflammation, but it may have some autoimmune components as well.

Ankylosing spondylitis is an autoimmune arthritis of the spine that causes pain and ultimately very restricted movement.

MULTIPLE SCLEROSIS is an insidious and slowly developing degenerative neurological disease that usually begins with infrequent symptoms that may recur and worsen over a decade or so. The immune system damages the nerve coverings, and the symptoms and problems are based on which nerves or areas of the brain are stripped of their myelin protective covering. People can lose their ability to walk, see, or even breathe.

DIABETES MELLITUS TYPE 1 is an autoimmune illness that attacks the cells in the pancreas that produce insulin, the key hormone for controlling blood sugar levels. When your body can't make insulin, too much sugar stays in your blood and doesn't get into your cells where it's needed. If blood sugar is too high, the eyes, kidneys, gums, teeth, and nerves can be damaged. A person with type 1 diabetes must take insulin to maintain life. People with type 1 diabetes are also at a greater risk for heart disease.

LUPUS, SCLERODERMA, AND SJÖGREN'S SYNDROME are connective tissue disorders in which antibodies are made to cells and tissues and can damage joints, skin, kidneys, and other organs. This causes inflammation that can bring about a wide range of symptoms such as joint pain, skin reactions, fatigue, and other health complaints. These serious autoimmune conditions are difficult to diagnose and treat, often requiring strong drugs. Reducing inflammation, lowering stress, and maintaining peace of mind may be helpful for any autoimmune condition.

CHRONIC INFLAMMATION

What's behind the symptoms of all those allergies and autoimmune diseases? One of the factors, scientists say, is chronic inflammation. Inflammation is an essential and helpful natural process of the immune system in response to injury or irritation, but it's not beneficial for allergies, asthma, and autoimmune illnesses. Yet even outside of these medical conditions, inflammation can get out of hand and continue when it's no longer needed. In Chapter 1, you learned that chronic inflammation is considered a

---

CRP: A USEFUL DIAGNOSTIC TOOL

Monitoring acutely elevated *CRP (C-reactive protein)* is now considered a useful way of tracking risk for heart disease. But this protein can be elevated with any kind of infection, other inflammations, and even pregnancy. So to evaluate cardiovascular risk, many other factors, like cholesterol levels, need to be looked at. Another indicator for generalized inflammation is determined by a lab test called the sed rate or ESR (erythrocyte sedimentation rate). The rate goes up with acute infection, inflammation, and arthritis. The test can help your doctor track your levels of inflammation.

AUTOIMMUNE ILLNESSES: OUR THEORY

Though there's a genetic propensity toward autoimmune disease, genetics are not destiny. The new field of epigenetics tells us that your life and your environment play a part in how your genes are expressed.[35] You may have inherited tendencies toward an overactive, misguided immune system, but you won't necessarily get sick.

What can set the immune system off against you? As your body fights invading microbes, it activates T cell immunity and antibody formation, making weapons against whatever it can find to fight. For example, the expression of Hashimoto's thyroiditis, in which antibodies are made against thyroid cells, may be a fight to eradicate a microbe that's made its way into the thyroid gland, leading to inflammation and, eventually, illness.

Candida yeast overgrowth, the gut biome, and epigenetic changes are other factors that play a part in overactive immunity. Many doctors—especially integrative physicians—believe that yeast overgrowth causes physical and mental problems, like digestive gas and bloating or brain fog. When *Candida albicans* or other yeasts grow out of control in the digestive tract, it upsets the balance of gut microbes, complicated by immune responses against that organism—and by the changes made to the genes of gut microbes and your own immune cells. The gut microbiome plays a huge part in the development (and prevention) of autoimmune diseases.[36] The gut biome is partially influenced by diet and environmental agents, which can alter epigentice control of the genes.

We still don't know the exact triggers of autoimmune reactions, but we believe that by becoming aware and tracking microbial imbalances in your body, especially in your gut, you may discover the role they play in setting up serious health problems like autoimmune illnesses. Lab tests can assess the digestive microbes and predict whether a certain constellation of microbes is leading to hyperactive misguided states. Research shows that people with rheumatoid arthritis, for example, have a distribution of gut microbes that differs from healthy controls. Cause or effect? We don't know yet. Perhaps this knowledge can help us understand why some people with RA improve when they go on a vegetarian diet.[37] But we still don't know for sure if their improvements are because of changes to their microbes or to epigenetic factors. It's a long road to fully discover how diet and the environment influence the gut microbiome and result in autoimmune diseases.[38] We have a lot to learn, but it could turn out that the gut may hold the answer to ultimate balanced immunity.

major factor in cardiovascular disease, diabetes, obesity, chronic pain, and perhaps even cancer and Alzheimer's. Because the inflammatory response is not turned off, chronic inflammation is another expression of a misguided or hyperstimulated immune response. A good thing to remember is: Acute inflammation keeps us alive and is part of the very first immune response, while chronic inflammation can make us seriously ill.

In the laboratory, various blood markers can be measured to determine the level of inflammation in your body. Indicators may suggest the presence of a chronic inflammatory response due to an infection, injury, allergy, or other underlying hidden inflammation, like in your blood vessels. Although many blood tests for inflammatory markers are in the clinical research evaluation stage, they are still used to follow the results of anti-inflammatory strategies like changing diet, stress reduction, exercising more, and losing weight. In addition, new approaches to treatments may target some of the inflammatory markers such as IL-6.[39] If you have an infection, those markers will be elevated. For women who are pregnant or on hormone replacement therapy, some of these blood inflammatory markers may be elevated, too.

THE UNDERACHIEVING IMMUNE SYSTEM

Although hyperactive immune responses account for many of the more contemporary concerns, like autoimmune diseases, for most of human history, it was a different story. An underactive immune system, leading to infectious disease, was the big problem, but that's less of a concern today in the developed countries. Of course, when there are deadly or virulent germs or epidemics, many more people are susceptible, even if their immune systems are functioning normally. Although some people are born with genetic defects limiting their immune abilities to fight off microbes, that's pretty rare. For most of us, our likelihood of catching infectious diseases is more about lifestyle choices—things you can change to improve your health and keep from getting sick. Poor diet, poor hygiene, too much stress, sleepless nights, and age all play a part in who gets more infections. Both babies and elders are more likely to get infectious diseases because of undeveloped or diminished immune functions. People who are immune compromised because of genetics, drug treatments such as steroids or chemotherapy agents, or illnesses like AIDS are at much greater risk for infections, too, usually from microbes that have lived previously in peace with them.

That's why it's even more important for them to keep their immune health strong. In later chapters, we'll look in more detail at the effects of nutrition and stress and what we can do to remedy those crucial issues for your health.

Infection

We all get infections once in a while. Of course, not all of them are due to immune weaknesses. Some people catch everything that's going around, while others stay healthy and strong no matter what's in the air or on their fingers. Whether you get sick or not depends on many factors besides the state of your immune health—from your stress level, lifestyle, and nutrition to the virulence of the microorganism that's trying to invade your body. Perfectly healthy people, after all, may come down with the flu during a major influenza epidemic. Your overall state of health, however, *does* influence whether you get an infection from any of the many microbes you're exposed to as well as how quickly you recover. Plus, the germs in your gut—if they're balanced properly—can help keep you well. And don't forget: Catching infections is also about exposure. During the winter cold season, your friends and co-workers can sneeze a slew of viruses into the air, spraying you with germs and increasing your risk of getting sick. Still, there are lots of steps you can take to avoid infection.

The Basics

Your best defenses are tried and true: Wash your hands, stay out of crowded places, and be vigilant around others who are sick. You may even see people wearing face masks during the height of the flu season. In the summer, avoid potentially contaminated picnic foods that can make you sick no matter how hardy your immune system. Do you go to public swimming pools and showers? Be proactive there, too, and watch out for the possibility of athlete's foot, a fungal infection living in damp, warm places. Wear flip-flops and wash and dry your feet well.

The Nutrition Connection

One of the best ways to strengthen your immune system and fight off infection is to eat a diet that's rich in fresh fruits and vegetables and that contains enough protein. A deficiency of specific nutrients can make you more susceptible to infections, and taking supplemental nutrients may enhance your immune system. In Chapter 4, you'll learn which specific nutrients are essential for immune health plus which superfoods work to keep your cells healthy.

Immunization

Controversies continue to rage: Do we have too many vaccines? Are some of them unsafe? What are the long-term effects on the immune system, the incidence of allergies and autoimmune issues, and overall health? But the fact remains that people refusing immunizations become more vulnerable to infections that are now preventable. And that increases the risk to children, pregnant women, and people receiving cancer treatments who have not been immunized. What we each do affects those around us.[40] Before the development of vaccines, people developed immunity by being infected by often-deadly organisms. If they survived the infection, their immune system was strengthened by the experience and they'd be protected for their lifetime against that microbe. The issue of survival with life-and-death or serious illness as the outcome is often the concern for people without immunizations. Immunizations were developed so that people didn't have to risk potentially dangerous or lethal infections to develop immunity. And by protecting ourselves, we help protect others who can't be immunized.[41]

In spite of the efficiency of a very effective immune system, people still get sick from infectious microbes, which are amazingly intelligent in their abilities to change themselves to escape destruction by our cells or our medicines. Flu viruses change their identities every year. So-called new microbes, including SARS or bird flu, are appearing, while old illnesses, once almost wiped out by immunizations and public health measures, are again becoming a global problem. Consider, for example, the recent increase in whooping cough,[42] also known as pertussis. In 2012, the United States had the highest rate of whooping cough since 1955 with 48,000 cases and 18 deaths, most occurring in infants. In fact, the increase in whooping cough, now a preventable illness, has been attributed to parents' refusal to have their children vaccinated against it.[43] Other viruses can also cause recurrent infections, like herpes of the mouth or genitals, or shingles appearing decades after a chicken pox infection.

Your Aging Immune System

At both ends of life, people tend to have less effective immune responses, and so they're more likely to get infections. Your immune system often begins to slow down as you get older. What does this mean in practical terms? First, your immune memory suffers. Just like you may be able to remember your senior prom but forget where you put your keys an hour ago, your immune cells can better remember immune responses to old infections—but they may not have a hearty response to a new invader. Often, they need a boost to fight and remember new microbes. So for some folks, getting vaccines for pneumonia and shingles is often a wise preventive measure. This educates your immune system to be ahead of the game when it comes to new infectious threats. What you can do to boost your immune system is also part of this book, wherein you will learn about nourishing your cells while spicing up life for them and your health.[44]

As you age, the healing process, in general, slows down. So avoid what you know slows your healing immune system: Don't smoke or drink too much alcohol. Eat well, get some exercise, and lessen your stress. Just as it may take older people longer to walk the block, their cells are slower, too.

Very young people need a robust immune system to handle the many new pathogens they come in contact with. During the first year of life, children's immune systems must adapt to thousands of new microbes in their environment. That's the time when they're most vulnerable to infections. Until recently, their increased risk to infections was thought to be due to an undeveloped immune system. But scientists at Cincinnati Medical Center have unearthed intriguing new data that suggest otherwise. In order for new beneficial bacteria to populate the baby's belly, the research suggests, the baby's immune system suppresses its activity to allow the new beneficial germs to get a foothold in the gut. So rather than an undeveloped immune system leading to infections in newborns, it's their immune system's ability to turn itself off that allows the new microbes a way in. In other words, new bugs in their belly need to take hold to ultimately help the babies stay well.[45]

From the moment of birth, babies are exposed to thousands of germs and other antigens in the environment, enabling their immune systems to respond. Newborns are immune to some diseases because they have antibodies from their mothers, transferred in utero.[46] This passive immunity lasts only a few months. Even so, most young children don't have maternal immunity to diphtheria, whooping cough, polio, tetanus, or hepatitis B. Thus, at an early age, they're given vaccines to jump-start their immune protection.

Fast-forward from the nursery to the kindergarten classroom. Kids share lots of germs, and although we may see more respiratory infections in children, they also recover fairly quickly, if they're healthy to begin with.[47]

(continued on page 60)

IS CANCER AN IMMUNE CONDITION?

No! Cancer is a disease caused by gene errors.[48] Those cancer-causing errors, mutations, or epigenetic changes occur throughout our lifetime, typically to the growth-regulating genes called *tumor suppressor genes* and oncogenes. New research shows that epigenetics are involved, too—that means the gene structure doesn't change or mutate, but the on-off switches do. These switches regulate which gene is expressed and which is silenced.

Inherited cancer genes, like the BRCA1 and BRCA2 varieties made famous by Angelina Jolie, are not common. Inherited cancer genes account for only 5 to 10 percent of all breast cancer cases. Women or men who have inherited these genes have a greater risk of breast cancer, but it is only the risk for cancer. Not all people who inherit these genes will develop the disease. About 55 percent of women who inherit one of these genes will develop breast cancer by the age of 70, and fewer than 40 percent develop ovarian cancer.[49] Most people who develop cancer didn't inherit "cancer genes," but the expression of their genes changed over their lifetime.

Remember the key to how the immune system works? It recognizes differences of "self" and "not self." Most cancer cells remain self—although their genes and growth patterns have changed, their cell identity remains the same.[50]

On the other hand, cancer is a disease in which abnormal cells reproduce out of control. Your body makes abnormal cells all the time. Fortunately, those cells with cancer potential are eliminated most of the time. However, they are not typically eliminated by immune cells but rather by a very potent DNA repair system. Your cells have more than 150 gene repair genes,[51] as your cells always aim for survival.

When the DNA of a cell becomes damaged, it results in a mutation. Damage can be caused by free radicals, by chemical carcinogens, and even by the cell itself making a mistake in copying its DNA for a new cell. In the normal process inside the cell, the cell has a kind of spell-checker that can correct any DNA coding errors. If the damage can't be repaired, the repair agency (spell-checker) triggers a gene program for cell death—or cell suicide—called *apoptosis*. Once the DNA repair system does its job, the abnormal cell and its DNA are removed so that they can't create any problems. But sometimes the repair agency genes are damaged so that they can't fix the DNA problem or program the death of the cell. Once a cell with a mutation slips by the repair agency, it's prone to more DNA or gene errors. It doesn't become an actual cancer cell until there are two to six gene errors or mutations, all to growth regulatory genes. The most well-known repair system is the p53 pathway of genetic surveillance.[52] Unfortunately, a mutant form of this tumor-suppressor gene is present in about 50 percent of human cancers.[53]

Most genetic mutations occur after you're born, over your lifetime, and may be caused by smoking, radiation, viruses, carcinogens, obesity, hormones, free radicals, lack of exercise, and chronic inflammation. Luckily, your body has many different DNA repair systems to protect you.

The DNA in the nucleus of your cells contains all the information for them to make every protein your body needs. The genetic code of DNA holds the instructions or blueprints, whereas switches surrounding the DNA turn the genes on and off. These switches are called epigenetic, and they can change the expression of a gene without changing the code.[54] Ongoing research suggests that you can influence those epigenetic switches through your lifestyle and perhaps even your thoughts. So it's possible that food and lifestyle choices can prevent or alter the expression of your genes.

But there's an important relationship between cancer and immune health: A person with cancer often has diminished immune responses, due either to the chemotherapy or radiation treatments or to the disease process itself. Many cancer treatments kill the fastest-growing cells, which happen to be the white blood cells (the immune protectors), the cells in the gut, and the hair follicles. It becomes even more important for people challenged by cancer to strengthen their immune systems by eating well, nurturing strong relationships, and keeping a positive outlook.

YOUR IMMUNE SYSTEM
AND COMMON INFECTIONS

When you're stressed or overworked and lacking sleep, you can become sick more easily than when you're strong, energetic, and feeling your best. Even when your immune system is working well, if you're exposed to bad bugs (the ones you haven't met before or those that are particularly virulent), you may be assaulted by microbes that multiply as your immune warriors get into action. It seems touch and go for those days that you have symptoms of an upper respiratory infection from a cold virus.

COLDS AND FLU are the most common health and infectious issue—runny nose, stuffy head, headache, and fatigue. Whether or not those invading warriors take over your body has a lot to do with your state of health, your body's terrain. Do you get whatever's going around, or can you resist most of the germs your family, friends, and co-workers share? Many of the symptoms you experience during colds or other infections are actually your immune system doing its work, inflaming and activating your tissues. In Chapter 7, we'll go over simple but effective prevention tips that include washing your hands, especially after being in public touching common pens or door handles, and keeping up your nutritional support.

STOMACH FLU OR FOOD POISONING is the next most common everyday ailment affecting all age groups. Pay attention to what and where you eat, and be cautious with foods that were mishandled, are old, or look or smell funny. Trouble is, we don't always know what food has gone bad. It takes a while for your immune system, very active in your gut, to sort out what's friend or foe among all those billions of bacteria. Luckily, there are many natural remedies like herbs and probiotics to help reduce and rebalance these intestinal issues. Most often, you don't need antibiotics, since they can upset your gut even more.

URINARY TRACT INFECTIONS (UTIs) are more common in women and relate to increased sexual activity and overall hygiene as well as hydration. If not treated early, UTIs often require antibiotics to protect the kidneys. Your immune system has to rally to fight off the infection by sending hordes of white blood cells to your bladder where there's inflammation in the inner membrane, causing pain and burning with urination. As with colds, the symptoms are often based on the reactions of your immune system's struggles.

UPPER RESPIRATORY INFECTIONS (URIs) include sinus and bronchial congestion and coughs, which have a tendency to go deeper and lead to persistent mucus production and irritation, especially as a result of stress and poor lifestyle or, more commonly, smoking. URIs are often treatable with rest and time for your immune system to do its work; if that path is not successful, then antibiotics can help. These deeper and longer-term problems can be prevented by addressing viral infections and colds early so they don't travel deeper.

HERPES INFECTIONS, both genital from sexual activity and oral cold sores from general contact and kissing, are quite common through many age groups, young to old. Both types of herpes can become chronic infections, because the microbe lies dormant in a local nerve and activates again in some unknown cycle, often as a result of stress. Medication can lessen the outbreaks and even prevent them if taken regularly in low doses.

THE TAKEAWAY

Your immune system is essential in protecting you from disease and keeping you healthy and strong. But sometimes your genes, your environment, and your lifestyle conspire to throw your amazing immune system out of balance, making it work too hard or not hard enough. As medical research continues to provide a better understanding of the causes of allergies, autoimmune illnesses, and chronic inflammation, great advances may be in store. In the meantime, there's plenty you can do to strengthen your immune system and live a balanced and healthy life.

We've explored the basics of the immune system in Chapter 1 and the problems of immunological dysfunctions in this chapter. Next, let's turn to the usual treatments offered by most Western medical practitioners. Armed with that information, you'll be better prepared to make decisions about your immune health. That's what *Ultimate Immunity* is all about.

CHAPTER 3

The Usual Treatment

By now, you probably have a newfound respect for your amazing immune system, which fends off dangerous invaders and works hard to keep you healthy and strong. You've learned about your multitasking immune cells, and you've caught a glimpse into what happens when they work too hard or not hard enough. That's when you end up with anything from allergies to autoimmune disease to infections. Your immune system is the foundation of good health and often the culprit when your health goes downhill.

When that happens and you head to the doctor, chances are you'll come home with a prescription.

Treating symptoms with medicine isn't new—doctors and other practitioners have been doing that for millennia. Since ancient times, people have relied on folk medicine, using plants to treat their ailments. Herbal medicine is the original health care. Then consider, for instance, the use of willow bark to calm fever and ease pain. Yet a century or so ago, chemists discovered willow bark's active ingredient—salicin— and the modern pharmaceutical industry was born. Scientists isolated salicin and turned it into aspirin, which sells to the tune of 50,000 tons worldwide, with Americans taking 29 billion tablets a year.[1] And aspirin was just the beginning. New drugs are being developed every day, and many of them are based on herbal remedies that go back thousands of years. Scientists have made incredible breakthroughs, developing medications that ease pain, alleviate symptoms, and often save lives. But sometimes, those pills and potions treat the outward appearance without getting to the root cause of the disease, which is often your out-of-balance immune system.

MIRACLE DRUGS

A miracle drug, the antibiotic penicillin, discovered in 1928 and ultimately developed for use by 1942, has saved hundreds of millions of lives. In World War I, 18 percent of those who died succumbed to bacterial pneumonia; in World War II, on the other hand, the death rate fell to less than 1 percent because of penicillin.[2] Ironically, when Alexander Fleming was awarded the Nobel Prize in 1945 for his discovery of penicillin, he warned of the dangers of its overuse. Since then, his warnings have come true, as antibiotic-resistant strains of bacteria continue to evolve. Developing a strong immune system has become more important than ever.

Since the time of penicillin, scientists have been making rapid progress in developing medications to treat symptoms and diseases. When you look at the number of drugs developed and approved by the FDA[3] from 1938 to 1940 (1,782 new drugs) and from 1942 to 1943 (1,000 more) and compare that total to the new drugs in 2010 (just 93) and in 2013 (55),[4] you can appreciate the explosion of drug development because of the war and the new, exciting pharmaceutical field. Scientists developing penicillin as a drug had to figure out how to purify it from the mold and then produce vast amounts so that it could be a medically useful commercial product. Other scientists learned how to extract hormones from animal and plant sources to treat thyroid problems and how to use liver extract to help with fatigue and anemia. But along with remarkable scientific strides, science has moved farther away from nature and into synthetic chemicals, taking the active ingredients in plants, isolating them, and changing them a bit to create a brand-new patentable medicine to sell to an enormous market that's always hungry for a new cure—at a high cost and healthy profits (maybe not so healthy for you, though).

So if you follow doctor's orders and take those pills, you'll likely eliminate the symptoms that have been troubling you, but the meds won't treat your misguided immune system or the lifestyle imbalances that led to the problem. Since knowledge is power, let's take a look at both the benefits and risks of the drugs that doctors prescribe as the usual treatment.

MEDICINES TODAY

In this chapter, you'll learn about which conventional medications are recommended for the many immune-related problems. In later chapters, we'll guide you to more natural treatments and preventive measures.

In some ways, your own immune molecules (such as cytokines) act as a drug, too: They fix things, jump-start an immune response, or prevent problems from occurring. Sure, they have a lot to do with protecting us from dangerous invading microbes and maintaining balance, but they can create problems as well. If an underactive immune system results in too-frequent colds, or if hyperactive or misguided immune responses trigger allergies or an autoimmune disease, you look for relief from any irritating or painful symptoms.

Western doctors are trained to diagnose what's wrong and to prescribe drugs to alleviate symptoms or correct abnormal levels of health risk factors like high blood pressure or elevated cholesterol. Knowing the correct diagnosis and then choosing the right medication out of the thousands of current choices isn't easy; clearly, experience and wisdom help. Diagnosing and correctly treating symptoms are important goals in mainstream medicine. But even more crucial is learning to keep your body healthy and vital so that you do not need doctors and drugs quite as much. The best scenario is when your doctor can identify, treat, and correct the real causes of ill health.

CASE STUDY:
Treating Allergies

Mary M. lives under redwood trees and has been plagued with allergy symptoms and lots of sneezing and coughing. At one point, her cough was so bad her doctor prescribed prednisone, an immune-suppressing drug, to relieve her symptoms. Within 2 days, she was much better. But a year later, her symptoms returned. The prednisone provided instant relief, but no one can stay on it permanently, since it increases risk for other problems—ulcers, bone loss, and more infections. What can a person with persistent allergies do besides rely on prednisone to suppress immune responses? See Chapter 7.

CASE STUDY:
Treating Bladder Infections

Betty is a 49-year-old woman with a bladder infection that arose after a romantic getaway weekend with her husband. This is a common scenario for the development of a bladder infection, or cystitis. After a culture and sensitivity test on her urine, the lab identified the bacterial organism present (*E. coli*) and determined which antibiotics (sulfa) would likely eradicate or suppress the organism's growth. Since Betty didn't think she was allergic to the sulfa medicines, she started her course of treatment. But on the second day, she broke out in an itchy rash, a common side effect of antibiotics. Now, even though her urinary symptoms improved, she still needed a longer treatment, so I stopped her sulfa meds, prescribed another antibiotic, nitrofurantoin (Macrodantin or Macrobid), and had her continue to drink fluids and take Benadryl to relieve her itchy rash and help her sleep at night. Betty eventually got better, but the side effects made her recovery long and uncomfortable.

Current conventional medical approaches focus on diminishing the symptoms to provide relief. But the underlying cause may be an immune system that isn't working at its best. Scientists are making strides in understanding how the immune system works and fails—and to successfully treat it when it breaks down. Until then, sometimes the best that can be done is to treat the discomfort you are experiencing, making your symptoms go away, at least temporarily. But the problems can surface again and potentially lead to more problems later.

How Pharmaceuticals Work

There are many types of drugs with various functions and actions. Drugs, regardless of their origin, can work in several ways.

CHANGE BIOLOGICAL FUNCTIONS. Some drugs have physiological effects on body functions, such as loosening constipation (laxatives) or slowing bowel function in diarrhea (Kaopectate or Lomotil) or blocking allergy symptoms (antihistamines).

BLOCK PAIN AND LESSEN INFLAMMATION. Some drugs are effective in relieving pain by blocking pain centers or the brain's experience of pain (acetaminophen and codeine). Since most pain is due to inflammation, many pain drugs are also anti-inflammatory (aspirin and ibuprofen).

ATTACK AND CONQUER. Some drugs kill the invader or prevent it from growing; strong antibiotic medicines such as penicillin or ciprofloxacin are examples of this kind of drug.

REPLACE MISSING INGREDIENTS. Some drugs replace ingredients that your body needs and has in short supply. Examples are thyroid hormones as well as insulin for diabetes, which replaces that hormone when your body stops producing enough of it. Other hormones that may be replaced through medication are estrogen and testosterone, especially in a person's later years.

What can drugs do for you? They are often useful at alleviating pain, reducing inflammation, and resolving infections. Some drugs focus on one primary problem or function, like an antihistamine (Benadryl, for example), which blocks the histamine/allergy response and can dry up a runny nose or reduce the itching from skin allergy. However, even with the relief they provide, many pharmaceutical agents may result in harmful side effects requiring additional drugs or even cause new problems. Have you seen the drug ads on TV lately? The adverse effects that pharmaceutical companies are required to disclose—from dry mouth or sleepiness from Benadryl to an ulcer from prednisone—might make you think that the cure is worse than the disease.

DRUG THERAPY

How much do you know about the drugs that you and your family take regularly? What about any new ones that are prescribed for you? These days, 48 percent of adults are taking at least one drug daily.[5]

Choosing the Right Medication at the Right Dose

Before you fill a prescription, have a conversation with your health-care provider. Ask this important question: What are the benefits versus the risks for any suggested treatment, especially drugs? It takes awareness—and cooperation—to find the right medicine and the lowest effective dose that will provide the greatest benefit with the fewest side effects. How can you make that decision? Look first at the condition you need to treat and then apply the following principles:

PRINCIPLE 1: TAKE THE SMALLEST DOSAGE NEEDED TO GET THE RESULTS YOU AND YOUR DOCTOR WANT. Start low and move up if needed. This way, you're likely to experience the fewest side effects. It may be an ideal approach with drugs that lower blood pressure, with statin medicines for lowering cholesterol, or with drugs like Claritin for allergies or Celebrex for arthritis.

MODERN MEDS AT A GLANCE

Here's a quick overview of the prescriptions you're likely to receive when you visit your health-care provider for an immune issue. Each targets the symptoms, sometimes making them disappear for a while. But none of them get at the root cause of your complaint—an immune system that isn't working quite right.

COMPLAINT OR SYMPTOM	THE DRUGS	HOW IT WORKS	POSSIBLE SIDE EFFECTS*
Allergies	Antihistamines like Benadryl, Allegra, Claritin, or Zyrtec	Blocks/reduces histamine and allergy reactions	Sleepiness, fatigue, dizzy, dry mouth
Asthma	Albuterol inhaler, Singulair, Intal, or inhaled or oral steroids	Dilates the bronchial tubes and reduces inflammation	Agitation, skin rashes, GI upset, and more for oral steroids (see page 85)
Skin rashes/ eczema	Cortisone creams; oral steroids if bad	Reduces allergic and inflammatory reactions	Thin skin, reduced immune response
Inflammation	Anti-inflammatory drugs like aspirin or ibuprofen	Blocks prostaglandins or changes pain threshhold	GI irritation, allergy
Autoimmune illnesses	Steroids, immuno-suppressive drugs	Reduces inflamma-tion from immune hyperactivity	Many, including acne, bone loss, GI upset, and low immunity
Hashimoto's thyroiditis	Thyroid hormones	Supports proper thyroid function	Sensitivity to excess thyroid, heart palpa-tations
Rheumatoid arthritis	Anti-inflammatory drugs like ibuprofen, aspirin, or acetamin-ophen; immunosup-pressive drugs; plus others	Reduces inflamma-tion, swelling, and pain	GI upset, burning, blood thinning
Chronic pain	Analgesics (pain); acetaminophen; Vicodin and other codeines; and anti-inflammatory drugs	Relieves pain or blocks pain centers in the brain; lessens the pain message and reduces inflammation	Gastric irritation, constipation, ulcers, liver irritation
Colds and flu (viral infections)	Advil, antihistamines, and/or acetamino-phen	Reduces symptoms like aches and pains, headaches, etc.	GI upset, fatigue, allergic skin rashes
Bacterial infections	Antibiotics	Kills bacteria or blocks their reproduction	Varied, Such as GI upset, allergic skin rashes

Note that most drug side effects occur fewer than 10 percent of the time and often much less frequently; side effects occur less often with lower drug dosages. A good policy is to use—or to ask your doctor to prescribe—the lowest effective dosage for any condition. Often these levels work, and if not, the dosage can be raised.

PRINCIPLE 2: PAY ATTENTION AND MONITOR ANY SIDE EFFECTS. Be ready to work with your doctor to adjust doses as needed.

PRINCIPLE 3: THINK LIFESTYLE FIRST, NATURAL THERAPIES NEXT, DRUGS LAST. When you incorporate lifestyle changes plus use natural therapies, you're more likely to see benefits, with or without pharmaceuticals.

THE USUAL TREATMENT: DRUGS AND IMMUNE-RELATED HEALTH PROBLEMS

Now let's look at some common conditions related to your immune challenges and imbalances and see what kinds of drugs are commonly prescribed. You'll learn about how these medicines work—and how they can sometimes go wrong.

THE TOP 10 MOST PRESCRIBED DRUGS

In 2011, the number of prescriptions filled at retail pharmacies in the United States was almost 4 billion,[10] and nearly 80 percent of those were for generic drugs. Here are the top 10 prescriptions filled.

1. Hydrocodone combined with acetaminophen (generic Vicodin and Norco)—131.2 million

2. Simvastatin (generic form of Zocor), a cholesterol-lowering statin drug—94.1 million

3. Lisinopril (brands include Prinivil and Zestril), a blood pressure drug—87.4 million

4. Levothyroxine (generic form of Synthroid and Levoxyl), a synthetic thyroid hormone—70.5 million

5. Amlodipine (generic form of Norvasc), a blood pressure drug—57.2 million

6. Omeprazole (generic form of Prilosec), an antacid—53.4 million (not including over-the-counter sales)

7. Azithromycin (brands include Z-Pak and Zithromax), an antibiotic—52.6 million

8. Amoxicillin (various brands), another antibiotic—52.3 million

9. Metformin (generic form of Glucophage), a diabetes drug—48.3 million

10. Hydrochlorothiazide (HCTZ, various brands), a water pill used to lower blood pressure—47.8 million

---

Everyday Infections

Infectious illnesses—those conditions that get passed along from one person to another—are a common health and immune-related problem. Think they're caused by germs? Yes and no. Although many illnesses *are* related to the microbes you meet up with, your general health and your personal internal environment, including the health of your immune system, offer the best prevention and protection.

When you decide to seek help because your symptoms from an infection got worse—or just hang on too long—your doctor usually finds it easy to make a diagnosis. You've got an "itis"—bronchitis, cystitis, or sinusitis ("itis" means inflammation at a particular site). So your doctor may write you a prescription for an antibiotic, the main option. That will likely work pretty well if the growing and invasive microbe causing the "itis" is a bacteria, since an antibiotic zaps those bugs. Antibiotics for bacterial infections are one of Western medicine's great triumphs. Sadly, though, you can't resolve all your health complaints with an antibiotic prescription.

If your infection stems from a virus, for instance, which is a more likely culprit than a bacteria, antibiotics don't work. Then your doctor's best advice to you is to get

---

THE TOP TEN MOST EXPENSIVE DRUGS

1. Lipitor, a cholesterol-lowering statin drug
2. Nexium, an antacid
3. Plavix, a blood thinner
4. Advair Diskus, an asthma inhaler
5. Abilify, an antipsychotic drug
6. Seroquel, an antipsychotic and tranquilizer drug
7. Singulair, an oral asthma steroid drug
8. Crestor, a cholesterol-lowering statin drug
9. Actos, a diabetes drug
10. Epogen, an injectable anemia drug

Americans spend a lot of time and a lot of money at the pharmacy. These ten range from the $7 billion plus for Lipitor down to the $3.3 billion for Epogen. Clearly, we can do better and save money for ourselves and the health-care system if we can prevent some of these problems. That's what this book is all about.

plenty of rest, drink lots of fluids, and try some over-the-counter remedies or your favorite remedy from the health food store or from your family's healing tradition.

Your doctor will likely interview and examine you, then consider whether any tests are needed to further evaluate your situation. Tests may include a throat or urine culture or a blood test, like a CBC (complete blood count) to look at the numbers and types of your infection-fighting white blood cells to see how your body is responding. Often, with a bacterial infection, your white blood cells are elevated, especially the phagocytic neutrophils, while with a viral infection, white blood cells stay lower with more lymphocytes than neutrophils present.

Let's take a look at some common infections and see how they're treated in a Western, pharmaceutical way—and how risky the side effects may be.

Colds and Influenza: Viral Infections

These common upper respiratory viral infections tend to run their own course, with the healthy body handling them perfectly well. Cold symptoms are usually a runny nose, cough, low-grade fever, sore throat, and difficulty sleeping—and your only recourse is to suffer through them and let your body do its healing (or control symptoms with over-the-counter medications or natural remedies), since no antibiotics or antivirals will hasten your recovery. In adults, the course of a cold is usually shorter than in children, for whom it can last a couple of weeks. Influenza is another story. Though it has some of the same symptoms as a cold, it also comes with intense body aches and high fever; thus, it is a systemic illness that affects your whole body.

THE USUAL TREATMENT. Several drugs, including Tamiflu, target influenza viral infections, although the data from clinical trials of young and older adults show that, at best, it shortens the duration of the infection by 1 day.[11] Generally, the medications recommended for a cold or the flu simply treat the symptoms—lessening nasal congestion or cough and countering aches and pains. Nasal decongestants in the form of a capsule or nasal spray contain phenylephrine or pseudoephedrine. Prescription cough suppressants include codeine and hydrocodone (both narcotics) cough syrups; over-the-counter medications include dextromethorphan and diphenhydramine. Guaifenesin is another OTC medication used for coughs to loosen mucus. Plus, pain relievers like ibuprofen can be helpful. Never take aspirin for the flu.

THE SIDE EFFECTS. Tamiflu can cause nausea and vomiting as well as allergic reactions including an itchy skin rash or trouble breathing. Nasal spray decongestants can have rebound effects, worsening the congestion. Oral decongestants are stimulants that can raise blood pressure, so avoid OTC decongestants if you already have high blood pressure.[12] Codeine-based cough remedies can cause sedation and constipation. Guaifenesin can lead to nausea, vomiting, dizziness, or rashes. Pain meds can result in GI upset and abdominal pain.

Otitis Media (Ear Infection)

Ear infections, more common in children, can happen at any age. They often occur after colds, as germs and fluids get into your ear canal through the eustachian tubes and cause inflammation, swelling, and pain that sometimes interferes with hearing. Your doctor can easily check your ears to see if there is an infection or redness. Sometimes, especially with kids, ear infections are related to an allergic response to a food such as cow's milk, which can cause congestion in the ear canals.

THE USUAL TREATMENT. Your doctor is likely to prescribe antibiotics, such as penicillin, amoxicillin, Cipro, or Keflex, which are often very effective for bacterial infections. These drugs can protect your ears from deeper infections that may damage the eardrums, tissues, and bones that support hearing; such damage could result in hearing loss. Because some people have recurrent ear infections, they tend to take antibiotics too often, even though many ear infections are viral based or symptoms of fluid pressure and pain due to noninfectious agents.

THE SIDE EFFECTS. These strong antibiotics can upset the digestion by direct irritation or by altering the microflora of the gut. They can also cause allergic skin rashes or, in women, vaginal yeast infections—all relatively common.

Bronchitis, Sinusitis, and Other Upper Respiratory Infections (URIs)

These are painful, often recurring problems that can come from bacteria, viruses, and even yeast (fungi). They can also result from exposure to cigarette smoke or other irritants, or from mucus congestion from the diet (mucus becomes a site for germs to harbor and grow and get into your system), which, along with weakened immunity and lower protection, sets the stage for deeper infections. Then you may experience a cold virus or bacteria. Also, during detoxification and cleansing diets, symptoms similar to URIs may occur. For some people, these URI problems may become chronic, inflamed conditions such as chronic bronchitis or sinusitis.

THE USUAL TREATMENT. When you show up at your doctor's office with an upper respiratory infection, you'll most likely leave with a prescription for an antibacterial or antiviral medication—and sometimes, you'll be back for a second or even a third go-round. Here's an overview of what to expect: Possibly the antibiotic helps, at least a little, if there's some bacterial component to the congestion and inflammation, along with the viral infection. You get a bit better, but when you finish the course of antibiotics after 7 to 14 days, your symptoms may return, leading to a second or third course, which affects your whole body, including your gut.

THE SIDE EFFECTS. As with any antibiotic treatment, side effects can include digestive upset, allergic skin rashes, headaches, and fatigue from taking these powerful medicines. Antibiotics lower the active beneficial intestinal flora and can cause yeast overgrowth and subsequent poor digestion, gas and bloating, and even diarrhea or constipation. Vaginal yeast infections in women are also common during antibiotic use.

Bronchitis

With any URIs, the bacteria already present may cause more infectious inflammation and congestion a bit deeper into the bronchiole tubes. These secondary respiratory infections are treated most often with Zithromax Z-Pak or with tetracycline medicines on occasion, partly because they can help to reduce mycobacteria, a bacterial variant that can also lead to respiratory infections. Inhaler medicines like albuterol or steroid sprays may be used if breathing is tight or compromised.

Chronic Bronchitis

If the respiratory symptoms keep coming back, that's a clue that your illness may be caused by something other than an infection—it may be related to irritation from smoking, an allergy, chemical exposure, or even some material you're exposed to at your workplace. One common example of a recurring respiratory illness is chronic bronchitis in smokers or those who work around chemicals. In cases like these, your doctor is likely to take a different approach to treatment and attempt to control your symptoms with inhalers containing albuterol and/or steroids. Albuterol opens and widens the airway for better breathing, whereas a steroid inhaler helps reduce the airway inflammation. Oral steroids also may be used for chronic bronchitis, a condition that can be worsened when an infection accompanies it, requiring another course of antibiotics. As with any condition, it's important to target the cause and lessen your exposure to whatever the irritant may be.

Sinusitis

Sometimes, infectious agents get into the sinuses, which are deep cavities in the bones of your face near your nose, eyes, and forehead. When a bacteria, virus, or fungus get in there, it causes mucus, inflammation, and swelling, resulting in pressure to your head and face and often severe pain. These are challenging to treat because there are microbes and congestion within the cavity, and the medicines only reach the membranes to reduce the germs there and don't make their way into the inner cavity of the sinuses. Sinus infections may take more than one course of antibiotics, such as amoxicillin, Cipro, or even Nizoral or Diflucan for fungal infections (see "Fungal Sinus Infections"). Nasal rinses from hot showers or steams can help to loosen the congestion, and a lighter diet high in liquids and juices may also lessen the congestion. See Chapter 7.

Pneumonia

Pneumonia is often a complication from a respiratory infection, causing the infection, congestion, and inflammation to go deeper into the lung tissue, compounding the

ULTIMATE IMMUNITY

Carly Swatosh, 25

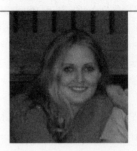

Ever been inside a typical kindergarten classroom? Then you know what it's like—a giant petri dish, constantly brewing up germs.

For Carly Swatosh, that petri dish is her workplace, where she teaches thirty 5-year-olds everything from their ABCs to the fine points of tying shoelaces. She loves her job, but when she first started 3 years ago, she found she was getting sick—a lot. "I was constantly exposed to germs," she says, "and I always seemed to have a cold or to be on the verge of getting one."

Then there was the stress: In addition to her full-time teaching job, Carly is working on her master's degree in education. That has left little time to recharge her batteries. And her favorite form of relaxation—hanging out at her parents' house, riding and grooming the horses, and playing with the dogs—was out. Whenever she was around animals, she'd suffer from severe asthma attacks, stuffy nose, rash, and hives. When it got really bad, she went to an allergist, who put her on two prescriptions and an inhaler to keep her airways open. Mostly, she had to stay away from the animals altogether.

Finally, she saw Dr. Haas, who tested her for allergies and put her on the Cool Down Program. Carly's program includes supplements like vitamin A, calcium, and lysine, plus drops (allergy desensitization) that curb her asthma and allergy attacks. She's also following the I-PEP program, and—just as important—staying active and finding time to recharge.

"I've learned how important it is to manage stress," Carly says. "I've gotten into the habit of going for a walk with friends in the evening, dancing with my kids at school, and remembering to just take a deep breath if I get anxious."

And the allergies and asthma? "It's amazing," says Carly. "Even though I'm not on any meds and I've given up my inhaler, I have a dog in my house and I have no problems. I can be around the horses and still feel great. And I hardly ever get sick anymore."

simpler bronchial tube infection. More serious than bronchitis, pneumonia may cause more fever and fatigue as well as shortness of breath. About half the cases of pneumonia are viral in origin, which are typically less severe than bacterial pneumonia; the latter is most often treated with antibiotics.[13] Viral pneumonia is sometimes referred to as "walking pneumonia," since people still have energy and can get around. A common pneumonia in the elderly is pneumococcal pneumonia caused by the pneumococcal bacteria, for which there is a preventive vaccine.

THE USUAL TREATMENT. For bacterial pneumonia, antibiotics are usually prescribed, and sometimes steroids are given to ease the inflamed lungs and challenged breathing. Intravenous antibiotics and even hospitalization may be required to help people get over pneumonia, which can take a week or two. As with most simple viral infections, the usual treatment is rest and good self-care.

THE SIDE EFFECTS. The usual reactions to antibiotics can be skin rashes, diarrhea, and digestive upset. If steroids are used, they can have a wide range of side effects from GI upset and ulcers to acnelike rashes; however, these reactions are infrequent with short courses of steroids.

Urinary Infections

Normally, the urine, bladder, and kidneys are sterile, with no bacteria or other germs present. When there's an overgrowth of bacteria in the bladder, most often it's a simple infection called cystitis (inflammation of the bladder), in which white blood cells move in to help fight off the bacteria. But when bacteria go through the urethra and climb up to the bladder and higher (up the ureters to the kidneys), it becomes a UTI (urinary tract infection). These terms are used interchangeably. UTIs are much more common in women than in men. Often, when women suffer from a urinary infection, it may be related to sexual activity, as bacteria are driven up through the short urethra into the bladder. Urinary infections can also occur in men, related to sexual activity or poor hydration, but for the germs to travel up their longer urethra, there's more likely another reason for the infection, such as diabetes, in which there's more sugar in the urine, helping to nourish the germs. Nephritis or kidney infection, much less common, occurs when the bladder infection is not treated and bacteria go up to the kidneys.

If you're plagued by recurrent bladder infections, you and your doctor will need to sort out why. You might even be advised to seek the advice of a urologist, a doctor specializing in bladder and kidney issues. There are lots of reasons your urinary infection may come back time and again. There could be a fistula (connecting path) contaminating the bladder from the bowel, or other structural factors.

THE USUAL TREATMENT. Most often, UTIs are treated repeatedly with antibiotics, such as sulfa medicines (Septra or Bactrim), nitrofurantoin (Macrobid), or the stronger Cipro, especially when it appears the infection has moved up to the kidneys. The antibiotics go into the bladder and urine and kill the bacteria. If the urinary infection is related to sensitivity to sexual activity, health practitioners may advise taking one pill of an appropriate antibiotic before or after intercourse and correcting any hygiene activities related to sexual activity. After menopause, hormones can also help strengthen the urinary and genital tissues in women, making them less susceptible to UTIs.

THE SIDE EFFECTS. Typically, bladder infection antibiotic treatment courses are shorter than they used to be, as clinical practice has shown that even a few days of treatment helps clear up most bladder infections. Still, antibiotics can create GI tract imbalances and immune stresses from the gut flora changes, as well as other side effects, such as skin rashes, headaches, and digestive upset.

Herpes Infections

These are common viral infections usually passed during intimate physical contact, such as kissing and sexual activity. There are two main types of herpes viruses: type 1, which usually results in an oral infection, and type 2, most often resulting in a genital infection. They can cross over, with type 1 becoming genital and type 2 contributing to oral infections. Blood tests for herpes antibodies (IgG and IgM) can tell which virus is present. To be specific, the IgG antibody shows whether you've ever been exposed to the virus in your past, and the IgM suggests either a new infection or a recent activation of the virus. Usually, people have only one type, but occasionally both viruses can cause problematic outbreaks. Herpes infections typically produce sores consisting of a patch of itchy or irritating blisters that can occur repeatedly, because the virus lies dormant in the nerves related to the area originally infected and is activated by stress, dietary imbalances, poor sleep, and other factors.

What sets off a herpes attack varies from one person to the next. But the factors most linked to outbreaks include stress, illness, surgery, vigorous sex, a woman's monthly period, and diet.[14] Its location may vary, too—it may recur in one area, or it may move around in the same nerve area where it resides, from near the mouth or areas around the genitals, which could even be in the groin or on the buttocks.

THE USUAL TREATMENT. There are relatively new antiviral drugs that treat both herpes infections (also used for shingles, a related virus). If recurrences of genital or oral herpes are frequent, your doctor may prescribe an antiviral medication such as valacyclovir (Valtrex), acyclovir (Zovirax), or famciclovir (Famvir) to take on a regular basis to help suppress future outbreaks. These drugs work by preventing viral reproduction and thus lessening the outbreaks, but they don't eradicate the virus itself. However, often over time, people can stop having outbreaks. Some people may have only one attack and no more, while others get it repeatedly. It may occur over a few years and then relent or may go on longer, with occasional outbreaks occurring years, even a decade, apart.

The immune system has a complicated approach to both eliminating the virus during the primary infection and then keeping the virus latent, unable to cause infections again. Remember, this virus lives in the neurons for a person's lifetime, and specific T cells keep it contained in the sensory neurons. Immune cells also produce interferons—cytokines that help keep the virus quiet and prevent it from infecting other cells.[15]

THE SIDE EFFECTS. These drugs are relatively well tolerated, but in some people, they can cause nausea, vomiting, diarrhea, dizziness, skin rashes, stomach pain, tingling, confusion, and headaches.[16]

Shingles

This is most common in people over age 50. The virus that causes it is basically the same varicella virus that causes chicken pox. If you had chicken pox as a kid, that virus is likely sleeping quietly inside you and could flare up when you're under stress, sleeping poorly, or dealing with other lifestyle issues that may weaken your body. Sometimes, though, doctors don't know why a shingles infection flares up, but they'll recognize one when they see it. Shingles often appear as a neuritis—inflamed and painful nerve endings, with a patch of blisters in one area, such as around the rib cage or abdomen—but wherever it occurs, the skin feels like it is burning. A shingles infection can last a few weeks and even a few months; sometimes, it keeps coming back.

There's a somewhat effective and fairly well-tolerated shingles vaccine, but it's not perfect. In one study of 13,000 people, the vaccine reduced the occurrence of shingles in half of those over 65. So far, only about 4 percent of older people are getting the vaccine.[17] People over 65 often have poor responses to vaccines unless they do something to enhance their immune responses, like practicing tai chi to reduce stress.[18]

THE USUAL TREATMENT. Shingles can often be treated (or lessened) effectively with medicines like acyclovir (Zovirax), valacyclovir (Valtrex), or famciclovir (Famvir)—the same medications used to treat genital herpes. These medicines may take time to achieve results and work the most effectively within the first few days of lesion outbreak, and they're not foolproof in eradicating the infection. The most effective "treatment" may be preventing it with the new vaccine.

THE SIDE EFFECTS. Side effects can occur as a skin rash, digestive upset, fatigue (along with the infection), and headache.

Infections from Hepatitis Viruses

Most hepatitis is caused by viral infections. The three primary strains (A, B, and C) generate antibody responses, which can be detected in the blood. Antibodies will also be present in the blood following an immunization against hepatitis A or B. Hepatitis refers to inflammation of the liver, and hepatitis A, B, and C are caused by different hepatitis viruses, each with different concerns and immune responses.

HEPATITIS A is an acute viral infection that's passed from one infected person to another, typically through food or water. It's called a "fecal to oral" route, which means that the virus is present in the intestinal tract and, through poor sanitation, can travel from the hands into food. Sometimes, feces from a person infected with hepatitis A can contaminate an entire water supply, although that's more likely to happen in undeveloped countries than in North America. Hepatitis A can cause fatigue and weakness, fever, or dark urine and light-colored stools (from the bile/bilirubin being blocked from entering the GI tract as bile makes stool dark, and the bilirubin coming out through the kidneys, which makes the urine dark). Although hepatitis A can be deadly, most people recover in a month or so. Unlike hepatitis B and C, hepatitis A doesn't become a chronic condition.

HEPATITIS B virus can be transmitted through blood-to-blood contact, primarily from shared needle use, most often from injections with street drugs, as well as through sexual contact. It often manifests as a chronic mild, low-grade infection, but it can become more severe and require a liver transplant. It is worsened by lifestyle, especially by alcohol and drug abuse, and exacerbated by any substances that are hard on the liver, which include most chemicals and even drugs like acetaminophen (Tylenol). The hepatitis B vaccine is highly recommended and even required by schools, though the likelihood of transmission in the United States before adulthood is nearly zero.

HEPATITIS C is transmitted through blood from drug use and shared needles and from virus-contaminated blood transfusions. Transfusion transmission is now quite rare, as all donor blood is checked for the hepatitis viruses. Seventy-five percent of people infected with hepatitis C will develop chronic hepatitis. In the United States, there are about three million people with chronic hepatitis C.[19] This form of hepatitis differs from the other two in that it can be asymptomatic and hidden for years. People may not even know they have hepatitis C and can be symptom free for decades. If the virus isn't cleared in the first 6 months, chronic hepatitis may result. In this case, immune cells can infiltrate the liver and attack the virus-infected cells, causing damage and chronic inflammation. About 15 percent of people who contract hep C clear the virus from their bodies and become virus free. How and why that occurs is still not understood. Hepatitis C infections can be more aggressive, especially worsened with alcohol use (as can all forms of hepatitis), and may require a liver transplant. It can be diagnosed with the HCV (hepatitis C virus) antibody test. Usually, this test is only indicated if a blood test shows the liver enzymes (ALT and AST) are elevated, indicating liver cell damage.

THE USUAL TREATMENT. For chronic hepatitis B and C, exceptionally strong medicines are prescribed, including interferon alpha and antiviral ribavirin. Interferons are a family of proteins made by the immune cells, usually in response to a viral infection. Commercially available interferons are produced through a special laboratory technology. How they work is still not fully known, yet the interferon drugs don't kill the virus; they boost the person's immune responses, leading to increased phagocytic and NK cell activity and decreased virus replication.[20] Sometimes, the drugs are offered on their own, but more often, treatment includes the antiviral drug ribavirin. Ribavirin interferes with the production of the virus's genetic material, thus suppressing its growth. In clinical trials, the combination of interferon and ribavirin lowered the viral load significantly compared to interferon alone.[21] Simeprevir (Olysio), a new drug on the market, is being used in combination with the others or instead of the ribavirin. Its mode of action differs in that it is a protease inhibitor, which means that it blocks a specific protein that the virus needs for replication. It is least effective against one specific strain of hepatitis C virus.[22]

THE SIDE EFFECTS. The biggest problem is that most people taking these drugs don't feel well for the first year or so. The most common side effects of alpha interferons include flulike symptoms, dizziness, muscle pain, fatigue, nausea, skin rash, photosensitivity, and abdominal pain. There is also an alarming potential side effect—serious psychiatric disorders. Ribavirin can cause anemia, and the combination (since ribavirin is rarely given alone) can lead to thyroid abnormalities. The most common side effects of Olysio include a rash, sensitivity to sunlight, itching, nausea, muscle pain, and shortness of breath. People are advised to limit sun exposure if taking Olysio. And since all these combinations include interferon, flulike symptoms are to be expected.

HIV/AIDS

HIV and AIDS are usually sexually transmitted, caused by HIV (human immunodeficiency virus). The virus can be transmitted by semen, blood, or other fluids. In the last 3 decades, research and drug therapy have transformed the death sentence of AIDS to a better-tolerated and manageable chronic infectious disease. AIDS (acquired immune deficiency syndrome) can be the end result of the HIV infecting the T helper cells and macrophages. This leads to the body's inability to fight off even simple infections. Yet not everyone infected with the virus goes on to develop AIDS.

THE USUAL TREATMENT. Today, there are a number of very effective medicines that work together to control and minimize the infection and its effects on the immune cells, specifically the T lymphocytes. AIDS occurs when the T cells are low to nonexistent and those infected cannot fight off general infections.

HIV is always treated with a combination of drugs, commonly abbreviated as ART—antiretroviral therapy. The drugs do not cure HIV or AIDS, nor do they prevent transmission of the virus to other individuals, but they seem to slow the virus growth and lessen the death sentence initially experienced with this virus. Thus, the ongoing development of these pharmaceuticals has been a great breakthrough. There are five main classes of drugs, plus combinations of these drugs: three that block different enzymes that the virus needs to make copies of itself (reverse transcriptase inhibitors, *protease inhibitors*, and integrase strand transfer inhibitors) and two that block the virus from getting into T cells (fusion inhibitors and CCR5 antagonists).[23]

THE SIDE EFFECTS. Adverse effects have been reported with all antiretroviral drugs; they are the most common reason for switching or discontinuing therapy.[24] Typical short-term side effects that may last for a few weeks after starting HIV drugs include fatigue, nausea, upset stomach, vomiting, diarrhea, headache, fever muscle pain, and occasional dizziness. Since a person may be on these medications for a lifetime, long-term side effects may appear months or years after starting treatment. These are much more serious and include liver damage, diabetes, a change in how the body uses fats, and osteoporosis.[25]

Allergies

Allergies are common—chances are, you or someone you know has them. An allergy is a hyperimmune, misguided reaction to environmental agents or foods. It may require experimentation and some testing to clarify what's causing your reactions. What you are allergic to and your responses are unique to you, and often your doctor will treat both the allergic reaction as well as the specific symptoms, like a runny nose, skin rash, or digestive problems. Some allergies you develop as an infant, while others may develop later in life due to various triggers—from eating too much of one food, excessive antibiotic use, intestinal parasites, gut immune dysfunction, or even stress.

THE USUAL TREATMENT. Allergies can be treated with over-the-counter and prescription drugs. For allergies that involve a runny nose or lots of congestion, treatment often begins with antihistamines like Benadryl, Claritin, or Zyrtec. Antihistamines work by preventing histamine from activating the cell, blocking histamine from connecting to specific receptor sites that trigger the cellular response.[26] Think of antihistamines as cloaking devices that don't let histamine get close to the potentially reactive cell. Remember, histamine is produced and released by mast cells as an early response to something your immune cells detect as foreign, and in the case of allergies, that "something" is an allergen. Some antihistamine medications also contain a decongestant; those typically have a "D" following their name, like Claritin-D. Allergic symptoms such as blocked and congested nasal passages often are alleviated by the decongestant, which relieves the swollen nasal passages and dries up the secretions. Coughing may require "expectorant" drugs like dextromethorphan found in many cough medicines, such as Robitussin, or in stronger cough suppressant medicines that contain codeine and its derivatives.

If allergy symptoms worsen or the initial meds don't work, corticosteroids like prednisone and cortisone may be prescribed. These suppress immune functions and inflammation. There are steroid sprays for nasal and respiratory allergies and asthma, and these most often are tried first. Drugs like Flonase are the mainstay for nasal allergy treatment.

For allergy symptoms like headaches or gastrointestinal upset, treatments include nonopiate pain relievers such as aspirin, ibuprofen (Advil), naproxen (Aleve), and acetaminophen (Tylenol). When there's irritation to a tissue, another family of chemicals produced, in addition to histamine, are prostaglandins, which contribute to pain and fever. Aspirin and ibuprofen prevent prostaglandins from being made.[27] These will also lessen inflammation. On the other hand, acetaminophen elevates the pain threshold,[28] preventing a pain signal from reaching the brain, so it's good for a headache but doesn't do anything for inflammation.[29] Your body might still have the pain, but your brain doesn't receive the message. Another drug, cromolyn sodium, is used for asthma, rhinitis, plus respiratory and intestinal allergies. This drug works by being a mast cell stabilizer, meaning it prevents the release of histamine and other chemicals from allergen-armed mast cells.[30]

THE SIDE EFFECTS. The older antihistamines like diphenhydramine (Benadryl) and chlorpheniramine (Chlor-Trimeton) can cause drowsiness and dry mouth and nose, part of the reason for using them, but sometimes they provoke too much drying. Newer antihistamines like Allegra, Zyrtec, and Claritin tend to not cause much drowsiness,[31] but they still dry people out. Decongestants (pseudoephedrine) and antihistamines containing decongestants, like Claritin-D, can cause nervousness, sleeplessness, dizziness, and increased heart rate and blood pressure. The steroid nasal sprays have fewer side effects than the oral corticosteroids, and these include nasal dryness, nosebleed, irritation of the nose or throat, headache, nausea, and cough. Long-term use of the nasal steroids can cause fungal infections of the throat, resulting from the dose and the level of steroids in the body. For more acute and extreme allergic reactions, like anaphylaxis (life-threatening reactions), injectable higher doses of steroid drugs are used. Higher amounts of steroids and their long-term use contribute to serious side effects, such as bone and hair loss, fatigue, muscle loss, impaired sleep, an anxious mental state, skin rash, stomach pain and ulcers, and weakened immunity.

Eczema

Eczema is an allergic skin disorder that's more common in children and often improves or disappears with age. For some, it's a lifelong condition; for others, it starts in the later years. Eczema, also called *atopic dermatitis*, is a dry, itchy rash; its cause is unknown other than genetic and environmental factors are contributors.[32] Some believe that although being an allergy, it may be an autoimmune disease. It's often a compounding issue in people who have celiac disease.

THE USUAL TREATMENT. This allergic/inflammatory skin rash is treated with steroid creams, which, if used consistently, lessen the itching and discomfort of the rash. Like other allergies, if eczema gets really bad, a course of oral or injectable steroids is used. Steroids work by suppressing the immune response. This then reduces the allergic reactions—but at the cost of lowered immunity.

THE SIDE EFFECTS. Medical treatment for eczema is primarily steroid creams, oral tablets, and injections and have the side effects of steroid treatment (see opposite page).

Asthma

Asthma can be caused by an allergy and/or by inflammation due to an irritant. It's often worsened by environmental irritants and allergies, smoke, respiratory infections, and emotional stress.

Asthma usually causes people to have "tight lungs" and experience the sense that they lack air; it's often accompanied by wheezing. Asthma can have seasonal allergic patterns and may be worsened when a cold occurs or with intense exercise. Anything that causes or exacerbates inflammation in the respiratory tract can set off an asthma attack—or intensify it.

THE USUAL TREATMENT. Steroid inhalers are the drugs of choice to reduce the chronic irritation from the allergic or irritant inflammation. Bronchodilators (inhalers) like albuterol help open the airway to ease the intake of air and oxygen and allow easier breathing. Steroids reduce the inflammation and allergies of asthma and thus lessen the symptoms and improve the ease of breathing. Another popular drug is Advair, which combines both drugs, the steroid with a bronchodilator like albuterol.

THE SIDE EFFECTS. For a look at the side effects of steroids, see the section on allergies and "What Exactly Are Steroids?" on the opposite page. Bronchodilators are usually well tolerated but can cause some anxiety and alter sleep.

WHAT EXACTLY ARE STEROIDS?

Corticosteroids ("steroids") are synthetic drugs that resemble cortisol, a hormone made by your adrenal glands. (These are not the male hormone steroids used by athletes!) Drugs in this category include cortisone, prednisone, and methylprednisolone, which work by reducing the activity of the immune white blood cells and taming inflammation by restricting the production of inflammatory chemicals. Low doses of steroids might provide significant relief from the pain and stiffness of rheumatoid arthritis, an acute case of poison oak or ivy, or acute back pain. Topical use is common for any kind of skin rash, particularly from allergies and eczema. Some of the main steroid drugs are oral prednisone (most common), dexamethasone, and hydrocortisone. Hydrocortisone (brand name Cortef) is a naturally occurring corticosteroid, rather than a synthetic.

The occurrence of side effects depends on the dose, type of steroid, and length of treatment. Some side effects are more serious than others. Side effects range from increased appetite and weight gain to mood swings (often an initial euphoria), acne-type skin rash, facial swelling ("moon faces"), blurred vision and risk of cataracts, muscle weakness, easier bruising, increased hair growth in women, high blood pressure, and worsening of existing diabetes. Gastrointestinal upset can occur, as can ulcers of the stomach lining. An increased risk of bone loss and osteoporosis is common.

Prolonged use of steroid creams can cause a weakening and thinning of the skin. Side effects generally don't occur following a localized injection for arthritis or tendonitis other than tissue breakdown when done repeatedly. But for higher doses or when taken over months, side effects often increase. Prolonged use is only for the most serious illnesses, because it puts the person at risk for more infections due to the way it diminishes the immune and inflammatory responses.

Food Allergies and Intolerances

Food allergies are far less common than other types of food reactions and intolerances.

True allergies are fairly obvious: We break out in a immediate rash from strawberries or have trouble breathing when eating peanuts. More frequent (and hidden) problems involve what's called a delayed reaction based on an IgG antibody response to a food (antigen), in which the body starts to react to an excess of certain foods. The reaction isn't based on IgE or histamine response as are "true allergies." The IgG delayed hypersensitivity reactions are common with dairy, eggs, and wheat or gluten, partly because these have more allergenic proteins and also because they are consumed so frequently in today's diets.

Some of these responses have to do with dietary choices, but many are related to gut health and immunity as well as what's called *leaky gut syndrome*, or increased intestinal permeability. Leaky gut involves a breakdown of the sensitive immune system at the membrane surfaces of the small intestine, where nutrient assimilation takes place. This may be due to a combination of factors—stress, tissue inflammation, microbial imbalance, and overuse of medications such as nonsteroidal anti-inflammatory drugs (NSAIDs, which are basic pain pills like aspirin or ibuprofen), steroids, and antibiotics. This unproven theory states that weaknesses or holes in the membranes allow larger-than-normal food breakdown products (and possibly microbes and microbial toxins) to go through the inflamed or damaged intestinal membranes. These large, foreign-looking molecules are free to circulate in the body, setting off the immune cells to mark them for elimination and triggering further cellular reactions and symptoms similar to allergies and inflammation. In addition, leaky gut may play a factor in the development or worsening of autoimmune conditions such as Crohn's or RA.

THE USUAL TREATMENT. This involves an elimination diet, which we detail in Chapter 4. In Chapter 7, we explore the more natural approach to healing the gut, which includes probiotics. Skin tests and blood tests may identify which foods may be causing reactions, although those tests are not completely accurate or conclusive. However, testing helps you decide which suspicious foods to eliminate. Then experience can guide you as you add these suspected foods, one by one, back into your diet. We'll explore this process more in Chapter 4. Drugs aren't typically used for food reactions other than severe allergies, for which antihistamines or steroids may be prescribed. An EpiPen (epinephrine injection), which your doctor can prescribe, is important to have handy for severe or anaphylactic reactions for those sensitive to that possibility.

THE SIDE EFFECTS. There are minimal or no risk of side effects to this elimination diet process, only the effects of eliminating foods and then retesting them. You'll feel better, with a clearer mind, better energy level, and potentially much fewer symptoms caused by the foods you eat.

Celiac Disease and Gluten Sensitivity

Gluten-free foods are all the rage, and they are useful for many people eliminating gluten products. Removing gluten products from the diet can aid weight loss, lessen digestive upsets, and lower the risk of diabetes and cardiovascular disease. Many more people have gluten intolerance than true celiac disease. Celiac disease is an autoimmune disorder (see Chapter 2), whereas the range of reactions to gluten can be from simple irritation to mild reactions, and from allergy to more serious autoimmune responses. That's why we discuss it here, between both allergies and autoimmunity.

There's a range of severity of gluten reactions, from mild to severe. There aren't many drug treatments, but for many people, working on healing the gut (see Chapters 4 and 7) can allow them to better tolerate reactive foods.

AUTOIMMUNE ILLNESS (AI)

Autoimmune disease is an immune attack against the self as your body mistakenly recognizes cells, proteins, or tissues of an organ system as "not self." There are autoimmune diseases that affect specific organs, like thyroid (Hashimoto's) and pancreas (type 1 diabetes), or specific tissues, like joints (rheumatoid arthritis) or the covering of nerves (multiple sclerosis). Most autoimmune illnesses result in antibody or T cell damage to the affected tissue, along with damage from inflammation. Autoimmune diseases affect millions of people in the United States and many more women than men. While each autoimmune illness is different, they tend to share some common symptoms—fatigue, dizziness, sometimes pain, and low-grade fever. Some symptoms can be mild, others severe. When symptoms are gone, that's called *remission*; sudden and severe onset of symptoms is called a *flare*.

THE USUAL TREATMENT. None of the drugs cure the specific diseases, although each illness may have a particular drug that works best to manage it for a while. Usual treatments are focused on first relieving symptoms and replacing any hormone or protein that has been damaged by the illness,[33] such as the thyroid (Hashimoto's) and insulin (pancreatic production in type 1 diabetes). If there's pain involved, anti-inflammatory and pain meds (aspirin, ibuprofen, naproxen, or narcotics like codeine or hydrocodone) are potential treatments. Other symptoms like insomnia, anxiety, or rashes are treated with sleep medications, antianxiety drugs, and so on. In addition, the major focus is reducing inflammation to prevent further damage and to reduce immune activation. When the symptoms can't be controlled, to prevent damage to an organ, or if the disease worsens, either immunosuppressive corticosteroids like prednisone, or more aggressive immunosuppressive drugs, such as methotrexate (mostly for arthritis) are used. Methotrexate does not specifically affect the immune cells; it interferes with the production of DNA in the cells. (We'll talk a bit more about methotrexate on page 90.)

None of these immunosuppressive drugs are disease specific, nor do they cure the illness. Most doctors believe that all AI treatments need to be personalized to each patient—based on the stage and severity of the disease, how long it's been present, and the immunological and biological problems that are creating and worsening the disease.[34]

THE SIDE EFFECTS. Anti-inflammatory pills irritate the gut and can cause gastritis and ulcers. Narcotic pain pills cause sedation, GI upset with nausea and constipation, allergic reactions, and potential abuse and addiction. Steroids can lead to ulcers, bone loss, skin rashes like acne, and many more issues. Of course, another side effect of prescriptions—especially some of the newer and stronger drugs—is the cost to you and/or your insurance company and the country's overall health-care spending. The new drugs require research and investment, and they are focused on specific diseases, so their monthly cost may be $1,000 or more.

Thyroid-Related Autoimmune Illnesses

Hashimoto's—Autoimmune Thyroiditis

This condition, due to inflammation from an antibody attack on your thyroid cells and tissues, often results in low thyroid function. The thyroid controls your metabolism, energy production, and body temperature. When there are not enough thyroid hormones (T3 and T4), people often feel cold, sluggish, and fatigued; gain weight; and experience hair loss, dry skin, and low libido.

THE USUAL TREATMENT. This generally involves adding thyroid support (prescriptions of natural or synthetic thyroid hormones), which can help with the low thyroid condition. The key is finding the right amount for each person, which is based on blood tests of hormones and TSH (thyroid-stimulating hormone), and even more ideally, adapting dosage based on how people feel.

THE SIDE EFFECTS. Thyroid replacement medicines, either natural (extracted from pig thyroid) or synthetic, have minimal side effects. Occasionally, people on thyroid replacement can feel "hyper" and have the sensation that their heart is racing, similar perhaps to the effect of too much caffeine. There are occasional intolerances or allergic reactions to both the pig thyroid extract and the synthetic hormones.

Graves' Disease

Another autoimmune condition, Graves' disease may cause hyperthyroid issues that often require more complicated medical management than Hashimoto's. When there's too much thyroid hormone, people often feel agitated and experience a fast heart rate; they may feel hot and sweaty; and they may lose weight. Beta-blocker drugs like propranolol (Inderal) and atenolol (Tenormin), both typically used for lowering blood pressure, can block the effects of too much thyroid and ease the heart stimulation. There's also a specific medicine called methimazole (Tapazole) that blocks the thyroid hormones and can control symptoms. This is usually well tolerated. A more intensive hyperthyroid condition may require radioactive iodine, which destroys the thyroid and thus requires that the person be given thyroid support for life.

Rheumatoid Arthritis (RA)

This is an autoimmune reaction in the joints resulting from heightened inflammatory response. Cells and antibodies attack the joint tissues, causing damage, inflammation, heat, swelling, and pain. Typically, RA occurs later in life, although there's also a childhood version. RA is worsened by stress and by inflammation that may result from certain food reactions. Both hands are often affected the worst, but RA can afflict any of the joints. One distinction between RA and OA (osteoarthritis): The joints affected in RA are usually symmetrical, whereas in OA, only one side may be involved, since a particular joint is more affected by wear and tear or injury.

THE USUAL TREATMENT. When RA causes pain and joint swelling, strong drugs are often prescribed, including anti-inflammatory and pain medicines, even narcotics, as well as steroids and stronger disease-modifying drugs like hydroxychloroquine (Plaquenil) and methotrexate. Plaquenil can prevent the swelling and pain of arthritis and is also used to treat lupus and other connective tissue autoimmune diseases. It's thought to work by interfering with communication between immune cells.[35]

Methotrexate is a chemotherapeutic agent that affects DNA production.[36] Though it's not known how or why methotrexate works in RA, it does lessen inflammation and slows progression of the disease. It's often the first disease-modifying antirheumatic drug prescribed.[37] As with most of these diseases, the treatment is based on the severity and duration of the symptoms.

In addition, newer biological drugs like injectable anti-TNF (antitumor necrosis factor)[38] may also be used for RA and other forms of arthritis, Crohn's, ankylosing spondylitis, and psoriasis. They can reduce inflammation and slow progression of the disease. TNF is a cytokine produced by the immune cells that triggers inflammation. By blocking it with anti-TNF, an antibody to this factor, inflammation is reduced.

THE SIDE EFFECTS. Side effects from all these drugs are common and include nausea, vomiting, diarrhea, hair loss, and immune suppression with methotrexate and steroids. Plaquenil can cause visual changes and, rarely, loss of vision. Since anti-TNF is given by injection, one of its side effects can be skin reactions at the injection site. The other significant adverse reaction to anti-TNF is increased risk of severe infections, especially fungal. Since these drugs tend to be used for years, more chronic troubles occur, such as stomach inflammation and pain from NSAIDs along with adverse steroid effects of more GI symptoms, ulcers, bone loss, skin thinning, and hair loss.

ITP (Idiopathic Thrombocytopenia Purpura)

This is an autoimmune issue that results when your body produces antibodies to your platelets, the cells responsible for blood clotting. The platelets are damaged by the antibodies and are removed by the spleen, causing low platelet levels in the blood. When platelet counts go lower than 50,000 platelets per microliter, there can be problems of easy bruising and bleeding. Platelets can also be damaged from drug reactions.

DRUGS OR BIOLOGICS?

A drug is manufactured by a definitive chemical synthetic process. The chemical ingredients are known, and the structure of the drug is easily analyzed and defined. A "biologic," on the other hand, is produced by a living system such as a microbe, plant, or animal cell. It results in a much more complex mixture of large molecules not easily defined.[39]

THE USUAL TREATMENT. Children may develop ITP after a viral infection and usually recover fully without any treatment.[40] If there's no sign of bleeding in adults and the platelet count isn't too low, drug or other treatment is unnecessary. Sometimes steroids are used to reduce immune destruction in more chronic or severe cases. For serious ITP, if the steroids don't work or aren't tolerated, what's recommended is the surgical removal of the spleen (splenectomy) to prevent further loss of platelets. Newer drugs include medications that help your bone marrow make more platelets, such as romiplostim (Nplate) and eltrombopag (Promacta). In severe ITP, biological therapy that reduces the immune response with rituximab (Rituxan) will be used if steroids fail. The goals of any treatment of ITP are to prevent the lowering of platelets and lessen the complications of bleeding, with brain hemorrhage the worst result.

THE SIDE EFFECTS. Taking steroids, of course, poses risks, and a splenectomy can place a person at permanent higher risk of certain infections. Possible side effects of drugs that influence the bone marrow's production of platelets include headache, joint or muscle pain, dizziness, nausea or vomiting, and increased risk of blood clots; side effects of Rituxan may be low blood pressure, fever, sore throat, and rash.

Because bruising and bleeding are major issues in ITP, your physician will likely tell you to avoid taking drugs that affect platelet function, such as aspirin and ibuprofen. Antioxidant supplements that affect bleeding, like vitamin E,[41] should be considered carefully, and participation in high-impact sports should be weighed against its risks.

Psoriasis

Psoriasis is thought to be an autoimmune skin condition resulting in red, raised patches often with a silvery sheen. Typical areas affected are around the elbows and knees, as well as the scalp. The condition seems to be exacerbated by stress, as are most autoimmune conditions.[42] There can also be joint involvement as psoriatic arthritis, which may require stronger systemic treatments.

THE USUAL TREATMENT. There are many psoriasis treatments. Creams, coal tars, and light therapy are common applications, as are steroids both topical and oral. Common creams are salicylic acid, calcipotriene (related to vitamin D), coal-tar ointments and shampoos, vitamin A (retinoid), and steroid creams, which help with the itching. UV light therapy is another popular treatment, either alone or combined with the drug psoralen, the latter called PUFA therapy. UVB light therapy is more recently popular and safer. Biologic drugs, as they are termed, such as adalimumab (Humira), infliximab (Remicade), and etanercept (Enbrel), are strong immunosuppressant drugs (TNF blockers) used for extreme cases. Methotrexate is also a drug choice for immunosuppressive treatment of psoriasis.

THE SIDE EFFECTS. These range from fairly mild for all topical treatments to quite extreme for the stronger immunosuppressive medicines. The popular PUVA treatment has carcinogenic risks. Topical creams can cause dryness and irritation of the skin. Humira has a long list of concerns, as do the other chemo and immunosuppressant medicines, ranging from fever and chills, muscle aches, bleeding, fatigue, and GI symptoms to getting sick from infections.

Multiple Sclerosis (MS)

This is often a debilitating autoimmune nervous system disorder in which the immune system attacks the myelin sheath that protects the nerves of the brain and the spinal cord. When the myelin is damaged, signals that travel along those nerves to other parts of the body can be slowed down or blocked.[43] This can cause various symptoms and medical problems affecting vision, bladder, bowels, and mobility.

THE USUAL TREATMENT. Treatments usually involve managing the symptoms, dealing with an attack, and preventing the progression of the disease. Some people have no symptoms, and this condition remains relatively mild for them. When the illness flares, steroids are often the first drugs used to reduce inflammation and prevent progression. Treatment strategies[44] to slow disease progression include beta interferon (Avonex, Betaseron); daily injections of glatiramer (Copaxone), which block the immune system's attack of the myelin; plus a variety of very potent drugs such as teriflunomide (Aubagio) and natalizumab (Tysabri), which are often a last resort when everything else fails to slow the disease. Beta interferon works to help prevent inflammation and damage to the myelin, and people who take this tend to have fewer brain lesions and less disability,[45] though it doesn't work for everyone.

THE SIDE EFFECTS. Beta interferon's effects can include GI upset, flulike symptoms, heartburn, hoarseness, loss of voice, and dizziness. Since the treatment options are so complex, if you are challenged by MS, we encourage you to talk to your doctor about the next best strategy. The whole list and side effects are too extensive and too detailed to discuss here and beyond the scope of this book.

Lupus (Skin, Joints, Cell DNA)

Lupus is an autoimmune disease that primarily affects women. It's estimated that there are 1.5 million people in the United States with lupus, with more than 16,000 new cases each year.[46] Diagnostic blood tests include a positive ANA (antinuclear antibody), which measures autoantibodies made against nuclear material in the cells. Positive ANA can occur with lupus, RA, scleroderma, and in healthy people as well.[47] (Some people show a mild to moderately elevated ANA test without AI problems.)

THE USUAL TREATMENT. Like the other AI diseases, treatment depends on the symptoms and severity of the illness. Common medications used to manage lupus include NSAIDs such as naproxen and ibuprofen, antimalarials like hydroxychloroquine (Plaquenil), and systemic steroids. Symptoms can be due to many immune reactions, from skin rashes to joint pains to damage of the kidneys, heart, and other organs. The treatment is with steroids and other immune-suppressing drugs.

THE SIDE EFFECTS. These are many and varied, and all have been discussed above.

Other Connective Tissue Diseases

Scleroderma (skin and tissues), Sjögren's syndrome (eyes and salivary glands), polyarteritis nodosa (arteries), and others are autoimmune diseases that primarily affect women. Although these are much less common than lupus, they are often severe and debilitating. Treatments are generally the same drugs used for RA and lupus.

THE TAKEAWAY

Western medicine and modern pharmaceuticals can be both problematic and lifesaving. Most doctors are trained to prescribe drugs primarily to treat diseases. Other practitioners (naturopathic physicians, for example) are trained to use primarily natural therapies. Some medical doctors are trained in multiple healing systems. These more integrative and functional medicine approaches are blended into this book.

When someone is injured or acutely ill, Western medicine approaches are often wisely the first choice. But for chronic problems, a more integrative program with lifestyle changes, natural medicines, and drug options may offer better choices. We have reviewed the wise approach to drug therapies. Now we'll explore the ways that diet, foods, and supplements can help to remedy many conditions.

CHAPTER 4

Healing *with* Nutrition

O ur earliest ancestors had the right idea when they hunted and gathered fresh food from the wild; so did later generations who learned to grow and farm the foods native to their surroundings. There were no exotic imported foods, no manufactured foods or artificially preserved meats from distant places. Our ancestors "shopped" local and ate fresh. Indigenous plants and animals were not only their primary sources of sustenance but also their sources for healing. In time, people learned that certain foods could produce specific beneficial results. Sailors, for example, might not have understood that it was a vitamin C deficiency that caused scurvy, but they learned that eating citrus fruits brought them relief and prevented another episode.

Generation after generation has experimented with foods, and now once again we view natural earth-based diets as healthy and see many nutrients as medicinal. We've all heard the stories that vitamin C has the power to protect us from colds and even cancer, and that vitamin B_{12} will give us an energy surge. But until there are scientific studies that prove these ideas, they remain part of medical folklore.

These days, constant exposure to advertising can make us think that we need manufactured food products and bottles of supplements—there's always one more ingredient, the hype tells us, that we must add to our diets. We seem to have forgotten the simple pleasure of enjoying food in its natural state, and we spin our wheels wondering if we're getting enough obscure nutrients rather than recalling the simple, ancient wisdom of our ancestors: Eat fresh and local for a healthful, balanced diet.

Food is essential for life and for building good health and immunity. Although it's something that you have tremendous control over, you don't always make good choices. There are a lot of reasons for that. Stress, mood, and relationships can significantly influence the kinds of foods you select. When you're feeling lonely, stressed, tired, or anxious, you tend to make poorer decisions, like reaching for the pint of rocky road or the bag of greasy chips. All aspects of how you live your life are tied together to sustain your health—or to sabotage it. Choosing good food provides the foundation for ultimate health and well-being.

In this chapter, we'll look at which nutrients are essential for immune health and which foods provide those crucial ingredients. We'll also guide you toward improving your eating habits through a 5-day starter plan followed by a lifelong way of eating that will be enjoyable and healthy.

We'll focus on foods that provide immune support and reduce inflammation and its consequences—heart disease, cancer, Alzheimer's disease, and other chronic, degenerative conditions. Medical research on those illnesses supports the concept that less inflammation is better for good health. Remember: While some inflammation is essential to defend your body against infectious microbes and injury, long-term inflammation contributes to the development of many chronic diseases through inflammatory molecules that cause tissue injury, oxidative stress, and cellular imbalances.

What exactly gives a food its anti-inflammatory or immune-supportive power? In this chapter, we'll show you how the key components of superfoods promote immune balance. You'll learn that while each whole food may be particularly high in a specific nutrient, it contains many other beneficial ingredients. Everyone knows that carrots are loaded with beta-carotene, but did you know they also contain vitamin C, a touch of calcium, and a dash of iron? And all those nutrients are important to your immune health. You'll learn that it's not only the specific foods but the variety of foods in your diet that makes a difference in your overall health (and in your immune health in particular). We even provide suggestions for flavoring your food with immune-supportive spices and herbs like easy-to-grow rosemary—an herb known to diminish inflammation—as well as turmeric and curries, two additional inflammation-busters, and garlic, which has natural antibiotic properties.

We can quote lots of statistics and scientific studies about foods and their characteristic nutrients, but in the end, if you're forced to eat foods you don't like just because they're "good for you," you're not enhancing the quality of your life. Far better to choose a dozen or so healthy foods you truly enjoy so that your new, healthier eating plan is more fulfilling and easier to sustain. We want to empower you to choose the best foods for you—starting now.

While writing this book, I moved into a new cottage with a huge yard. One of the first things I did was to plant herbs that are important to my cooking repertoire—rosemary, sage, thyme, mint, and oregano. Living in an area with lots of freezing nights, I waited to plant my winter vegetables, including kale and broccoli. When I first met Elson several decades ago, I remember one of his first questions to me: "If you were on an island, what seven key foods would you have to have?" For me now, one of those foods is kale. What about you? What would you select?

This chapter offers two perspectives: the scientific evidence regarding "superfoods" that contain nutrients important to immune health, and the health benefits and pleasures of food. We invite you to go on a personal exploration to discover your own best foods for natural immune health. The menu plans, guidelines, and delicious recipes (see Chapter 8) will help you find new ways to feel fulfilled by your food choices. We want you to have great experiences and fun in the kitchen, preparing and enjoying healthy and tasty food that benefits everyone.

Before we dive into the eating plans, let's start with the basics of nutrition to explore how specific nutrients affect immune functions and determine which foods contain beneficial amounts of these vital ingredients.

NUTRIENTS AND IMMUNITY

What you eat affects the health of your immune system and that of the rest of your body. Your cells require many nutrients that they can't make, so you must provide them yourself from the foods you eat. These are called "essential" nutrients, which include vitamins, minerals, certain amino acids, and fatty acids. Although not known to be essential, many phytonutrients—natural plant substances, such as flavonoids and *carotenoid* pigments that give each plant its color, aroma, and taste—can provide benefits to your immune and other cells.

Food is the best place to start for building good health. Sometimes, though, you need more of a particular nutrient than a food can give you. In that case, you could benefit from adding nutritional supplements. For instance, immune cells need zinc to produce antibodies—about 20 or 30 mg a day—while healthy doses of antioxidants like vitamins C and E help keep inflammation in check.

A daily multivitamin/mineral supplement (appropriate for your age and gender—see "Using Nutritional Supplements Wisely" starting on page 133) may provide your cells with the overall nutrient boost they need. There are some contradictory studies on the possible benefits of "multis" and other supplements. Those conflicting study results are due to several factors: small numbers of people assessed, their health status, the quality and dosage of the supplements being evaluated, and how well the supplements are assimilated. But we know this for sure: We need all the essential nutrients for optimal function, and choosing the right products, if you decide to go in that direction, is an individual exploration. Even though this can be a complex process, we'll do our best to simplify it for you.

When it comes to supplements, be aware that while a little may be useful, too much may be harmful. Too much zinc (more than 30 to 50 mg a day) can inhibit immune function and cause digestive upset. We'll get into these specifics later in this chapter and also in Chapter 7, where we'll discuss natural approaches for immune problems.

Limiting your exposure to toxins from air, water, and food is also essential to your immune health. Toxic chemicals like pesticides, pollutants, perfumes, and heavy metals (lead and mercury are two main concerns) can damage your cells and the enzymes and proteins that activate your cells' life-supporting biochemical processes.

The bottom line: To support your health, consume fresh, vital, pesticide-free food while avoiding or limiting "treats" and "junk," such as sweetened sodas, cakes, and candy and fried, oily, and processed foods. Watch out for anything with added sugar. Eat whole foods—more vegetables and whole grains instead of refined grains and white flour products. Eat less red meat, dairy, and wheat to reduce or prevent inflammation. In general, a hypoallergenic diet (one free of *your* known allergens) that doesn't cause inflammation gives your immune system the best support.

And one more thing: Enjoy what you create. Approaching food in this new way may call for a new mind-set and a shift in emotionally based eating habits, like craving sweets and other junk foods. But you'll find new treats that don't come out of a box, can, or microwaveable container by expanding your horizons with healthy, delicious foods.

Nutrient Basics

Let's take a close look at some of the nutrients necessary to a healthy functioning immune system and then identify key foods that contain those nutrients. By the end of this chapter, you'll be able to choose 20 to 30 foods that will help you build a health-enhancing, immune-balancing diet.

You'll recall how we mentioned that your body can't produce certain nutrients on its own. The only way to get them is from your food (or as supplements). And some of these vitamins and minerals provide *essential* support for immune processes as well as other metabolic functions. Vitamins A, C, and E, plus some of the B vitamins and vitamin D are all needed for many of your body's tasks. Minerals that support immune functions include zinc, selenium, manganese, magnesium, and iron. Much of today's understanding of the importance of any nutrient, as it relates to immunity or other body systems, comes from observing the effects of deficiencies in humans or findings from animal studies.

Interestingly enough, it's also possible to be deficient in a nutrient that your body produces, such as coenzyme Q10 and alpha lipoic acid. These are needed for immune activity, for energy production, and for balancing inflammation. We'll get to the details in a minute.

And speaking of inflammation, three key antioxidant vitamins that help protect your cells and molecules from inflammation are A, C, and E; just remember that an ACE is the top card to have in your hand.

Vitamin A and Beta-Carotene

Vitamin A and beta-carotene are in the same fat-soluble vitamin family. Vitamin A is found only in animal foods (butter, eggs, liver, and other meats), while beta-carotene

---

IMMUNE-SUPPORTIVE NUTRIENTS

Vitamin A and beta-carotene	Vitamins B_5, B_6, and B_{12}	Coenzyme Q10
Vitamins C, E, and D	Minerals zinc, selenium, iron, and magnesium	Alpha lipoic acid
		Omega-3 fatty acids

---

and other carotenoid compounds are present in brightly colored fruits and veggies—mainly yellow, orange, red, and green foods like carrots, papaya, mango, kale, and pumpkin. Your body can convert beta-carotene into the amount of vitamin A that it needs—and when it has enough, it stops. Both vitamin A and beta-carotene have antioxidant and anti-inflammatory effects.[1] Vitamin A also supports healthy tissue membranes, mucous membranes (like those in your mouth and nose), and cell membranes to keep them strong, which lessens your vulnerability to infectious organisms. Additionally, vitamin A aids in wound and skin healing while generally stimulating immunity (T helper activity, NK cell functions), T and B cell functions, and macrophage activity.[2]

Vitamin C

Vitamin C (ascorbic acid), another crucial immune-supportive nutrient, is a water-soluble vitamin found in many fruits and vegetables, especially citrus fruits, rose hips, peppers, and most berries. You should enjoy bursts of C a few times a day. Drinking orange juice or a glass of water with a squeeze or two of lemon or a bit of vitamin C powder (buffered, or not, with minerals like calcium and magnesium) a few times a day may help you and your immune cells. Drinking the nonbuffered vitamin C before meals helps to support digestion, since citrus fruits have mild citric and ascorbic acids as part of their makeup. Your upper intestinal tract benefits when an acid medium helps digest proteins and fats and absorb minerals, like calcium and iron. Stress and infections both lower your levels of vitamin C, so those may be appropriate times to consider a supplement to boost your C.[3] Vitamin C supports T and B cell functions, phagocytes, skin health, and wound healing, plus it's a potent antioxidant.[4] One note: Although controversial, a new study suggests that taking high amounts of supplemental vitamin C may increase the risk of kidney stones,[5] so don't overdo it.

Vitamin E

This has immune-supporting functions, primarily as an antioxidant, though it has received mixed reviews in studies looking at its protective role in lowering risk factors for cardiovascular disease. One explanation for the conflicting results is that different forms of vitamin E were used in the studies, with many employing the less active synthetic vitamin E (dl-alpha-tocopherol acetate) rather than the naturally occurring, more bioactive chemicals found in food that include d-alpha-tocopherol and mixed natural tocopherols. An interesting note is that when people over age 65 took a 200-mg alpha-tocopherol supplement (the Recommended Dietary Allowance is 30 mg), their responses to some vaccines increased. Older people don't respond as well to vaccines as younger people, but taking vitamin E boosted their response, meaning they made more antibodies to the virus.[6] Some foods that contain the whole family of vitamin E include wheat germ and sunflower oils, peanut butter, avocado, almonds, sunflower seeds, and even spinach.[7] Vitamin E supports T and B cell functions, is anti-inflammatory and an antioxidant, enhances immunity,[8] and even influences immune genes in older people.[9]

Vitamin D

Essential for life, vitamin D is the "now" vitamin, popular in the press because of the excitement about its newly discovered functions and the disease protection it appears to offer. It's believed that 70 percent of adults and children in the United States are deficient in vitamin D,[10] probably because they don't spend enough time in the sun or eat foods containing this important nutrient. Vitamin D may be a preventive panacea—protecting you from cancer, cardiovascular disease, dementia, and even the flu. People with low D levels are at higher risk for some cancers and autoimmune diseases. Vitamin D is found naturally in oily fish like sardines, tuna, and salmon, plus it's in egg yolks and mushrooms. It's also used to fortify foods like milk, butter, and cereals. Your body produces vitamin D from your skin's exposure to sunlight, so it's often called the "sunshine vitamin." Building blocks for vitamin D are converted to the active form your body needs with as little as 15 minutes of sunshine a day, without sunscreen, in the summer. The sun's energy turns a chemical in your skin into vitamin D_3, which is carried to your liver and kidneys to be transformed to the active form of vitamin D that can be stored in your fat tissue. Skin exposed to sunlight through windows indoors or in a car won't produce vitamin D from this exposure. Those living in northern climates and those with darker skin are particularly at risk of becoming deficient, and once that happens, it takes a while to rebuild adequate levels. Ask your doctor to measure your vitamin D level, particularly the 25-OH (hydroxyl) molecule. Evidence is accruing that supplemental D_3 is beneficial for people with MS, lessening the progression and perhaps even preventing the illness in genetically susceptible folks.[11] Vitamin D plays an important role in inflammation and T cell activation. It also helps with the production of antibodies and cytokines.[12]

B Vitamins

Three B vitamins that specifically support immunity are B_5 (pantothenic acid), B_6 (pyridoxine), and B_{12} (cobalamin). B_5 and B_6 are found in most whole grains like brown rice, oats, and whole wheat. Many cereal products are enriched with B vitamins. B_5 and B_6 assist with antibody synthesis even as they help your cells produce energy from the food you eat. B_{12} is found only in animal foods and is often added to cereals and breads. Very limited amounts of B_{12} can be found in fermented foods, like sauerkraut and tempeh (from soybeans). Vegetarians, especially vegans, usually need to take a supplement. B_{12} helps with B cell proliferation[13] and is needed for the production of healthy red blood cells.

Zinc

Zinc is the most "immune-essential" mineral, and a zinc deficiency puts you at risk for infections.[14] It supports many enzymes related to immunity, especially antibody production, cytokine activity, phagocyte activity, and antioxidant capacity. As part of the antioxidant team, zinc works with vitamin E and selenium. It also plays a role in NK cell activity plus T and B cell proliferation and functions. Although zinc is found in whole grains, beans, nuts, and seeds, it's highest in oysters, mussels, other seafood, and meat. It's more easily absorbed from animal than plant sources. The body doesn't store much zinc, so you need a steady dietary source—at least 15 mg a day, but 20 to 30 mg would be better. (Taking much more than 30 mg of zinc a day regularly, however, can actually depress immune function.) Many over-the-counter cold remedies contain zinc. Whole grains contain chemicals called phytates that can impair zinc assimilation, so don't take zinc when consuming products containing wheat.[15]

IMMUNE TIP

Have you lost your sense of taste or smell? A zinc deficiency could be to blame. White spots on your fingernails, skin rashes, or loss of appetite are other clues you may need to up your zinc—but not too much. The loss of the ability to smell can also be an early indicator for neurodegenerative diseases like Alzheimer's.[16]

Selenium

Selenium is a trace mineral needed in tiny amounts—just 200 mcg a day. (A

Does your breath smell like garlic when you haven't touched the stuff for days? Do you have a metallic taste in your mouth? Could be you've taken too much selenium. Brazil nuts contain a high amount of selenium—about 90 mcg per nut or 500 mcg per ounce. If you eat a lot of Brazil nuts, you may be overdosing on selenium. Mottled, blotchy teeth are another sign, but the taste test tells the story before your teeth do.

microgram, or mcg or µg, is one-millionth of a gram. Most vitamins and minerals are required at a milligram level, which is one-thousandth of a gram.) As with other minerals, selenium is a soil nutrient, meaning it has to be in the soil where the food plants, such as rice and Brazil nuts, are grown. Higher amounts of selenium are found in nutritional yeast (yeast also produces B vitamins). Other sources include seafood, some cereal grains, and meats. Selenium is important to phagocytosis, lymphocyte activation, and antibody production.

Selenium is essential for antioxidant activity; it collaborates with vitamin E to produce the key antioxidant *glutathione*, which protects your cells from free radicals and supports detoxification.[17] Like other nutrients, a selenium deficiency impairs your health, whereas taking too much may be toxic. You should not exceed 300 mcg a day, and the best form is selenomethionine (selenium bound with the amino acid methionine for better absorption).

Iron

This essential nutrient helps transport oxygen to all your cells, so it's required for energy production. Two forms of iron are found in foods. The form in animal foods like beef, liver, and oysters is more easily absorbed by your body than the form found in plants and fortified foods. Vegetarian sources of iron include lentils, beans, spinach, and raisins plus fortified cereals and oatmeal.[18] An iron deficiency may cause you to feel tired and have frequent infections. In contrast, too much iron can be irritating or even toxic. The body stores iron in tissues and organs and recycles iron from red blood cells into new ones, so the risk for toxicity can be high, especially if you're taking supplements.

Anemia is common, especially in women, but the only people who may need to supplement with iron are women during their menstruating years (18 mg a day is the recommendation) and people who donate blood frequently. Men and postmenopausal

QUICK GUIDE TO NUTRIENTS AND FOODS

VITAMIN A/ BETA-CAROTENE	B VITAMINS	VITAMIN C	VITAMIN E	VITAMIN D
Carrots	Brown rice	Grapefruit	Almonds	Butter
Mango	Nutritional yeast	Kiwifruit	Oils	Egg yolks
Papaya	Nuts	Oranges	Salmon	Fortified milk
Squash	Oats	Rose hips	Walnuts	Liver
Sweet potato	Wheat germ	Strawberries	Wheat germ	Sunshine

ZINC	SELENIUM	IRON	MAGNESIUM
Chicken	Brazil nuts	Beef/liver	Almonds
Egg yolks	Brown rice	Lentils	Avocado
Oysters/mussels	Nutritional yeast	Raisins/molasses	Brown rice
Pumpkin seeds	Salmon	Soybeans	Leafy greens
Red meats	Wheat germ	Spinach	Soy/tofu

women need just 10 mg a day or less. Iron plays a role in phagocyte activity and cytokine production,[19] but since it's an oxidant/irritant in certain forms, too much compromises health by promoting bacterial growth and triggering inflammation. The immune cells can hold on to their iron unless a bacteria compromises them and uses the iron for themselves.[20] Avoid iron supplements if you have—or are at a high risk for—infections.[21]

Magnesium

This mineral has been shown to be effective in lessening chronic inflammation, especially in postmenopausal women.[22] You can get magnesium from green leafy vegetables, grains, nuts, and legumes.

The chart above offers a snapshot of these key immune-enhancing nutrients and the foods that contain them.

Antioxidants

Many of the nutrients we've already talked about act as antioxidants in addition to their other functions. Antioxidants are super-important to immune health because they protect cells against damage caused by oxidants (aka free radicals), those potentially irritating molecules that undermine health at a cellular level. When apple slices turn brown in the air, that's oxidative damage—which we can avoid with a squeeze of lemon juice. The vitamin C in lemon juice is a potent antioxidant and prevents free radical damage. We need a variety of antioxidants to protect us from free radicals. Foods containing high levels of antioxidants include those with natural red and blue pigments (flavonoids, flavones, and anthocyanins), which also appear to lower inflammation. Dark chocolate, green tea, blueberries, red grapes, and red cabbage are examples.[23] The potency of an antioxidant in food or supplements is sometimes expressed as an Oxygen Radical Absorbance Capacity (ORAC) value.[24] Herbs considered to have anti-inflammatory and antioxidant activity include cloves, cinnamon, oregano, rosemary, and many more.[25]

CHOCOLATE: THE WORLD'S BEST SUPERFOOD?

Dark chocolate is a powerful antioxidant and anti-inflammatory food.[26] In one study of people at high risk for cardiovascular disease, those who ingested 1½ ounces of cocoa powder mixed in a 16-ounce glass of skim milk every day for 4 weeks showed significantly less expression of inflammatory molecules.[27] The conclusion from this small study is that compounds in cocoa can lessen inflammation and hence decrease risk of heart disease. Scientists also recently discovered that the good bacteria in your gut love dark chocolate, too, and they ferment it into powerful anti-inflammatory compounds that help you.[28] In another study in which 30 people ate 1½ ounces of dark chocolate every day for 2 weeks, both gut microbial activity and stress hormones were reduced.[29] Research also showed that polyphenol-rich chocolate as well as some fruit increase the beneficial gut microbe bifidobacteria.[30] Alkalized cocoa powder, however, loses its antioxidant activity, so look for labels that say "nonalkalized" cocoa. In addition to the cocoa, however, many chocolate products contain a lot of sugar, milk solids, and chemical emulsifiers that don't support health. And milk chocolate doesn't seem to possess the same powers as dark chocolate. Raw cacao nibs and natural dark chocolate are likely the best immune-healthy treats.

Coenzyme Q10 (CoQ10) and Alpha Lipoic Acid (αLA)

Important for healthy cells, these two nutrients provide antioxidant activity along with other benefits. Unlike vitamins and minerals, which we must obtain from food, our bodies produce CoQ10 and αLA, but our diets can improve or compromise that production. CoQ10 is part of the energy production system that occurs inside the mitochondria in your cells, while αLA is a superantioxidant that supports liver detoxification and can balance most other antioxidants after their electrons have been stolen by free radicals. αLA is also essential for glutathione (GSH) balance in your cells. Glutathione is the most essential cellular antioxidant; one consequence of chronic infections is a decrease in this protective molecule, especially in HIV infections. Conversely, when 33 men and women with HIV received αLA supplements, their blood levels of GSH were restored to normal levels and their T cell functions improved.[31] To achieve the beneficial effects of CoQ10 and αLA, you may need to take them as supplements. To help prevent liver toxicity or nerve damage from diabetes, you can supplement with αLA (100 to 300 mg a day). CoQ10 production is compromised in people taking statin drugs, so supplementing with 50 to 100 mg, up to 300 mg daily, helps prevent both CoQ10 deficiency and the muscle pain associated with statin drugs.[32]

Omega-3 Essential Fatty Acids

Omega-3 oils from fatty fish, olives, and flaxseeds support your body in many ways and provide a range of protection from inflammation. Your body can't make polyunsaturated fatty acids, so they're another group of essential nutrients that you must obtain from food or supplements. Omega-3 polyunsaturated fatty acids are the ones most important to immune and cellular health.[33] Omega-3 oils play a critical role in preventing inflammation, while too much omega-6 increases inflammation. (Most vegetable oils and oils used in fried and processed foods are omega-6s.) Omega-3s may prevent the production of proinflammatory cytokines and have been useful in delaying or preventing the progression of some autoimmune and cardiovascular illnesses, which are worsened by chronic inflammation.[34] The typical American diet includes much more omega-6s than omega-3s, while a Mediterranean-style diet, which we adapt in this book in our Immune-Power Eating Plan (I-PEP), favors a healthy balance that includes more omega-3s. The Mediterranean diet includes whole

ULTIMATE IMMUNITY　　SUCCESS STORY

Claudia Edwards, 66

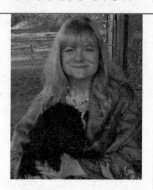

After a career that spanned 30 years and three continents, Claudia decided it was time to spend her years relaxing in nature's beauty. She moved to a house in the Blue Ridge Mountains in western North Carolina and looked forward to the next chapter of her life. But 2 years later, those plans went up—literally—in smoke. A fire damaged her home and possessions and left her feeling uprooted and traumatized. "The chemical exposure and the carbon monoxide left me with a lot of swelling," she recalls, "and I had huge immune problems, from inflammation and congestion to joint pain and digestive upset."

Instead of enjoying her life and hobbies of music, art, and literature, she was living in hotels and consuming refined flour and sugary foods such as bread, cereal, and pastries. Her energy plummeted—she could barely walk down the hall—and insomnia became a way of life. Even with two medications, she couldn't get a good night's sleep. Her elevated blood pressure continued to rise, and she was taking a medicine for that, too. All those breakfasts and after-noon snacks of cookies and brownies, combined with the emotional struggle of dealing with the insurance company and a lack of exercise, led to a 75-pound weight gain and feelings of hopelessness and despair.

At the end of her rope and barely hanging on, she relocated back to California and met with Dr. Haas, who'd been her trusted physician years ago. He put her on the I-PEP diet and Cool Down plan and in 8 months, she was down 50 pounds. "I went from being unable to walk half a block to taking a brisk walk for an hour a day," she says. Finally, her allergies were under control, her sleep improved, and she could concentrate, read, and focus once again. From being depressed and lethargic, she's gone back to being her former, optimistic self.

Now, 4 years after the event that changed her life, she has a new one, filled with "love and laughter." "Healing my immune system was at the heart of my recovery," Claudia says. "This included nourishing myself physically. Learning to choose healthy foods went hand in hand with my spiritual and emotional healing."

grains, fresh fruits and vegetables, fish, olive oil, and garlic, as well as an occasional glass of red wine.

Omega-3 fatty acids come in three forms. Two of them—EPA (eicosapentaenoic acid) and DHA (docosahexaenoic acid)—are found in oily fish such as salmon, sardines, tuna, and anchovies, plus omega-3-enriched eggs. Macrophages use DHA to produce switches that turn off inflammation.[35] ALA (alpha-linolenic acid), the third form, is found in vegetable oils like olive oil, flaxseeds, walnuts, chia seeds, hemp seeds, pumpkin seeds, and dark, leafy vegetables. Your body can convert some ALA to the other two forms. So to protect yourself and your cells from too much inflammation, make sure you have a few doses of omega-3s every day.

Protein and Amino Acids

Your body is about 70 percent water. Remove that water and almost all that's left is protein. Proteins are large molecules found in every part of your body, and they run all biochemical processes that keep you alive. Some proteins are simply structural components like the collagen in your skin or keratin in your hair. All antibodies are proteins, and so are immune cytokines and many hormones. The cell's communication antennae (receptors) are proteins, and so are the cellular markers of your identity.

The biggest responsibility of proteins? They act as enzymes, serving as conductors of every metabolic and immune process in your body. You've got about 100,000 different proteins in your body, and at least 5,000 of them are enzymes.[36] Enzymes catalyze all biochemical reactions needed for life, lowering the amount of energy required to make the reaction possible.

Proteins are made of smaller building blocks called amino acids; there are 20 different amino acids. Your cells can produce most of them, but eight are *essential amino acids*—that means you must obtain them from your food. Meats and eggs contain all the amino acids used to produce proteins in your body, but most plant foods lack one or more essential amino acids. Two plant powerhouses that contain all essential amino acids: soybeans and quinoa.

Research shows that a protein deficiency can cause a depletion of immune cells, which prevents your body from making antibodies and other immune-related molecules like cytokines. Immune functions are severely compromised by inadequate protein intake.[37] In the elderly, this is even more of a problem. Since immune functions often slow down as you age, if your diet lacks adequate protein, your health can suffer severely.[38] In a 9-week study of 12 healthy elderly women, those given a low-protein diet lost lean tissue, muscle function, and T cell functions, and their antibody responses were lower than those given a diet with adequate protein.[39] Protein malnutrition lowers T cells, making infections more likely and deadly, particularly in hospitalized patients.[40]

To do their work, many proteins require vitamins and minerals, and when it comes to enzyme activity, those needed nutrients are called cofactors. A deficiency in any of the cofactors can cause the enzymes to slow or fail, and that can contribute to health problems. In addition, you need adequate antioxidants to protect proteins from ongoing free radical damage. It's easy to see why food is such a crucial part of a vast collaborative system to ensure your health and survival—everything's connected.

The bottom line: You need to eat some protein every day to provide all the amino acids your body requires. Not getting enough puts your immune system and health at risk. Nutritionists recommend about $^1/_3$ ounce or 10 grams of protein for every 20 pounds of body weight. So if you weigh 120 pounds, you need about 60 grams of protein daily (about 2 ounces). Check out "Finding High-Quality Protein" below.

FINDING HIGH-QUALITY PROTEIN

We get protein from animal foods like beef, poultry, fish, eggs, and dairy; plant foods like lentils, chickpeas, soybeans, and black beans; whole grains; veggies; and fresh water algae. Here's a quick guide with some examples of how much.

FOOD EXAMPLES	GRAMS OF PROTEIN
1 lean 6-oz hamburger	48
1 can (6 oz) water-packed tuna	40
4 oz broiled wild coho salmon	27
1 cup cooked chickpeas	14
1 cup cooked quinoa	11
$^1/_2$ cup tofu	10
1 cup fat-free milk	8
1 large egg	6
1 cup cooked kale	2.5

Proteins in your food are broken down through digestion into their amino acid building blocks. The small amino acids are then assimilated to produce the proteins your body needs to form muscle, hemoglobin, cytokines, hair, hormones, skin, enzymes, and more. Many amino acids serve other functions besides being part of proteins. Glutamine and glutamic acid, for instance, act as neurotransmitters. In addition, glutamine,[41] arginine,[42] and cysteine on their own stimulate immune functions.[43] A few specific amino acids provide support for several key immune functions, as you can see in the chart below.

AMINO ACIDS AND IMMUNE FUNCTIONS

AMINO ACID	IMMUNE FUNCTIONS
Glutamine	Enhances lymphocyte function during trauma and surgery
Arginine	Essential for T cell proliferation
Cysteine	Used to produce the cell's primary antioxidant, glutathione

In this section, we've learned how nutrients, antioxidants, proteins, and amino acids can significantly benefit our immune function. Now let's take a look at another key part of the system—probiotics—as they affect your gut microbiome. Probiotics play an important role in helping your body absorb important ingredients by keeping your intestinal bacteria in check.

PROBIOTICS: A KEY TO IMMUNE BALANCE

Probiotics are live microbes (mostly bacteria, but also some yeasts) that balance the microbes in your gut. Your gastrointestinal tract and its specific microbiome may contain hundreds of different species of bacteria—billions of "bugs" in all—that work to maintain good digestive and immune health. If this delicate balance is thrown off by illness or antibiotics, diarrhea and other intestinal symptoms may result. Probiotics restore intestinal balance by crowding out the disease-causing microbes and lessening or halting diarrhea.[44] These "good bacteria" can prevent or improve many health conditions, especially those affecting your gastrointestinal tract. Probiotics also protect your immune system,[45] since your gut microbes aid the development and regulation of immune cells in your gut.[46] "Good guy" probiotics recruit T and B cells to the area and help stimulate immune responses, making it tougher for bad bacteria to cause illness.

IMMUNE-SUPPORTIVE NUTRIENTS
AND FOOD SOURCES

NUTRIENT (SUGGESTED DOSE)	IMMUNE FUNCTIONS	GOOD FOOD SOURCES
Vitamin A (3,000–10,000 IU) **Beta-carotene (10,000–25,000 IU)**	Immune stimulant Increases T helpers T and B cell proliferation NK activity Aids wound healing and macrophage activity Antioxidant	A: Liver, fish oils, animal foods only Beta-carotene: Deep green, yellow, orange, and red vegetables and fruits, such as broccoli, apricots, cantaloupe, carrots, mangos, sweet potatoes, winter squash
Vitamin C (ascorbic acid) (500–2,000 mg)	T and B cell growth T cell function Antioxidant	Citrus fruits, berries, kiwifruit, cranberries, red peppers
Vitamin B$_5$ (pantothenic acid) (250–1,000 mg)	Antibody response: helps in release of antibody from plasma cells	Whole grains, legumes, nuts, seeds
Vitamin B$_6$ (pyridoxine) (25–50 mg)	With B$_5$, essential for antibody synthesis	Whole grains, nuts, wheat germ, nutritional yeast
Vitamin B$_{12}$ (cobalamin) (200–1,000 mcg) Vegetarians risk deficits.	B cell proliferation	In animal foods: yogurt, liver, beef Tempeh and nutritional yeast may have some
Vitamin D (1,000–5,000 IUs as vitamin D$_3$)	Antibody and cytokine synthesis	Egg yolks, liver, fortified milk, butter, cereal grains, sunlight
Zinc (30–50 mg) Excess zinc (300 mg/day for 6 wk) decreases immune functions. Zinc citrate is good.	T and B cell growth NK cells T cell function Antibody response	Oysters, shellfish, seafood, almonds, root vegetables, pumpkin seeds

Where do we find these beneficial probiotic organisms? In yogurt, for starters, but look for yogurt that contains live and active cultures. Or try kefir and buttermilk. You can find probiotics in some soft cheeses, like Gouda.

Do you suffer from dairy allergies? Then turn to probiotics in nondairy yogurts made from rice, soy, or coconut milk. Alternatives to yogurt include fermented foods like brewer's yeast, miso, unpasteurized sauerkraut, the spicy Korean food kimchi, and tempeh from fermented soybeans. Even sourdough bread is a source of the lactobacillus

NUTRIENT (SUGGESTED DOSE)	IMMUNE FUNCTIONS	GOOD FOOD SOURCES
Iron **(10–20 mg)** Excess iron impairs bactericidal activity and enhances bacterial growth. Amounts vary for women and men. Iron chelates like iron glycinate may be better tolerated and absorbed over the common iron sulfate.	T and B cell proliferation T killer cell function	Meats, molasses, spinach, lentils, leafy greens, raisins
Selenium **(100–200 mcg as seleno-methionine)**	Antioxidant Supports glutathione production	Brazil nuts, nutritional yeast, brown rice, wheat germ, fish
Magnesium **(250–500 mg as magnesium citrate or glycinate)**	Anti-inflammatory effects Supports enzyme and cell activity	Greens and more greens, nuts and seeds, whole grains
Alpha lipoic acid **(150–300 mg)**	The antioxidant's antioxidant Increases T cells in HIV Protects liver from poisons	Small amounts in spinach, broccoli, yeast, red meat, potatoes Can't get enough from diet: 7 lb spinach = only 1 mg
Essential fatty acids **(omega-3s) (300–600 mg each of EPA and DHA)**	White blood cell function Anti-inflammatory	Oily fish like salmon and mackerel; flaxseeds; whole grains
Protein **(10 g per 20 lb body weight)**	Primary source of all antibodies and cytokines, enzymes, some hormones	Fish, meat, eggs, beans, quinoa
Probiotics (Millions or preferably 5 billion–10 billion live organisms per capsule)	Aids development of immune cells and Balances gut microbiome	Yogurt, miso, sauerkraut

probiotic.[47] Whatever the source, always look for "live and active cultures" on the label.

While probiotics from food contain live microbes, some scientists recommend prebiotics, foods that nourish the good bacteria already in your belly. Some examples: asparagus, Jerusalem artichokes, oatmeal, legumes, honey, bananas, and red wine.[48]

Although probiotic supplements can provide relief from recurrent bouts of diarrhea,[49] people with compromised immunity, like those undergoing cancer treatment,[50] should use them cautiously. That's because in the United States, probiotic supplements, though they're generally safe, aren't regulated for safety, purity, or potency as they are in Europe, Australia, and Japan.

For most people, though, probiotics are safe and effective for treating a variety of concerns, including diarrhea, GI infections, and vaginal bacterial infections.[51] Research shows that they may support immune regulation, assist immune response in allergies,[52] and help treat autoimmune illnesses[53] and even obesity.

Probiotics enhance your healthy gut microbes, which then educate your immune cells to do their jobs. They help regulate the immune balance of T cells to favor less allergic eczema in children and in people with food allergies. And gut microbes seem to play a role in obesity. Researchers have found that obese women have different and fewer kinds of gut microbes than thin individuals. In a 24-week Canadian study of 125 overweight men and women, the first half of the experimental period was devoted to losing weight, and the second to maintaining body weight. Fifty percent of participants received probiotics capsules, while the others received a placebo. At the end of 12 weeks, the probiotic group averaged a 10-pound weight loss, compared to 5 pounds for the control group. (No weight differences were seen among the men.) In the maintenance period, the control group's weight stayed the same, while the probiotic group continued to lose weight—their total weight loss was double that of the control group. In addition to losing weight, the probiotic group experienced a decrease in obesity-related gut microbes and appetite-stimulating hormone.[54]

Spice Up Your Immunity

So far, we've touched on the nutritional elements of foods that offer immune support. You may be wondering whether your new, healthful diet will be bland and monotonous. Absolutely not. You may soon rediscover the tasty, natural flavors of fresh foods. Plus, adding herbs and spices is an easy way to create variety and expand the flavors of your meals—and load up the immune-boosting properties of your food, too. Herbs are typically leaves, roots, and stems used in cooking or for medicinal purposes. Spices usually come from bark or seeds, are intensely aromatic, and are generally added to dishes in much smaller amounts. Most of our common herbs and spices originated in Asia or the Mediterranean region, where many were healing folk remedies generations before manufactured drugs or supplements were derived from them. Scientific research and analyses of the plants have provided measurable evidence of how, or if, these herbs and spices work in any healing capacity. Large clinical studies of these plants are still relatively rare, so we offer the following dietary ideas with a word of caution. As tasty additions to your foods, there is likely no risk. Herbs and spices can simply season your food, or they can be taken as nutritional supplements when necessary. In general, they provide antioxidant and/or anti-inflammatory functions—both essential for good immune health. But if you consume them as supplements, exercise caution. Many substances with anti-inflammatory and antioxidant activity can alter blood clotting, and some herbs can interact with prescription medications.

Herbs can help the body and alleviate symptoms of various medical conditions, but since this isn't a book on herbal medicine, we've provided a simple basic review of those herbs and spices that may improve your immune functions and your meals. In Chapter 7, we'll talk more about using these as supplements. Here, we offer suggestions for spicing up your dinner—and your immune health.

Cayenne Pepper

Hot and spicy cayenne pepper is a member of the nightshade family, which includes potatoes, tomatoes, other peppers, and eggplant. The heat-producing component in the cayenne fruits is *capsaicin*, and patches or gels containing capsaicin can be used to soothe localized pain. It turns out that capsaicin is a potent inhibitor of pain-producing *substance* P made during inflammation.[55] Substance P when released by neurons worsens pain sensations. Cayenne peppers are also powerful antioxidants, as you would expect from the bright red color.[56] Remember, most highly pigmented foods contain antioxidants.

Cayenne, used sparingly, stimulates blood circulation and stimulates secretions to clear a stuffy nose. Some people sprinkle a little ground cayenne in their socks to warm their feet in cold weather or take it in capsule form for its warming effects. Also, be cautious with amounts used of spicy peppers, cayenne, and even black pepper until you know your level of sensitivity. Some people are very sensitive and reactive or don't like the warm or hot feeling that peppers generate.

Cinnamon

Cinnamon comes from the dried bark of a tropical species of evergreen tree grown in Asia. The cinnamon more commonly sold in North America comes from the related cassia tree. It helps prevent infection and may stimulate immune activity. There's considerable research indicating that cinnamon can prevent clumping of blood platelets by blocking the release of inflammatory fatty acids from cell membranes. It also inhibits the formation of other inflammatory substances.[57] Some research suggests it helps regulate blood sugar[58] (a factor in inflammation), has antioxidant activity,[59] and may reduce pain. Try it on your morning oatmeal.

Clove

Eugenol (clove oil) is widely used in dentistry as a local analgesic agent, so you may already be familiar with the smell and taste of cloves. Both an anti-inflammatory and antioxidant,[60] sweet and fragrant cloves have been used to prevent gum pain—in addition to giving gingerbread and the Indian drink chai their signature aromas and flavors.

Garlic

This potent and pungent cooking staple provides antiseptic and antioxidant activities. In one study, garlic was shown to prevent colds or at least shorten the duration of the symptoms.[61] Allicin, a potent sulfur compound found in garlic and onions, provides both their powerful pungent aromas and supports antioxidant and anti-inflammatory activity.[62]

MAKE YOUR OWN GARLIC OIL

Chop 5 to 10 cloves of garlic and place them in a small bottle of olive oil, or pour 4 to 8 ounces of olive oil over the garlic in a bowl or container. Let it sit for a couple of days to allow the garlic to infuse in the oil, and then put it in the fridge for several days. You can add other herbs, like rosemary, to the oil as well. Use this in cooking or rub it on your chest to soothe cough and congestion. *Note:* Don't store garlic in oil at room temperature for more than a day or two, as garlic-in-oil mixtures could cause some bacterial overgrowth, with the growth of botulism being the biggest concern.[63]

Ginger

The pungent root of the ginger plant decreases inflammation[64] in ways similar to aspirin, and it's an antimicrobial against bacteria and fungus. Some sailors, pregnant women, and people undergoing chemotherapy have found that ginger helps prevent or soothe nausea and motion sickness.[65] Nausea and vomiting are complex processes controlled by the central nervous system and influenced by psychological issues. Studies show mixed results especially with chemotherapy-induced nausea, although ginger has reduced its severity. It's been shown to be helpful in preventing pregnancy morning sickness.[66] It also aids circulation and heat generation in the body. Ginger is readily available in ginger ale, as capsules, and in candied form. Fresh ginger livens up the flavor of whatever you're cooking or drinking, so try it in your morning oatmeal or evening stir-fry. Or use freshly grated ginger to make tea as a wonderful cold remedy. Avoid ginger if you're taking blood thinners or aspirin.

Licorice

Most people think of licorice as a chewy candy, but its health benefits date from ancient times. Licorice, another root, has been shown to have powerful cortisone-like activity, which means it can help diminish immune responses and inflammation. It works well in the gut to lessen the symptoms of an inflamed stomach. Research indicates that at medicinal doses, it is antimicrobial and an antioxidant.[67]

Shiitake Mushrooms

This fungus has been used in Chinese medicine for more than 6,000 years[68] and offers another tasty and health-promoting food to your anti-inflammatory repertoire.[69] This mushroom lessens the likelihood for heart disease by preventing immune cells from sticking to the thin walls of your blood vessels (the stickiness is a consequence of inflammation). Rich in vitamins B and D, shiitake mushrooms should be gently sautéed for a few minutes to enhance their flavor. Soak dried shiitakes for a few minutes and then rinse; they cook better when hydrated. Add a few to chicken soup or a veggie sauté for more flavor and immune support.

Taken at a medicinal level, shiitake extracts can both suppress and activate immune functions, so consult with your health practitioner before supplementing with high amounts.

Onions

This flavorful, versatile addition to meals contains several immune-boosting chemical components. One is quercetin,[70] a bioflavonoid also found in red wine, green tea, apples, berries, and buckwheat. Quercetin is not only anti-inflammatory[71] and an antioxidant, it also acts as an antihistamine. Eat onions daily.

Oregano

A powerful antimicrobial herb, oregano is effective in treating some fungal, bacterial, and parasitic infections.[72] Oregano has more antioxidant activity[73] than apples, oranges, or blueberries! The popular seasoning is commonly used in Italian dishes like pizza, spaghetti, and minestrone soup.

Rosemary

The highly aromatic needlelike leaves of rosemary contain substances that increase circulation, improve digestion, and are anti-inflammatory. Some studies suggest it may reduce the severity of asthma attacks.[74] In animal studies, an extract made from rosemary leaves was shown to have powerful and measurable antioxidant and anti-inflammatory effects.[75] In a study at the University of Florida, white blood cells isolated from 10 people were incubated with hydrogen peroxide, which causes oxidative damage to DNA. Blood cells from people who consumed capsules of rosemary (or ginger or turmeric) for a week were protected from this oxidative damage. The rosemary also lowered the inflammatory markers in the cells.[76]

Thyme

Thanksgiving stuffing, fragrant with thyme and onions, may actually protect us from infections during the holidays. Thyme contains some of the same components as oregano and is especially high in *thymol*, which gives thyme its antimicrobial properties against bacteria and fungi. Also an antioxidant, thyme has been shown to prevent oxidative damage to DNA in human lymphocytes.[77] In other words, it protects genes. It also contains quercetin, found in onions, which inhibits histamine.

Turmeric (Curcumin)

The slightly bitter, bright yellow-orange turmeric root contains curcumin, a main ingredient in curries. Used for its intense yellow color (think mustard), curcumin is a powerful anti-inflammatory that may protect the liver from toxins. Preliminary research suggests it may delay the onset of Alzheimer's disease, lessen the pain and inflammation of rheumatoid arthritis, and even prevent some cancers.[78]

Herbs and spices add flavor complexity to cooked foods, and now you know that many herbs provide health benefits as well. Though much of the scientific research on the biological properties of these seasonings was performed using extracts, oils, or supplement dosages, at the food level, herbs and spices add pleasure to your eating experience and may improve your health on many levels. In Chapter 7, we go into more detail about the benefits of and advisements on taking these and other herbs as supplements. Remember: If you have allergies, asthma, or an autoimmune illness, don't supplement with herbal products that are said to stimulate your immune activity. Your immune system is already stimulated.

Now that your spice rack is stocked, let's take a look at some of the foods you can enhance with your new seasonings.

FOODS: WHAT TO BUY
AND WHAT TO BYPASS

If you've ever experimented with your diet, you know that separating good foods from bad foods isn't always easy. Some foods really *are* superfoods because they're especially rich in immune-supporting nutrients that you could healthfully eat every day—not just when you're tackling a weight or other health problem.

Then there are foods that can trigger or enhance inflammation because of their chemical makeup, such as fatty red meats or other foods containing saturated or hydrogenated (trans) fats. Some foods trigger histamine release, which increases allergy and inflammatory symptoms. For example, "azo" dyes and benzoates—common food additives—can trigger the release of histamine from your cells. This is another good reason to avoid prepackaged foods with all their added chemicals. Avoid these foods or eat them in moderation to lessen inflammation.

In building your new menu, stay away from any foods that you know cause allergic or other unpleasant reactions, and avoid too much refined flour and sugar, which can add weight and lead to inflammation.[79] Some foods simply cause irritation when eaten in high quantities—like black or cayenne pepper. Pay attention to what happens in your body when you eat various foods. Some spinach is good, but consuming heaping helpings of raw spinach, kale salad, or juices made from these greens can cause an excess of oxalic acid in your body and increase your risk for kidney stones. Strive for balance; don't overemphasize any one food. Eat a variety, rotate your ingredients, and learn which foods to steer clear of.

Key Foods to Bypass

The foods to avoid? That depends partly on your genetics and your previous diet—you'll want to stay away, for example, from foods you've overindulged in in the past. Based on your weight and overall health, it may be wise to limit foods such as simple sugars, fruit juices, or refined carbohydrates like pasta or rice. For some people, simple carbs tend to cause them to overeat. Plus, you may have specific allergies and other reactions to foods. Does red wine give you a headache? Does cheese make your nose stuffy? These are all considerations in finding your own special diet and knowing yourself. Let's look at these factors in detail.

Allergens and Reactants

Your healthy-eating goal: an anti-inflammatory diet. So avoid foods that cause allergic sensitivity, inflammation, and other kinds of immune reactions. When it comes to inflammation, red meat and fat[80] are the most common culprits. Data from the Nurses' Health Study[81] of more than 3,500 nondiabetic women revealed that the more red meat they consumed, the higher their blood markers for inflammation. Substituting another meat, like chicken for the red meat, showed healthier blood profiles. The following chart summarizes foods that commonly trigger inflammatory responses and should be eaten only in moderation.

INFLAMMATORY FOODS

FOOD	POSSIBLE ADVERSE ACTIONS
Aged cheeses, fermented soy products, sauerkraut, red wine, vinegar	All contain histamine, causing allergic-type reactions; many also have beneficial probiotics.
Whole-fat dairy, eggs, peanut oil, red meat	Increases inflammatory chemicals called leukotrienes from saturated fats.
Omega-6 fats from soy, corn, safflower, palm, sunflower oil (used in many processed foods)	Can activate inflammation and throw off the beneficial effects of omega-3 oils.

If you have food allergies or sensitivities, you already know which foods to avoid. Allergic reactions can trigger an immediate IgE antibody and histamine release or, sometimes, a delayed reaction through the IgG antibody, both of which cause significant discomfort in the skin, gut, and respiratory tract. If you're sensitive to gluten, whether it's an allergy, intolerance, or autoimmune response, you know you must

KEEP IT PERSONAL

Every culture has its own repertoire of traditional foods, so don't forgo all your family favorites. If corn or beans are part of your heritage, eliminating them from your diet may starve your soul's need to connect to your cultural roots. Often, those childhood comfort foods are the ones that you can digest and assimilate well. When planning your new menu, keep in mind the answers to the following questions:

- Which foods nourish you physically and emotionally?

- Do you have a favorite comfort food? If so, what is its origin or significance? Does it stem from your family's heritage? Or from a lifelong tradition?

- Do you have a beverage that nurtures you? What is it? What do you currently drink the most?

- What are the dozen or so basic foods that you wouldn't want to live without?

There are no right answers—just information about yourself and what nourishes you, so you can tap into that place when you need comfort.

avoid or limit wheat products, too. Fortunately, lots of gluten-free products—from pancakes to soy sauce—are now available in the marketplace.

There are also substances that act like psychoactive "drugs," including sugar, caffeine, and alcohol. You may enjoy the effects of consuming these druglike ingredients, which often stimulate or sedate, but beneath the surface, they're putting stress on your body and immune system.

The biggest challenge you'll probably face when creating a healing menu is eliminating common (but less-than-healthy) foods to which you've become attached, like bread, pastries, chips, coffee, and red meat. Following the elimination diet on page 123 will help you discover if you feel better when you take a break from your usual way of eating. You'll also clarify which foods bother you if you consume them again. If you suffer from symptoms and chronic illnesses related to foods, this step can be life changing.

Lectins: Potential Troublemakers

Some foods, by their very nature, can contribute to chronic illnesses and digestive problems.[82] You learned in Chapter 2 that your reactions to different foods could be due to allergies, or they could be nonallergic sensitivity reactions. Now there's another culprit: *lectins*. Lectins are specific food proteins whose chemical makeup resembles the surface of certain microbes. Your cells may detect them as dangerous food molecules, so lectins can contribute to the mysterious food reactions that aren't allergies. Mainly found in plant foods, especially seeds and beans, some lectins are severely toxic and can't be eaten at all, while others, like red kidney beans, need to be cooked for a long time to be safe. (Never eat raw kidney beans; as few as four or five raw, soaked beans can trigger symptoms of food poisoning.) Wheat gluten is another lectin, which may explain all the complex reactions gluten can initiate.

LECTIN-LOADED FOODS

Beans: lima and kidney

Grains: wheat germ and gluten

Legumes: peanuts and soybeans

Dairy foods

Nightshades: tomatoes, potatoes, and peppers

Many responses to foods that aren't true allergy could be due to lectins. So knowing which foods have the potential to trigger digestive upset may help you make better food choices. Part of being a good food sleuth is paying attention to your body, its energy level, and any reactive symptoms when you eat a new or questionable food. If you suspect that your body has been irritated by the food, eliminating it from your diet might make sense. The good news about lectins: You can destroy their ability to cause trouble through cooking.

Key Foods to Consume

Now comes the good part: the delicious foods and meals that can support your body and overall health. The emotional aspects of changing what you eat can be challenging, especially if you wave good-bye to some of your favorite foods. But rather than focus on that buttery croissant that you've given up for breakfast or the sugary dessert you forgo at dinner, keep your focus on all the good things to come—the healthy foods and the way your body will feel when it's nourished by them.

Overall, eat as close to nature as possible. Eat a rainbow of foods but not from artificial colors; eat organically grown foods whenever possible. Think gardens and orchards. Embrace fresh vegetables in steamed, roasted, and stir-fried dishes. Consume a few pieces of fresh, mostly seasonally based fruit daily, and mix it up. Have citrus fruits, apples and pears, berries, and occasionally tropical fruits. Find the best proteins for you—the cleanest of meats, poultry, and fish. If you're a vegetarian, think legumes and sprouted beans, plus nuts and seeds, such as almonds, walnuts, sunflower seeds, and pumpkin seeds; raw and organic are the best choices. Avoid GMO (genetically modified organism) foods. And always drink plenty of water.

The list on page 122 would make a great shopping list to get you started.

Go Wild for Fish

The American Heart Association recommends eating fish several times a week for all their health benefits.[83] But what fish should you choose? Most people have heard warnings about seafood being contaminated with environmental chemicals and toxic metals. Tuna and swordfish, for instance, can contain high levels of mercury. This is especially of concern to pregnant women and nursing mothers. In addition, the ocean contains other environmental chemicals and potential radioactive fallout from the

IMMUNE-HEALTHY, NUTRIENT-RICH FOODS

These are the healing foods of the I-PEP diet. Turn to this list again and again as you create delicious, healing meals.[84]

Vegetables—beets, broccoli,* Brussels sprouts,* cabbage, carrots, cauliflower (brassicas or cruciferous), chard, garlic, green beans, kale, kohlrabi, leeks, onions,* peas, potatoes (some varieties), shallots, shiitake mushrooms,* spinach (dark, leafy greens), sweet potatoes, tomatoes, zucchini

Fruits—apples, apricots, banana, blueberries,* cherries, figs, some grapefruit, lemon, mango, oranges, papaya, pineapple, pomegranate, raspberries

Proteins—eggs, Greek yogurt, lean red meat, legumes, oysters, poultry (free-range, organic), salmon* (wild), sardines, some seeds and nuts (raw and organic), sprouted beans

Nuts—almonds* (high in omega-3 oils), avocado, Brazil nuts, coconut, walnuts (high in omega-3 oils)

Seeds—flaxseeds,* pine nuts, pumpkin, sunflower

Legumes and their sprouts—azuki, black, chickpeas, mung

Grains—buckwheat, millet, quinoa*; some oats and rice

Seaweeds—arame, hijiki, nori

Cultured and fermented foods—kefir and yogurt, kimchi (a traditional Korean dish commonly made with fermented cabbage), nondairy fermented products like tempeh and tofu (both soy)

Spices and herbs—basil, cayenne (ground red pepper), chives, cinnamon, curry, garlic, ginger, onions, oregano, turmeric

Beverages and treats—acai, bee pollen, dark chocolate, goji berries, nutritional yeast, tea (green* and black)

Water for good hydration, preferably spring water

*These are our 10 key foods to fight inflammation, though many of the others also have anti-inflammatory abilities.

Fukashima nuclear incident, while rivers and lakes may be contaminated with runoff from pesticides and other agricultural chemicals. And what of farm-raised versus wild fish, like salmon? Depends on the farm and how conscientious they are about chemicals and feed. Typically, farm-raised fish live in crowded waters, so more chemicals and antibiotics may be used. Today, there are some organic fish farms, but wild is usually best. It's a good start to know where your fish comes from. Be sure to choose smaller species (the larger the fish, the more toxins it may contain) and vary the kinds you eat. Focus on these varieties:

- Wild salmon
- Small, oily fish like sardines and mackerel
- Wild cod, sea bass, and halibut[85]

Check out this link to determine which fish to eat and which to avoid: womenshealthmag.com/nutrition/types-of-fish-to-eat.

Choose Grass-Fed Beef

If you wish to include meat in your diet, research indicates that grass-fed cattle—pastured when possible—has a higher omega-3 fatty acid and antioxidant content (vitamins A and E) than grain-fed beef. The health advantage: This altered composition of the grass-fed meat favors less inflammation than conventionally raised cattle.[86] Studies show that eating lean red meat doesn't cause any increase in markers of inflammation.[87] Avoid processed meats and those high in saturated fats, which do contribute to inflammation.

THE 5-DAY ELIMINATION, HEALING PLAN

We'll start with a short-term transition diet to help you move from how you eat and live right now toward a new eating program aimed at maximizing immune health. Later, we'll get deeper into the specifics of our diet: the Immune-Power Eating Plan, or I-PEP.

Knowing where to start on your journey toward healthier eating habits is half the battle. So here's what to do: Begin by eliminating certain inflammatory and allergenic foods—that's the focus of the 5-Day Elimination, Healing Plan. Start simple by avoiding substances like sugar or caffeine or just one food like bread. If you're feeling especially motivated, take on a more encompassing food elimination program or even a nutritionally supportive 5-day juice cleanse to lighten your body and give you energy. You choose the starting point that sounds best for you.

The Immune Power 5-Day Cleanse

Juice cleansing can be a powerful healing tool, but it's not for everyone. Nor do you need to do this before embarking on the 5-day elimination plan. We include it here for those of you who would like to start your healing journey in this more adventurous way. Cleansing can also be done *after* the 5-day elimination program that follows. Since juice cleansing contains calories and a lot of nutrients, most people can handle it for a few days. Those who do best are overweight to start with and have good physical energy. People with chronic problems like pain, high blood pressure or cholesterol, allergies, or digestive issues are also good candidates. However, if you are fatigued, underweight, pregnant, anemic or iron deficient, or suffering from a chronic, debilitating disease such as cancer or are on chemotherapy medications, avoid this cleansing option.

Here's the easy recipe close to the formula people know as the Master Cleanse, but with less maple syrup. Just mix together the following ingredients—adjust the cayenne to your taste, but don't omit it. If you don't like the hot flavor, take a capsule of cayenne for every 2 glasses of cleanse.

2 tablespoons fresh lemon juice
1 tablespoon pure maple syrup
$1/_{10}$ teaspoon cayenne (ground red) pepper (not chili powder)
8 ounces water

Drink 8 to 10 glasses throughout the day—that's 1 or 2 glasses every hour to two. Don't sip throughout the day, but schedule your glasses at regular intervals. Rinse your mouth with water after each glass so as to not damage your tooth enamel. During the day, you can drink herbal teas as well.

Follow the cleanse for 5 days. You can also add a separate drink of fresh vegetable juices that include greens like

IMMUNE TIP

Before eliminating foods from your diet, start a journal of the foods you suspect will have to go. If you decide to eliminate coffee, for instance, write down any sensations or discomfort you experience after drinking coffee. Then, on day 1 of the elimination diet, note what you're feeling, and do this for at least 5 days. Three weeks is the milestone you want to reach to experience the full effects of eliminating a food. During the first few days of your coffee strike, you may actually feel worse, with headaches and fatigue, but these symptoms will pass if you don't give up.

kale, plus celery, cucumber, and carrots. You can dilute with water and drink a few glasses throughout the afternoon and evening. After you complete this powerful 5-day cleanse, transition into the 5-day elimination plan with a day consuming nice vegetable soup, and then transition into I-PEP. For more information on cleansing and elimination diets, see *The Detox Diet*.[88]

Almost everyone can benefit from a lightening and enlightening diet, an important part of your transition to healing. You'll feel better when you make good choices and eat foods that feed your cells—and when you avoid foods that undermine your health by causing irritation and inflammation. If you have nagging chronic symptoms or are in the throes of a serious health problem, this transition may slow or reverse the progression of your symptoms and disease.

Making the Transition

The 5-Day Elimination, Healing Plan primarily focuses on adding more fresh vegetables and fresh juices while taking a break from the five habitual substances that can undermine your health: sugar, caffeine, alcohol, wheat, and dairy. Some people see additional improvement by eliminating red meats and fried foods.

If your three worst habits happen to be lots of sugar, caffeine, and alcohol, it's time to give your body a break from these substances. You'll drop some weight and feel lighter, too.

This elimination program is similar to many cleansing diets, such as Dr. Haas's *Detox Diet*, that emphasize steamed fresh vegetables and alkalinizing the body to reduce the acidic toxins that contribute to inflammation. Many symptoms (such as

---

Note to Readers: The 5-day elimination plan is a simple eating program featuring less than you typically eat with different choices than your usual fare. The lighter diet with a vegetable focus is a core of the I-PEP, which expands your diet by adding more food choices to each meal and snacks. Most people consume too much food in general, so we've made both these eating programs lighter overall. If you are underweight and need more nourishment, please consume more food and make sure you get your snacks in, too. If you are overweight and want to drop a few pounds yet still stay nourished, these can work for you as long as you follow the weight-management guidelines under "Lighten Up: Lose Weight with I-PEP," page 132.

IN A NUTSHELL: YOUR 5-DAY ELIMINATION, HEALING PLAN

Wake up: Begin with hydration: 1 to 2 glasses of water with a squeeze of fresh lemon ($\frac{1}{4}$ to $\frac{1}{2}$ lemon per glass) soon after you wake up

Breakfast: One or two 6-ounce portions of fruit and grain

Midmorning snack (optional): 1 small handful of nuts or seeds

Lunch: Large bowl of salad with optional protein, plus 3 to 4 ounces beans or 3 to 4 ounces fish or poultry (Mostly veggies and less protein means more detoxifying.)

Afternoon snack: 1 to 2 pieces of fruit

Dinner: Steamed or roasted veggies with optional protein or one or two 6- to 8-ounce servings of a simple vegetable soup*

Throughout the day: One or two 8-ounce glasses of water 30 minutes before lunch and dinner, as well as other times during the day, away from meals

*Lunch and dinner foods can be swapped: For one meal, consume fresh, raw greens, and for the other, lightly cooked veggies. You can add several teaspoons a day of olive or flaxseed oil to your veggies or salad with some lemon and/or seasoning herbs.

headaches, allergy congestion, and digestive symptoms) may be alleviated with this new eating approach.

Get ready to give your digestive tract, liver, body, and mind a mini-holiday! Make your selections from the immune-healthy, nutrient-rich food list on page 122 and follow the 5-day eating plan here. Have fun with this and know that you are going to feel

SUPPLEMENTS FOR THE ELIMINATION PROGRAM

If you generally take few or no supplements, consider a daily multivitamin/mineral to ensure you're getting all essential nutrients. Or take an antioxidant supplement with extra vitamins A, C, D, and E along with selenium and zinc. If you normally take more than half a dozen supplements, consider simplifying these now. Stick with a multi, vitamin D, antioxidants, probiotics, and some omega-3 oils. Keep it simple, like your diet.

EASY GUIDE TO 5-DAY ELIMINATION

DAY	1	2	3	4	5
Breakfast	Lemon water first Fruit and whole grain or fruit with nuts/seeds if on a low-grain plan	Lemon water first Hearty Oatmeal (page 239) and seasonal fresh fruit (dried or frozen in winter)	Lemon water first Nice Rice (page 240)	Lemon water first Quinoa with raisins	Lemon water first Millet with sliced apple and sunflower seeds
Snack	Herbal tea or water with nutrients or a piece of fruit	Strawberries (organic), blueberries, or raspberries	Apples or pears	Banana and mango	Oranges or tangerine
Lunch	Mixed Greens Salad (page 249) or Roasted Vegetables Deluxe (page 263); optional protein	Greens (lettuce, kale, arugula) with cucumber, shredded carrot, and chickpeas	Steamed mixed vegetables with 3–4 oz chicken breast	Roasted veggies from last night and 3–4 ounces black beans	Mixed Greens Salad (page 249) with 1 can sardines
Snack	Fruit or drink, green tea or 3–4 oz protein snack if protein not consumed at lunch or dinner	Apple or two	Grapefruit or orange	Pear and few walnuts	Green tea and sliced fruit
Dinner	Seasonal mixed vegetables and, if needed, small amount of protein	Steamed veggies with potato, broccoli, chard, and green beans with hummus dip	Roasted veggies with carrots, mushrooms, garlic, Brussels sprouts, and zucchini	Salmon (3–4 oz) with green beans, garlic, carrots, and cauliflower	Baked veggies (choose 3–4) with small portion of chicken breast
Snack	Celery, carrot, and/or cucumber or a fruit like apple and a date or two	Apple and date	Orange	Celery and/or carrot sticks	Grapefruit

better. You'll stop missing those nutrient-poor foods in a few days. It does help to get your partner, friend, or family member to do this with you. Emotional and food support are often helpful with new eating programs.

Here's your step-by-step guide to the 5-day elimination plan. It's easy. You'll find some of the simple, delicious recipes in Chapter 8.

In the chart on page 127, Day 1 gives you the general guidance, so repeat that day or explore each day for your actual 5 days of eating. If you feel especially tired, or if you need more protein, add 3 to 4 ounces of protein like fish, poultry, or legumes to lunch or dinner or to the midafternoon snack.

Next up: the centerpiece of this easy plan—I-PEP.

THE IMMUNE-POWER EATING PLAN (I-PEP)

When we began this journey toward better health, we talked about eating foods from nature. Geography and climate affect what grows where and when, but consider all the options in your surrounding areas: Think gardens, orchards, farmers' markets, and growing your own; think color, taste, and aroma. Think the pleasure of good food!

QUICK TIP: FOCUS ON YOUR KEY FOODS

What are the best foods for you and your body, and can these correlate with what you like? Base your decisions on how you feel after consuming certain foods, on your ancestral diet in part, and on what you know to be healthy. Make a list of 7 to 10 foods that you know are good for you. Tune in to what foods are part of an everyday healthy diet and ask yourself the following question: If you were to live on your own island for 1 year and had to prepare healthy, enjoyable meals with basic foods, what 7 to 10 foods would you choose? You know you need nutrients, fiber, protein, oils, and some greens. My choices today would be salmon, apples, broccoli, avocado (or almonds for essential fatty acids), arugula, grapes, and carrots. These are core foods, and it's a good starting point when shifting to a healthy individualized eating plan. We can all have lemon and olive oil as extras since they are so good for us. So have some trees on your island for shade and food!

Nutrition is the core of your health and one of the cornerstones for building and maintaining lifelong well-being. On this program, you'll eat more fresh foods—especially vegetables, which contain many of the nutrients essential to life, such as vitamins, minerals, and phytonutrients, plus good fiber for healthy digestion and elimination. Good fat and protein sources are equally important—think low-fat meats, legumes, nuts and seeds, and olive oil. Fruits are good, too, but because of their high sugar/carbohydrate load, they shouldn't dominate your diet.

After you've completed the 5-day elimination plan, it's time to put the 2-week I-PEP into action. You'll notice improvements in your health and your feelings of vitality within a couple weeks—but remember: This is a plan you can live with forever.

I-PEP IN A NUTSHELL

I-PEP DAILY OVERVIEW

Eat slowly and chew well. Snacks are optional—if your energy is good and you're managing your weight, you may skip a snack, but grab one if you need one.

Proteins: Two or three 4- to 6-ounce portions

Veggies: 4 to 6 cups, especially greens

Legumes: 4 to 8 ounces

Grains: One or two 6-ounce bowls

Nuts and seeds: 2 to 4 ounces

Fruits: 2 to 3 pieces or, especially, $\frac{1}{2}$ to 1 cup berries

Wake up: Start your day with water and lemon (the juice from $\frac{1}{4}$ to $\frac{1}{2}$ lemon per 8-ounce glass of water).

Breakfast: Grain with fruit, plus 1 small handful of added nuts/seeds, to promote slower digestion and sugar absorption. Choose from less-reactive grains such as quinoa, millet, rice, and oatmeal.

Morning snack: 1 handful (or 1 to 2 ounces) of nuts or seeds like almonds, walnuts, or sunflower seeds or another piece of fruit

Lunch: Salad or vegetable combos with 3 to 4 ounces protein, like fish, poultry, or legumes

Afternoon snack: Veggies like celery, carrots, or cucumber with hummus; rice cake with nut butter and sliced organic apple or banana (1 piece of fruit)

Dinner: Protein and veggie focus with optional rice or quinoa (8 to 12 ounces total)

Evening snack: 1 to 2 pieces fruit

I-PEP 10-DAY MENU

DAY	1	2	3	4	5
Breakfast	Hearty Oatmeal (page 239) Green tea	Yogurt with mango, shredded ginger, ground flaxseeds Piece of gluten-free toast with nut butter Herbal tea	Veggie Frittata (page 242) Corn tortilla Tea—herbal, green, or black	ProBowl smoothie with OJ, banana, blueberries, other fruit, yogurt optional (page 240), plus a green powder Green tea	Nice Rice (page 240) Herbal tea
Snack, optional	1 apple and/ or handful of nuts	Kale Chips (page 276) or rice cake with nut butter and sliced banana	Sliced cucumber with hummus	Roasted carrots and/or other roasted veggies with optional dip	$1/2$ baked sweet potato with olive oil and sesame seed sprinkles
Lunch	Mixed Greens Salad (page 249) with chicken	Carrot Ginger Soup (page 255) and small green salad	Warm Red Cabbage Salad (page 251) plus optional 4 oz. chicken	Sweet potatoes with tofu Spinach salad	Asian Ginger Slaw (page 250)
Snack, optional	1 apple and peanut butter or almond butter	Pumpkin-Carrot Bar (page 279)	Leftover piece of meat loaf from previous night	Popcorn with olive oil and nutritional yeast	4–6-oz smoothie made with juice or rice milk with banana and protein powder
Dinner	Baked Dill Salmon (page 274) Baked sweet potato	Veggie Turkey Meat Loaf (page 271)	Risotto with Mushrooms, Asparagus, Manchego, and Thyme (page 275)	Tuscan Minestrone (page 261) Simple Kale Salad (page 252)	Quinoa Tabbouleh (page 248) Tuna or halibut
Snack or dessert	Moya's Flourless Chocolate Torte (page 292)	Blackberry-Ginger-Apple Crisp (page 291)	Triple-Ginger Cranberry Bar (page 278)	Rice cake with nut butter and apple, banana, or date	Baked Apple (page 287)

I-PEP 10-DAY MENU (CONT.)

DAY	6	7	8	9	10
Breakfast	ProBowl (page 240) with grated ginger Herbal tea	Tofu with Tumeric (page 241)	Fruit salad with yogurt Green tea	Hearty Oatmeal (page 239) with fruit, nuts Almond milk	Veggie Frittata (page 242) Corn tortilla Green tea
Snack	Baked Apple (page 287)	Fig and Almond Energy Bites (page 277)	Rice cracker with almond butter	Kale Chips (page 276)	Fruit option
Lunch	Simple Kale Salad (page 252) with feta cheese and avocado	Chicken-Lime soup (page 257)	Polenta with Tomato-Lentil Sauce (page 265) with kale and tahini dressing (page 284)	Wild sardine and rice salad	Turkey Chili (page 266) or Rainbow Veggie Rice (page 267) Rice crackers
Snack	Veggie sticks (celery, cucumber, carrot, zucchini) with hummus dip	Fruit option in season	Leftover green salad	Spicy Tofu leftover from previous night	Rice cake with almond butter and apple slices
Dinner	Chicken-Lime Soup (page 257)	Roasted Vegetables Deluxe (page 263) with choice of protein Citrus Shrimp and Garlic (page 269)	Spicy Tofu (page 262) with broccoli Coconut Rice (page 264)	Veggie Burger (page 270) with salad greens and gluten-free bread or rice crackers	Rainbow Veggie Rice (page 267) with chicken
Snack or dessert	Banana-papaya Fruit Freeze (page 288) or other freeze	Triple-Ginger Cranberry Bar (page 278)	Fruit Freeze of your choice (page 288)	Your choice	Moya's Flourless Chocolate Torte (page 292)

LIGHTEN UP: LOSE WEIGHT WITH I-PEP

Shifting your body composition, losing weight, and keeping it off requires more than just "going on a diet." It takes a conscious effort, lifestyle changes, including food, and adherence to a complete program of diet, exercise, and stress relief. The following tips can help you succeed.

- Avoid all flour and sugar products, even whole grain baked goods.

- Limit total grains to one to two portions a day, not more than 10 to 15 percent of your daily food calories.

- Center your diet on vegetables; they should comprise at least 50 to 60 percent of your intake, and, of those, only 25 percent or less of starchy veggies like potatoes, carrots, and beets.

- Add good quality proteins to your vegetables. (Refer to the list on page 108.)

- For best digestion, don't drink water during meals. Drink one to two glasses of water when you wake up and 30 to 40 minutes before meals to reduce your appetite as well as satisfy you.

- Chew your food well. Slow down as you eat to feel more satisfied with less food.

- Stop eating in the early evening, and finish your dinner by 7:00 p.m. at the latest. Eat dinner even earlier in winter.

- Get enough quality sleep to support your body functions and protect your health.

- Find your favorite activities and do them often. Incorporate walking, stretching, aerobics, and weight work.

Ultimately, you are your own best doctor and dietitian. You may sense that certain foods don't agree with you, whereas others make you feel really good. With greater awareness of your responses, you can choose wisely and thrive.

Nutritional needs vary depending on your gender, age, and lifestyle. If your goal is to receive the nutrients your cells require for the thousands of functions they do every day, then you might wish to consider adding supplements to your diet.

USING NUTRITIONAL SUPPLEMENTS WISELY

Many people choose to bolster their balanced nutrition with an appropriate multi-vitamin/mineral, and we support this even though research is mixed regarding the long-term health benefits of taking nutritional supplements. For instance, while a recent study appeared to demonstrate that multivitamin and mineral supplements can reduce infections in people with type 2 diabetes mellitus, other studies have revealed little or no benefit from long-term use of supplements.[89] Two recent studies showed that taking a daily multi didn't improve aging brains or the health of heart attack survivors, and headlines suggest that multivitamins don't help your health. That conclusion, though, is based on incomplete studies and not on good science.

The quality of the products and how easily nutrients are absorbed and utilized can make a big difference in the effectiveness of supplements. Some multis, for example, come from food sources; these tend to be more expensive than the lower-cost synthetic nutrients made with chemical fillers and food coloring. Many people may benefit from taking omega-3 fish oils or flaxseed oil; extra B vitamins; probiotics; and antioxidants such as vitamins A, C, and E plus zinc and selenium. There are specific nutritional approaches and herbal therapies that can help many conditions. (See Chapter 7 for a review of immune-related problems and their corresponding supplement suggestions.)

Which vitamin supplements are right for you? Start by asking yourself, "Am I eating a nourishing, balanced diet?" You may be getting all, or most, of the nutrients you need from the foods you eat, but if you suspect your diet is lacking, talk to your health-care practitioner about supplements.

Supplements are not under FDA control, so there's no guarantee you're getting exactly what the label claims. (The FDA does oversee claims and keeps companies honest; it also can remove products that cause harm.) When you buy a supplement, you may be getting more than you bargained for, like lead in your calcium or insect parts in your spices, so it's important to look for reliable companies. Quality control companies, like ConsumerLab.com, can offer dependable guidance on a product's quality and safety. When choosing—and taking—supplements, follow these guidelines.

- **Assimilation is the key to effective supplementation.** How much of what you take actually gets into your blood and then your cells? This has a lot to do with efficient digestion and how easily the nutrient dissolves in the first place. Some nutrients, like vitamin C and the Bs, are more readily absorbed than minerals like calcium or iron. Taking the latter with a little orange juice can improve absorption.

- **Many minerals compete with each other** to be absorbed and to get into your cells, so *when* you take them is also important. Taking most minerals, like calcium, zinc, and iron, with an acidic juice (like orange or cranberry) will help your body assimilate them. Drug interactions can occur with some nutrients and, more commonly, herbs. Seek some guidance on nutrients that work well together and those that don't.

- **Your age and gender affect what's right for you.** Women tend to need more iron (during their menstrual years) and calcium (later in life); men may benefit from more zinc and magnesium.

Confused about which supplements to take? Here's an overview of some of the more commonly used supplements.

MULTIVITAMINS/MINERALS. A multi is like an insurance plan. It's usually best to choose a low-dose multi with levels close to the RDA (Recommended Dietary Allowance) rather than one with higher amounts.

VITAMIN D. Many people measure low in vitamin D, though numerous studies show its protective and even preventive effects against chronic diseases, including cancer, dementia, and multiple sclerosis. Vitamin D supplements are widely endorsed by both mainstream and alternative/complementary physicians. Recommended daily amounts of vitamin D_3 vary from 1,000 to 10,000 IU, with about 2,000 being the acceptable amount to maintain adequate levels. If your vitamin D levels are very low, you need to supplement more vitamin D over a longer time. Your doctor can measure your blood level (as 25-hydroxy vitamin D).

OMEGA-3 OILS. These are widely accepted and used as anti-inflammatory supplements that aid good tissue health and may offer some cardiovascular protection.

VITAMIN C. Although it's not the cure-all it once was thought to be, you need C for good tissue strength and for its antioxidant properties. Helpful levels range from 60 mg (RDA) to 2,000 mg (2 grams). Megadosing isn't common, but higher levels of intake, like 3 to 4 grams, may lessen some allergy responses.

VITAMIN E. To get the maximum benefits from this powerful antioxidant, choose good quality, natural-mixed tocopherols rather than synthetic acetates, and the potential benefits will likely show up better. (Remember this: Natural vitamin E has "d" in front of the name, as in d-alpha; "dl" means it's a synthetic product.)

CoQ10. Known as ubiquinone and the more bioavailable ubiquinol, CoQ10 is more expensive than many other supplements. It may be helpful as an antioxidant, for supporting energy in cells, and for calming irregular heart rhythms. Anyone taking statin drugs, which cause CoQ10 deficiency, should consider a supplement.[90]

CALCIUM/MAGNESIUM COMBINATIONS. These have become controversial, with varying opinions about their benefits and possible risks. In large clinical trials, such as the Women's Health Initiative, which studied more than 30,000 women, researchers looked at whether calcium supplements (1,000 mg/day for 7 years) would prevent osteoporosis or bone fractures. Although the effect on reducing fractures is still unclear, the surprising result was that there were more cardiac events in the women who took calcium supplements.[91] A similar finding came out of the Auckland Calcium Study, which studied more than 1,400 postmenopausal women. Until research provides conclusive evidence, obtain your calcium primarily from food sources[92] and take magnesium supplements alone or with any calcium supplement you take—or, better yet, eat more foods high in magnesium[93] and calcium. Remember that calcium and magnesium are interrelated: Levels of one influence the other. It's believed in the natural and functional medicine worlds that an adequate magnesium level is important to keep calcium in solution and not cause kidney stones or worsen hardening in the arteries. Ideally, of course, we get these vital minerals from good foods, such as leafy greens, nuts and seeds, and some dairy. Older people with bone loss probably need more calcium, and magnesium can be helpful for high blood pressure or for constipation. There are many forms or "salts" of calcium and magnesium; the citrates are common, but magnesium citrate can cause some trouble since it is a laxative. People with loose bowels can take magnesium glycinate, an amino acid chelate that allows good absorption and doesn't appear to cause loose bowels.

ANTIOXIDANT COMBINATIONS. Popular and readily available, antioxidant supplements are useful as added insurance. If you're already taking a multi, you probably don't need it, but it can be used when stress is high or during travel or for exposure to toxic chemicals. Antioxidant combinations often include vitamins A, C, and E and zinc and selenium. Green and red powders are also available that are high in antioxidants on the ORAC scale.

SPECIAL OR CONCENTRATED FOODS. These include nutritional yeast, seaweeds, blue-green algae, protein powders, nuts and seeds, and green juices and/or smoothies made from these items.

THE TAKEAWAY

You've learned a lot so far. But information isn't enough to motivate you to change. Think about the health problems that are challenging you now and what you'd like to change—and why. The next chapter guides you to transform mind patterns and stressful reactions that may put up roadblocks to your new health choices. Lifestyle and health aren't just about food and eating right. All factors play a part in the circle of your life.

As we move forward from food into stress and movement, think about what living a good life means to you and what you can do to make that a reality. Nutrition has a tremendous impact on your immune health and, ultimately, the well-being of your entire body. In Chapter 5, we'll learn how to beat one of your immune system's biggest threats: stress.

CHAPTER 5

The Stress Connection

Do any of these scenarios sound familiar? You're already late for an appointment when you get caught in a traffic jam. You're upset over an ongoing argument with a friend. You're starting a new job or just lost one. Your partner was diagnosed with cancer, and you're worried about treatment and outcome. Without question, these situations are stressful. The stress you feel could be temporary, or it could develop into a long-term problem that impacts your immune functions and health—the outcome is, in large part, up to you.

Stress happens. It can stem from something simple like giving a presentation or having a flat tire. Or it can be the result of ongoing issues like relationship troubles or job dissatisfaction. The circumstances themselves, however, aren't solely to blame for your stress level: Your *perception of* and *reaction to* the situation factor in heavily. For instance, if you have a chronic illness and some part of your body hurts, you may feel stress if you perceive that pain as a sign of the disease progressing. On the other hand, your stress level might be low if you knew the pain was from exercising too vigorously and unrelated to your illness. Your *perception* of what's happening in your environment or in your body is your mental and emotional response, and it colors how you manage the stressful situation. The way you manage stress has a direct effect on your overall health and that of your immune system.

Do you get colds frequently? Do you have allergy symptoms or reactions to food? Does your arthritis pain worsen with worry? Can you link your worst physical symptoms with something stressful happening in your life, like job concerns, the arrival of a new baby, or lack of sleep?

Stress certainly isn't to blame for every bug you catch, but it can make you more vulnerable to infections and can worsen the symptoms of allergies, chronic pain, or autoimmune illnesses. Your health and every disease and its healing are impacted by stress.

Stressful situations are a fact of life. The good news is that you can keep your immune system balanced and reduce stress by learning and practicing coping strategies designed to relax you and shift your mental state.

So what exactly is this all-encompassing thing called stress? One thing is certain: It's not only in your head, it shows up in your body, too. Ways that your body tells you you're experiencing stress include a racing heart, shallow breathing, tense shoulders, dry mouth, a clenched jaw, and sweaty or cold hands. Let's see how this happens.

THE BIOLOGY OF ACUTE STRESS

Experts in the field of body-mind medicine don't all agree on the definition of stress. Let's consider one definition: Stress can result from any situation for which you think you lack the resources to handle it—resources like energy, time, money, intellect, or mood. An injury or illness, extreme hot or cold weather, or even the anticipation or perception of a threat can trigger a stress response. The way you perceive the situation and what meaning you give it determine whether or not your body has a stress response, ranging from mild to very intense. Stress can be acute, immediate, and short lived or chronic, ongoing, and long lasting. It's the ongoing stress you have to watch out for.

Acute, fleeting stress is biologically different from ongoing chronic stress. Acute stress triggers fight-or-flight biochemical reactions, which prepare your body to fight or run away by activating every response you need for immediate short-term survival—especially increased energy production. During acute stress, your body slows down digestion or reproductive capacities. If you have only so many units of energy, they must all go toward protecting you in that immediate stressful situation. In the acute scenario, once the threat or challenge is met, your body automatically rebalances itself into a more relaxed mode.

Chemical Reactions

What actually happens during a stress reaction? Molecular energy in the form of a powerful chemical called ATP (adenosine triphosphate) is released to fuel your body, especially the larger muscles that help you handle an assault or run away from it. You may physically notice this stress response: When your blood moves to fuel the muscles in your legs, it moves away from your hands and feet, leaving them colder.

After that first surge of ATP, your body releases more stress hormones to rev you up and get you moving. It begins with adrenaline (epinephrine) and its cousin norepinephrine. These hormones trigger your immediate reactions that call on the energy your cells are churning out—you run away from an attacker or you quickly move to the right lane when you hear a fire engine roaring up behind you. Your muscles tense, your breathing accelerates, and sweat may pour out. Next along comes cortisol, which kicks in a few minutes later to regulate some of your less critical (for the moment) body functions, like appetite and digestion. That allows your body to focus its energy on the problem at hand and conserve energy for survival.

Once your body handles the danger, it automatically returns to a more relaxed state. Your racing heart slows down, your breathing deepens, your hands warm up, and you're ready to continue with the rest of your day.

It's a brilliant system. The trouble is, sometimes those hormones keep pumping, even when danger has passed. And too much cortisol for too long can diminish your immunity, elevate your blood pressure, lower your bone density, weaken your memory, and even add inches to your waistline.[1]

> **STRESS-REDUCTION TIP**
>
> Notice what happens to your shoulders and jaw when you even think about (let alone experience) a stressful situation. Pay attention to your body: Tense muscles and cold hands (when the room isn't cold) are telling you that you're undergoing stress. Now relax your jaw and shoulders to calm your mind; intentionally changing your physical tension sends your brain and mind a different message. One deep, cleansing breath often does the trick. As you breathe deep into your belly, let your energy drop from your head to your heart and then to your navel area, the center of your body. Then breathe out, and feel your body and jaw relax.

Cortisol is the chief culprit in terms of throwing off the balance in immune activities. Although cortisol may lower the number of active T cells and suppress your immune response, some cytokines also released during stress can increase inflammation. The chemistry and immunology of stress is complex, with 20 to 30 different mischievous molecules doing their dance up and down and all around. As usual, balance is critical.

Energy Crisis

A key part of the biochemical stress response is energy—lots more is used to get you out of a difficult or stressful situation. One sign that you may be experiencing ongoing chronic stress is that you're always tired. That physical and even emotional fatigue has a biochemical cause, and it's all about cellular energy.

When your cells and muscles are confronted with ongoing stress, they contract and become tense. When your muscles are experiencing tension, they begin to become starved for oxygen and produce less energy. In fact, those tense muscle cells make one-tenth the amount of energy molecules than when they're relaxed. This decreased energy production compromises your immune functions and other jobs your body must do to keep you alive and well. You need energy to produce more immune cells and to manufacture immune proteins like antibodies and cytokines. And, of course, your brain needs energy to help you think clearly and to balance your mood and memory.

All that mayhem going on inside your cells is bound to show up on the outside through symptoms we've touched on earlier. Those ongoing symptoms can wear you down, and you don't even know it until you're exhausted or get sick. That's when your body gives out and wants a rest. Illness is one way your body forces you to slow down. If you pay attention to how you are living your life and to the symptomatic clues *before* you get sick, you may be able to head off an illness at the pass.

Just like an army, though, our physical borders protect us from alien invasion. Breaches at these borders—a cut on the skin, an open mouth, a breath of air, the food we chew—are doorways where aliens can easily enter. Our sentinels at the border usually protect us, until the invasion gets out of hand. That's when ordinary stress turns into long-term, chronic, and toxic stress.

TOXIC STRESS

You face short-term stresses nearly every day, from being late for work to meeting with your tax accountant. Short-lived stress can actually motivate you to better prepare for these activities. But what if you habitually relive and rehash stressful events? When that happens, you're putting your body through trouble it was never designed to face. Daily repetitive stress can lead to chronic stress—the sort that contributes to ill health. This is especially true in people whose immune systems are already in a weakened state.

In a 2002 review, Janice Kiecolt-Glaser and Ronald Glaser of Ohio State University reported that mild depression may also suppress an older person's immune system.[2] Another study of 92 elderly people showed that those who had major depression and were not on antidepressants had a much lower response to the herpes zoster (shingles) vaccine.[3] That could explain why many people appear to have no protection with this vaccine.

Chronic, persistent stress and depression diminish your quality of life and contribute to many health problems. They can worsen conditions like chronic pain or trigger an asthmatic attack, a bout of diarrhea, or a headache. Even acute stress can do the same. In one study, for example, researchers followed more than 5,000 adults over 10 years for developing asthma. They found that higher stress levels doubled the risk for asthma, even after they adjusted for a number of different variables.[4]

The stress response, like your immune response, is essential to life, keeping you on your toes when danger comes along   in the

STRESS-AWARENESS CLUES

When you're waiting to give a presentation or engaged in an uncomfortable conversation, notice whether your hands feel warm or cold, sweaty or dry. Clammy or cold hands signal stress. Relieve it with a 5-minute walk, a 3-minute breather, or a couple of deep inhalations of lavender.

These are common stressors. Do any of them sound familiar?

- Unhappy relationships—personal or work related
- Loneliness
- Financial difficulties
- Worry
- Lack of sleep
- Lack of relaxation
- Chronic pain or illness

form of an out-of-control car racing toward you, an impossible deadline, or a life-changing discussion. But when you're chronically stressed, trouble follows, because your immune system stops working at its best.

Triggering Toxic Stress

Sometimes, when stress happens, we rise to the occasion like superheroes, overcoming obstacles in our way before calmly returning to our desk jobs. Other times, stress sticks, and we can't shake it. Why the difference? For decades, scientists have been studying just what it is that turns a run-of-the-mill stressor into a relentless stress monster that wears down your health and eventually makes you sick. They've found fascinating connections between stress and your health, especially your immune health. Here are some of the most important ones.

Life Events and Your Immunity

In 1967, psychiatrists Thomas Holmes and Richard Rahe began studying whether stress contributed to illness. They devised a scale of 43 life changes, weighting events with different values when they appeared to increase the likelihood of the person becoming ill. After the creation of the Holmes and Rahe Stress Scale, scientists began using it to estimate the effects of stress on a person's health. The scale compared stressful events like moving, losing a job, the death of a relative, going on vacation, and starting a new position. Scientists found that those with more "significant" events in a given time period were more likely to get ill in the coming year (see the following chart).

THE HOLMES-RAHE STRESS SCALE

From early work by psychiatrists Holmes and Rahe in 1967, it looked like it was the event itself that caused the stress. They weighted events that we all experience, like the death of a loved one, at the top of the stressful life events scale, and then placed divorce, illness in the family, and losing a job further down the continuum, with even a vacation listed as a possible stressful life event. However, since the chart's creation in 1967, researchers have learned that it's not simply the event that affects your health, it's how you interpret the event.

LIFE EVENT	VALUE
Death of a spouse	100
Divorce	73
Marital separation	65
Jail term	63
Death of a close family member	63
Personal injury or illness	53
Marriage	50
Fired from your job	47
Marital reconciliation	45
Retirement	45
Health changes of a family member	44
Pregnancy	40
Vacation	13

Of course, the death of a spouse is traumatic, but you'd likely experience different qualities or duration of stress depending on the circumstances surrounding the death. An unexpected death from a car crash, for instance, might be more acutely stressful than death following a long illness, which might be tinged with relief as well as sadness. Enter the new field of mind-body medicine.

The Mind–Body Effect

Not all life events are created equal. To determine how stressful life events—the good as well as the bad—impact immunity and health, mind-body specialists, scientists focusing on psychoneuroimmunology (PNI), have uncovered this scientific reality: It's not simply an event that causes stress, it's the way you interpret the event that affects your stress response, your sense of control, your resilience, your attitude, your behaviors, and, ultimately, your health. PNI is an integrative approach to health that encompasses your psyche or mind (P), neurochemistry (N), and the immune system (I). In this medical discipline, the many processes of your body and mind are viewed as connected, working together to help you thrive and stay healthy. PNI began gaining its credibility as a field of science and medicine a few decades ago when it was proved that:

- The immune organs are actually physically (anatomically) connected to the brain and nervous system.[5]
- Stress hormones affect immune responses, and immune responses affect the brain.[6]
- Mental attitudes like optimism or pessimism impact emotions, immune health, and behavior.[7]

Until that time, PNI, once called psychosomatic medicine, was on the fringes of medicine because scientists believed that the immune system was an independent operator, not influenced by either hormones of the body or moods of the mind.

Psychologist Robert Ader coined the term "psychoneuroimmunology" when he unexpectedly discovered that immune behaviors could be conditioned by the physical senses.[8] Ader was exploring "conditioned taste aversions," a phenomenon experienced by many cancer patients who had nausea after receiving chemotherapy. Ader and his colleague Nicholas Cohen set up a model in animals to learn more. In their study, mice prone to the autoimmune disease lupus were offered saccharin-flavored water at the same time they were injected one time with a potent immunosuppressive drug (Cytoxan). When the conditioned association was learned, the taste alone (with no injection of the drug) reduced inflammation, immune responses, and symptoms of lupus almost as much as the drug itself. In other words, Ader and Cohen discovered that the immune system can be conditioned in the same way Pavlov's dogs learned to salivate in response to a bell.[9] This opened a compelling field of research that illustrates that even human immune behaviors can be conditioned by physical senses[10] and, perhaps, by expectation.[11] In fact, some scientists believe that the placebo effect is also a conditioned response—you expect to get better from a drug or procedure given to you by your doctor in a medical setting you've visited before.

In the laboratory, it's easy to measure specific components of immune function and link them to experimentally induced stress events. A few pioneering examples: Married couples fight about money while being videotaped. Their blood is drawn before, during, and after the argument to follow stress hormones and immune markers. Both spouses showed increased stress during the argument, but the wife's stress hormones remained elevated while the husband's quickly returned to normal. The interpretation: She's reliving the argument while he has let it go.[12] Another study exposes healthy volunteers to cold viruses to see if they get sick.[13] They all showed immune responses to the virus, but only some got sick with symptoms—those with the most stress the week before. In a follow-up study, those with few social contacts

The Immune Diaries   Sondra

When I taught graduate courses in psychoneuroimmunology, I gave students an assignment to design their own conditioning experiment to test whether they could change their physiology by engaging their senses. One young man took homeopathic remedies to help manage his asthma, and they lessened his symptoms. So for his conditioning experiment, for 1 week, he tapped on his chest (the thymus area) whenever he took the remedies. After that, when he felt asthma symptoms coming on, he just tapped his chest and his symptoms receded.

So how can you test this in your life? Suppose you're taking anti-inflammatory ibuprofen for joint pain. When you take the drug, pair it with a unique scent like lavender, a taste of ginger ale, a tap on the chest, or a specific song. Use that same sensory strategy each time you take the ibuprofen for at least 1 week. To test the strength of your conditioning, try only the sensory strategy the next time you want to take the drug. Did it work for you? If so, you have now conditioned your body to lessen inflammatory pain. If it didn't work, you might need more time or a different sensory trigger. Write us and let us know how it worked and what you learned. However, please don't try this strategy with medications essential for your life without speaking to your doctor first. And with conditioned responses, you have to retrain your body every once in a while with the actual physiological trigger—in this case, ibuprofen.

got sick more easily.[14] Studies like these measure specific immune proteins or stress hormones in the blood and provide evidence that mental stress can influence immune responses. In real life, however, the situation is much more complex, and not simple cause and effect. We're not dealing with one behavior change or only one particular measurable immune reaction; we have an entire system within us. Nor are we dealing with only one specific physical or emotional stressor. To achieve better health, it's important to understand the complexity of the human response and use that knowledge to discover ways of taking better care of ourselves. It's all about lifestyle in the long run, not a one-time change.

MANAGE STRESS, BUILD RESILIENCE

The science is clear: Chronic, persistent stress wreaks havoc with your immune system and leads to a wide variety of health concerns. But how? A popular assumption is that stress depresses immune functions and makes you more vulnerable to illness. However, from a relatively recent review of 300 studies on the relationship between stress and immune health,[15] the following important conclusions were made:

- Acute, time-limited stress (like giving a public presentation) activated natural innate immunity—the quick responses of the natural killer (NK) cells, phagocytes, and inflammation—while slowing down longer-term lymphocyte responses. In other words, acute stress, which lasts from 5 to 90 minutes, activates your first line of innate defenses. This enables your body to immediately deal with injury and be protected from infection. Plus, no new cells or proteins have to be made, and that conserves energy for the important tasks at hand.

- Stressful life events were not reliably connected to any one specific immune modification. But chronic stressors, like living with a handicap or being unemployed, had consistent negative effects on almost all immune functions.

You can impact your health right now by engaging in strategies that reduce your chronic stress.[16]

Stress happens to everyone. But remember, it's not the challenging event that leads to toxic stress, it's the way you respond to it. Research clearly reveals that relieving stress and preventing it from becoming chronic will help keep you—and your immune system—healthy and strong.

Now, let's look at some of these science-tested strategies for preventing toxic stress responses by managing stress before your mind becomes attached to reliving it over and over.

It's important to note that the more strategies you've got in your stress-relief vault, the better. And the more you practice these techniques, the more effective they'll be. Yes, you certainly want to apply them when you feel stressed, but by integrating these strategies into your daily routine, you can use them to lower the amount of ongoing stress you experience. It's like building an "antistress" muscle—the more you practice, the more fit you become in managing stressful moments, so that you don't even react stressfully to old trigger situations. Stress buffers or relaxation strategies include meditation, exercise, laughter, music, friends, and play.

Don't forget—if you can't change the stressor or the situation, work on changing your mental and emotional attitude about it. You can learn to interpret difficult situations differently. You'll find valuable tools in the pages that follow.

Meditation

Whether you're thinking about work, worrying about your children, or plowing through that mile-high to-do list, your mind is constantly churning. If you aren't careful, those cluttered thoughts will multiply and take over. Meditation can help you stop that incessant mind chatter. It's an ancient practice that produces a state of deep relaxation and calms the mind, giving the brain a much-needed respite from the usual day-to-day mental activity.

Research shows that any form of meditation can diminish stress. In a pioneering study more than 40 years ago,[17] Herbert Benson, a cardiologist at Harvard looking for ways to lower the stress and blood pressure of his patients with hypertension, discovered what he called the Relaxation Response (RR). Benson based his exercise on the practice that the Beatles popularized—Transcendental Meditation. Benson trained his patients to sit quietly in a darkened room for 10 minutes repeating one word, the word "one." (It could be any word like "love," "peace," "friendship," "God," or a commonly used Hindu Sanskrit word, "om." You get the idea.) Benson showed that by practicing two times a day for 10 minutes, his patients reduced both their blood pressure and heart rates.[18] The RR, which can be learned and initiated voluntarily, is associated with decreases in oxygen consumption, respiratory rate (slower breathing), and blood pressure, along with an increased sense of well-being. On the other hand, the stress response is involuntary, with physiological changes that include increases in heart and respiration rates and blood pressure.

New research is looking more deeply into the positive effects of RR. In one 2013 study of longtime practitioners and novices, researchers wanted to see if there were short-term, immediate physiological changes during only one session of RR practice. The novices had weekly training for 8 weeks in techniques that elicited RR, including a combination of breathing, body scan, RR, and mindfulness exercises. They also listened to a relaxation CD once a day. The longtime practitioners reported regularly practicing meditation, yoga, and/or repetitive prayer over a time period from 4 to 20 years. On the test day, blood was drawn from the control subjects (including novice and longtime

---

RECLAIMING RELAXATION

The first essentials of any relaxation practice are a quiet environment, a comfortable position, a mental tactic, and a receptive attitude. A "mental tactic" is something on which to focus your mind. In Herbert Benson's Relaxation Response (RR), for example, it is repeating a word, like "one." In other practices, the mental focus is on the breath, a candle, or a sound. Being receptive means to observe what happens without judging your performance or expecting anything.

Here's how to do RR after you've set the stage with the basic elements. Try this once or twice a day, but wait at least 2 hours after you eat.

Close your eyes. Relax your muscles, beginning with your feet and moving up your body to your legs, belly, shoulders, neck, and head. (Or you could start with your head and neck area and move downward.) Breathe in through your nose, becoming aware of your breath. As you breathe out, say the word "one" (or "om" or any word you prefer) silently to yourself. Breathe in, breathe out with "one." Whenever distracting thoughts occur, ignore them and repeat "one" as you breathe. Do this for 10 or 20 minutes. Do not use an alarm or timer; you can open your eyes occasionally to check the time. When you finish, sit quietly for a few minutes, eyes closed, and then open them and go about your day.[19]

meditators) both before and after listening to a 15-minute relaxation CD. White blood cells were analyzed for various physiological markers. Both novices and longtime meditators showed a reduced expression of proinflammatory and stress genes. While both groups experienced positive changes, results were more pronounced in the longtime practitioners.[20] What was significant from these studies was that even a short 15-minute meditation practice changed the genes. Another recent study of longtime meditators showed that their production of proinflammatory proteins was reduced after a single 8-hour day of intense meditation.[21]

Other techniques can also elicit the RR, including progressive relaxation and hypnosis, and they all share some basic elements. Progressive relaxation[22] was developed in the 1930s by physician Edmund Jacobson to help his patients lessen their anxiety. The technique involves asking the patient to tense and relax each muscle group throughout the body; it is often the first stress management practice people learn. It's been used effectively for relieving stress and anxiety in almost every clinical condition, including ringing in the ears, chronic anxiety, asthma,[23] and prostate cancer.[24] Many of these practices were used originally in a religious or spiritual context but have been stripped of any cultural practices to make them more accepted by the West.

Even more popular than the classic RR practice and accepted into mainstream medicine is mindfulness meditation, a strategy first introduced by Dr. Jon Kabat-Zinn to help people with chronic pain. Mindfulness meditation begins with scanning your body to become aware of any places where you're experiencing stress, tension, or pain. Next, you engage in 30 minutes of mindfulness as you sit quietly and become aware of your thoughts without getting caught up in them. In his pioneering studies, Kabat-Zinn showed that people with chronic pain could diminish their discomfort with mindfulness and that they were still practicing it weeks after their training stopped.[25] Later studies by Kabat-Zinn and his team also showed that immune functions could be improved with this strategy.[26]

What's great about mindfulness meditation is that you can find free or inexpensive classes at many hospitals and health-care settings, or you can learn it on your own. Once you know how, it costs you nothing to improve your health.[27] Some meditation programs suggest using a sensory signal—like touching your fingers together or sniffing lavender—whenever you reach your relaxed state. Lavender has been used for centuries to reduce anxiety, and modern research is beginning to show the usefulness of the sense of smell for changing physiology.[28] When you use touch or experience a particular scent while learning a relaxation strategy, you are conditioning your physiology to relax. Soon the sensory stimulus alone will elicit relaxation or the meditative state. Meditation is becoming such a useful practice for reducing stress and hostility, it's even being taught to at-risk youth, resulting in less violent behavior in schools.[29]

Guided Imagery

One form of meditation suggests imagining a candle or a peaceful place. This is called imagery or visualization, an early and still active form of healing. Imagery isn't difficult to master. In fact, you may already be using imagery when you worry or imagine defeat or danger when none exists, exce pt in your mind. (Studies show that 90 to 95 percent of what people worry about never happens.[30]) One of the earliest research studies relevant to immune health was teaching imagery to children to increase their white blood cells. Their training was so specific that they could elevate the phagocytes (the innate primitive white blood cells) but not the lymphocytes (white blood cells that engage in learned specific immune responses).[31] Imagery has been used by athletes for decades as something called mental practice—imagining, for example, hitting the ball with your racket or outrunning your opponents in a race. Scientists are taking this mental practice a step further. When your body is immobilized for any length of time because of a broken leg, surgery, or chronic pain, for example, you usually lose function of the area. In a small study of 18 healthy young men, their forearms were immobilized with a cast for 3 weeks to simulate a fracture. They received four training sessions in which they imagined moving their wrist, and they were asked to do that mental exercise 15 minutes every day. Those who practiced the imagery lost no hand function due to the immobilization, while those in the control group did.[32] When you lose mobility for any reason, it's useful to know that you may be able to prevent loss of function or improve function by imagining your body doing what it can't do now.

Further evidence for the benefit of imagery: In a 12-week healthy lifestyle intervention study with obese teenagers, which provided education about diet, physical activity, and stress, the group that also practiced guided imagery showed much greater improvement in increasing their physical activity and trended toward reducing their food intake as well as producing lower salivary cortisol, a marker of stress.[33] Information alone doesn't necessarily help you change behaviors; engaging your mind does.

The practice of imagery requires that you first relax your body and mind. Next,

ULTIMATE IMMUNITY　　SUCCESS STORY

Elizabeth River, 69

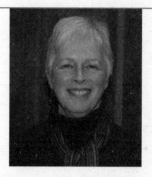

An interfaith minister who officiates at weddings and serves as a hospice chaplain, Elizabeth began her career and found her true calling at age 59 as she walked with others through important spiritual moments.

She realized, though, that her own health was jeopardizing her profession. "I've learned from hospice work that the thing you have to take care of first is pain," she says. "When you're in pain, you're completely consumed by it and can't think about anything else. Though I never thought of myself as a person who suffered pain, I began to realize that I was in constant discomfort—I had indigestion, heartburn, and bloating. That discomfort took away my attention and my energy from my work."

So she turned to Dr. Haas, who ran a series of blood tests and found that Elizabeth was reactive to dairy ("Cheese and crackers were my drug of choice," she says) and suffered from severe gluten intolerance. With Dr. Haas's help, Elizabeth learned that when she fed her body the wrong foods, it produced an immune reaction that led to extreme inflammation.

The doctor's advice: Go on a 3-day cleanse, completely eradicate gluten and dairy, and follow the Immune-Power Eating Plan.

The result: "It was astonishing," Elizabeth recalls. "In only 2 days, I had no heartburn, indigestion, belly pains, or headaches. And I began sleeping better—no more waking up in the middle of the night." In a week, she felt better in her clothes; in 3 weeks, she'd dropped two sizes; in a month, her waist had shrunk 5 inches and she'd gone from a size 12 to a size 8.

As a spiritual companion to those in their final days, Elizabeth's hospice work is demanding—seeing patients, updating charts, interacting with health-care providers and other clergy. Helping young couples celebrate a joyful wedding day provides a wonderful sense of balance. To give her the energy to do all this important work—and to enjoy her own life to the fullest—she's committed to strengthening her immunity with her new, healthier way of life. Besides following I-PEP, she does yoga, meditates daily, and goes for long hikes every chance she gets.

imagine a healing scenario, such as seeing yourself doing something you haven't been able to do because of an illness. You can also imagine the hyperactive immune cells calming down and coming into balance, or picture red-hot hyperactive immune cells cooling down. You can even write your own imagery script. This is where you learn to trust your intuition and inner wisdom. Additionally, you can find guided meditations online. Check out the following Web sites for some ideas:

- University of Michigan Comprehensive Cancer Center: mcancer.org/support/managing-emotions/complementary-therapies/guided-imagery
- Health Journeys: healthjourneys.com/what_is_guided_imagery.asp
- Inner Health Studio: innerhealthstudio.com/meditation-scripts.html

Using images is a powerful strategy for creating more peacefulness in your body, which enhances your health even if specific immune changes cannot be measured. The point is, reducing stress by knowing that you have effective ways to manage stress opens doors to better health. Remember that resilience means you have a sense of control over a situation. When you learn dependable ways to lessen stress—be it imagery, meditation, or listening to music—you have improved how you manage and cope with difficult situations.

The Immune Diaries   Sondra

A woman with numerous allergies and environmental sensitivities attended one of my immune health groups to see if she could learn to be less hyperreactive. Just the whiff of someone's perfume would cause a reaction, so there were hazards everywhere she went. Using imagery, she imagined that impenetrable boundaries surrounded her, and she practiced this imagery every day. When she had to attend a party in Los Angeles, one of the smoggiest cities in the United States, and stay in a motel near a refinery, she practiced the boundary exercise before and during her visit. When she returned to our group, she announced that she had no reactions to the polluted air. She was apparently protected by the shield put up by her mind, which calmed her body's hyperreactive state.

Freeze-Frame

The Freeze-Frame method, developed by the Institute of HeartMath,[34] can teach you to manage your thoughts and emotions with a simple five-step process. In a nutshell, you learn to "pause" a stressful moment that you're experiencing (imagine pausing a DVD you're watching) and disengage from it. Shift your attention to your heart and ask yourself to think with your heart, not the reactive mind, to refocus on something positive, then "restart" the moment and address it from a more balanced heart-based perspective. One wonderful story the institute tells is about a young boy who was bullied. His usual way of reacting was to fight. Having been trained in Freeze-Frame, he looked at the situation from "his heart" and remembered his birthday. No need to fight at all—he was able to simply walk away.[35] Doc Childre's book *Freeze-Frame: One-Minute Stress Management* will teach you much more about this useful method.[36] There's lots of useful information at the HeartMath Web site: heartmath.org.

Cognitive Behavioral Therapy

Have you ever closely examined your point of view about life? Do you tend to be a "half empty" or "half full" person? Your outlook on life might originate in your head, but it doesn't stay there. It influences your behaviors, emotions, choices, and health. If negative thoughts dominate your days, cognitive behavioral therapy (CBT) may help. At its core, CBT seeks to balance an overabundance of negative thoughts with ideas that are more realistic and fair. The process uncovers the reasons for your negative beliefs and attitudes and encourages you to shift to a reality that is more positive.

Receiving a diagnosis of cancer, for example, is one of the most stressful, anxiety-producing experiences, triggering every possible negative thought. So it's clear why people with cancer are often the research guinea pigs into ways to improve mental and emotional health. At the University of Miami in Florida, for instance, 199 women with early stage breast cancer participated in a 10-week program that combined imagery, relaxation, and CBT to decrease stress, negative mood, thoughts, and anxiety.[37] The question was whether altering these factors would improve recovery from breast cancer. Good news: This program resulted in a decrease in the expression of proinflammatory genes and cancer-related genes, with an increase in the expression of healthy immune response genes. So at all stages of life and health, engaging in regular stress management is a great strategy.

CBT can be undertaken with the help of a therapist, facilitated by professionals in groups or individually, or learned on your own. Some people can shift their thinking with CBT, while others do better with meditation. Explore what works for you. Psychologist Martin Seligman developed many techniques to explore in *Learned Optimism*,[38] and he's a pioneer in the field of positive psychology, which looks for what works rather than what's broken. To learn more, visit this Web site: shearonforschools.com/learned_optimism.htm.

Other Stress Busters

More and more pioneering studies are revealing how immune health can be improved even when you're stressed out. Final exams are common stressors for college students,

---

WORDS MATTER—ESPECIALLY WHEN YOU'RE TALKING TO YOURSELF

What do you hear yourself saying inside your head? Do your words encourage you or find fault? Does that inner voice hold you back, accusing you of some past deed, or does it support your potential success? Self-talk often relates to what you heard growing up and what you believe now. And since that ongoing "silent" conversation reflects your overall attitude, it has the power to influence your mood, your behaviors, your stress, and your immune health. Often, healing and relieving stress begins with changing the internal conversation, correcting and improving your basic attitudes and outlook toward life. Research is beginning to reveal that various practices can help you change your talk, such as meditation, imagery, and cognitive behavior therapy. Change your mind and you change your life.

You may not realize that an overwhelming sense of negativity colors your outlook on virtually every aspect of your life—you've been negative for so long that it's become your own reality. Use the "What's Your Outlook on Life?" questionnaire to gauge your overall perspective on life. It can offer a helpful starting point as you embrace a program of change. And try this link to the adapted Learned Optimism test: stanford.edu/class/msande271/onlinetools/LearnedOpt.html.

WHAT'S YOUR OUTLOOK ON LIFE?

Answer true or false to the following statements, and be honest!

1. I believe that things usually work out for the best.   T   F

2. I make time for myself to either relax or do things that I enjoy.   T   F

3. When something goes wrong, I learn from it and move on
   without finger-pointing or holding a grudge.   T   F

4. There are no stressful relationships in my life right now.   T   F

5. I have a circle of close friends, and I spend time with them
   regularly.   T   F

6. I have a lot to be thankful for.   T   F

7. I take pride in my work and feel that my life has purpose.   T   F

8. I look forward to trying new things.   T   F

9. I can't recall the last time I was truly angry with someone.   T   F

10. I view each day as a gift and a new beginning.   T   F

Scoring: If your "trues" outweighed the "falses," you're on the right track. But if most of your responses were "false," it's time to find a way to tip the scales in your favor. Cognitive behavioral therapy is a strategy that can help you adjust your attitudes.

and some students get sick during or right after exams. Researchers at Harvard University wanted to figure out why. They measured the amount of IgA in the saliva of these students (IgA helps protect against respiratory infections). Researchers learned that this protective molecule was lower during stressful testing times. What could increase this protective molecule? Watching funny movies appeared to help. In contrast, watching films about war or violence lowered the IgA further.[39] In fact, salivary IgA is one of the most reliable indicators in looking for immune changes with varying levels of stress.

A recent review of 111 studies including nearly 5,000 people provided more evidence of mind-body strategies and immune outcomes.[40] Half the studies were with healthy people; the other half encompassed those with HIV, cancer, or allergies. Relaxation training had the strongest scientific evidence of a mind-body strategy affecting immune outcome. And the immune measurement that most reliably changed was salivary IgA; it's also the easiest and least stressful measurement to obtain with a simple saliva test. These and other studies mentioned in this chapter establish the point that your mind plays an important part in your immune health. Of course, in the final analysis, the proof is in your health on a clinical level. Because your mind is so important in how you take care of yourself and handle stress, in this section we offered you additional strategies to gain mastery of your mind to relieve stress. Practice helps you discover which methods work best for you, and it's always valuable to have a few techniques in your back pocket. Check out the advice that follows.

Laughter: The Best Medicine

During particularly stressful times, like holidays or tax time, pay attention to what you watch on TV or online. Protect your immune health and mood by watching something funny rather than a show that's frightening or suspenseful or even the news. When it comes to relieving stress, a good belly laugh is just what the doctor ordered. Laughter melts tension, stimulates your heart, and soothes your muscles. It can improve your immune system,[41] relieve pain, and improve your mood.[42] Add a dose or two of belly laughs every day as part of your healing plan's lifestyle enhancement.[43]

The Friendship Factor

Having friends and social support helps diminish the devastating effects of stress.[44] Here's where we see a big difference between men and women. Women "tend to befriend" others and frequently develop deeper alliances with other women. They talk to their friends if they're stressed out; they may also bake a batch of cookies. Women can mitigate stressful moments by nurturing themselves and others. Men, in general, are unlikely to talk to friends about a stressful problem. They may exercise it out or isolate themselves in work and activities. This gender difference may be one reason women tend to live longer than men.

The importance of friendship in relieving stress is something that we've all experienced—and science is weighing in as well. In a major study, researchers at the University of California at Los Angeles showed that, especially for women, a social network of close friends offers a "tend and befriend" alternative to the body's normal stress response of "fight or flight."[45] That's because when women get together, they release the calming hormone oxytocin.

The Power of Music

Music, one of the oldest forms of stress reduction, can bring people together and strengthen friendships, an important part of reducing stress, because people in your life matter to your health. Listening to music, either alone or with others, helps you become more relaxed. Of course, it can invigorate you as well. A review of more than 400 studies on the effects of music on human physiology showed significant benefits on immune functions, mood, and reducing stress hormones.[46] Compelling evidence is accumulating that music can play an important role in health-care settings, ranging from operating rooms to outpatient clinics. Increasingly, it is being found that listening to music before and/or during stressful medical procedures[47] significantly lessens stress, which means quicker healing and fewer infectious episodes. Many hospitals now recommend that people listen to their favorite music before and during a surgical procedure to reduce their stress and anxiety and promote better outcomes. Can you imagine how stressful an amniocentesis is for a pregnant woman? Or having open-heart surgery? Now music is helping people have a more positive experience in medical settings.[48] Martin Seligman, the pioneer in learned optimism and positive psychology, reminds us in his new book, *Flourish*,[49] that music can help create overall well-being through pleasure and eliciting positive moods. The higher the positive emotion, the less inflammation as measured by cytokine blood levels.[50] In ongoing studies, music has been shown to help improve cognitive functions; also, it helps in getting speech back after a stroke. In general, listening to dance music is shown to increase levels of protective IgA and natural killer cells. And dancing, which combines music with movement, physical exercise, and stress release, is a potent stress-reduction strategy.

If using meditation to calm your mind sounds appealing, music is an effective and enjoyable way to reach a meditative state. Our minds become easily occupied with sound, and a strategy called "toning" can help you reach a meditative state. Toning involves the action of voicing extended vowel sounds, like "Aah" or "Ooo." No melody, words, rhythm, or harmony—just the sound of your vibrating breath. Toning is a simple yet powerful technique, accessible to everyone. It massages body and mind

KIRTAN KRIYA: SINGING MEDITATION

Another meditation practice shown to reduce stress and inflammation and improve memory is Kirtan Kriya. The origins of this practice, which is simple to do and gives your mind a focus, go back to yoga traditions in ancient India. It involves singing or chanting four sounds—"saa, taa, naa, maa"—while repeating four finger movements, called mudras. Because it uses chanting, mudras, and even visualization, researchers find that it's a "brain fitness" exercise in addition to one that reduces stress and inflammation. Caregivers of family members with dementia are at extremely high risk for chronic stress and depression, which is associated with chronic inflammation.[51] In a pilot study at UCLA, older caregivers (median age 60 years) practiced Kirtan Kriya for 12 minutes a day for 8 weeks. Cognitive functioning, stress, and depression all improved.[52] In related studies, the expression of genes associated with inflammation were also reduced.[53] In just 12 minutes a day, memory is improved, inflammation dimmed, and stress reduced.[54] Here's how to get started:

1. Repeat the "saa taa naa maa" sounds (or mantra) while sitting with your spine straight. Focus and imagine each sound flowing in through the top of your head and out the middle of your forehead (your third eye point). If that visualization feels too complicated, simply do the sounds (to your own tune) and the following "dancing fingers":

   On "saa," touch the index fingers of each hand to your thumbs.

   On "taa," touch your middle fingers to your thumbs.

   On "naa," touch your ring fingers to your thumbs.

   On "maa," touch your little fingers to your thumbs.

2. For 2 minutes, sing in your normal voice.

3. For the next 2 minutes, sing in a whisper.

4. For the next 4 minutes, say the sound silently to yourself.

5. Then reverse the order, whispering for 2 minutes and then singing out loud for 2 minutes, for a total of 12 minutes.

6. To end the exercise, inhale deeply, stretch your hands above your head, and then bring them down slowly in front of you as you exhale.[55]

from the inside out. Meditative toning can help you focus and relax, release negative emotions, and reduce stress.

There are numerous online sources for toning (including spiritsound.net) and meditative music (such as meditationmusicx.com). SoundsTrue.com is an exceptional site that offers free downloads. Just turn on your iPod to change your rhythm, lower your heart rate, and soothe your stress.

The Power of the Pen

Writing a term paper might have caused you stress in school, but writing down thoughts and feelings on your own time, in your own words, and without regard to style, grammar, or punctuation can be very therapeutic. Fascinating results came from psychologist James Pennebaker, who investigated the power of disclosure and confession on immune health.[56] As a clinical extension of the research he did with psychology students, he studied people with asthma and rheumatoid arthritis—both hyperactivated immune states. The people were told to write for 15 to 20 minutes a day for 4 days only. He asked them to write their thoughts and feelings about what was most stressful to them at the time, such as a recent emotional trauma. At the end of 4 days, lung function improved in the people with asthma, and those with rheumatoid arthritis had less pain. Six months later, from only 4 days of writing, those with asthma still had improved lung function and those with arthritis had less pain.[67]

Give it a try yourself. First, think of the health problem or symptom you'd like to change. Then, take 15 or 20 minutes to write your thoughts and feelings about what is most stressful to you right now. It could be an event from your past, a secret you're hiding, a shame you've kept inside, or even a recent fight with a friend. Write only your feelings and what's going on in your mind, not the story of what happened. Do this for 4 days only. You can then tear up what you wrote and never look at it again. Now watch what happens to your symptoms in the coming days and weeks. Keeping a journal will help you become aware of the small changes happening.

SLEEP YOUR WAY TO STRONGER IMMUNITY

We all have nights when we lie awake, tossing and turning because of something that happened that day—or something we're worried might happen tomorrow. Occasional bouts of restlessness are a fact of life. But if stress keeps you up at night more often than not, it's time to make changes. We know from studies of people with erratic sleep patterns that lack of sleep compromises immune and heart health, increases inflammation, and leaves people more vulnerable to infections. Think of medical residents, bus drivers, insomniacs, or new parents!

And—you guessed it—scientists are discovering just how important sleep is to the healthy functioning of your immune system. Sleep studies are done either experimentally in a lab, where people are deprived of their sleep artificially, or by observing people who regularly are sleep deprived, like this study of physicians on call. Modeling a real-life situation, this research of 15 medical residents deprived of 1 night's sleep showed more stress and inflammatory responses.[68] In contrast, a study of 23 healthy young adults, with an average age of 24, showed no immune changes after being deprived of sleep for 30 hours,[69] suggesting that our age and overall state of health and well-being influence whether a night or two of lost sleep will have any effects on immune health. What we do know is that the cumulative effects of interrupted sleep or poor quality sleep play havoc with the immune system, moods, and cognitive functions.[70]

Here are some tips to help you get those all-important zzzz's.

Melatonin

One evolutionary-based strategy that supports health is to sleep when it's dark and be active when it's light. Living according to nature's light and dark cycles can help balance your immune health. That's because an important chemical in your brain, *melatonin*,[71] helps regulate your responses to the daily rhythm of light and dark cycles. Your body produces melatonin in response to the sun going down. Research shows a significant relationship between melatonin and the functioning of your immune system.[72] In fact, it's been discovered that your immune cells can even produce melatonin.[73] This chemical's role in regulating your sleep cycle is understood, though its influence on your many immune functions is not. Research is beginning to show that melatonin can lessen inflammation, enhance cytokine production, and stimulate T cell responses, shifting the balance of Th1 and Th2 cells to favor the latter. Here's a refresher about this complicated part of immune balance: There are two kinds of T helper cells. Th1 favors the immediate immune protection against infectious microbes and the requisite inflammation that follows. Th2 favors the adaptive immune response and antibody production. High Th2 sounds positive—unless you have an autoimmune or allergic condition. Then too much Th2 is not a good thing. Taking melatonin as a supplement should be avoided by people with autoimmune illnesses since melatonin stimulates immune functions. As research continues, we should discover more about the many facets of melatonin and immune health.

If you work the night shift, your chemistry is thrown off, your body produces less melatonin, and your immune functions may suffer. Some people benefit from taking melatonin supplements to reset the process and activate some immune processes. Melatonin seems to work best when used to reset your diurnal light–dark sleep patterns when you travel to different time zones. And everyone can benefit from better sleep hygiene (see "The Top 10 Ways to Get a Better Night's Sleep," page 164).

Note: If you have hyperactive immune conditions like allergies or autoimmune diseases, or a disease involving lymphocytes like lymphoma or HIV, consult with your health-care provider before you take melatonin supplements.

Shifting Sleep

One of the many solutions to shift workers' disordered sleep cycles is to readjust their own melatonin production. People make lots at night when it's dark, but if you have to work at night, you need to counter the sleep-inducing melatonin—bright lights at work will help. When you want to sleep in the morning, your body's melatonin is

---

The Immune Diaries   Sondra

For years, I kept my writing studio in my bedroom and worked there at all hours, night and day, with my computer, printer, and telephone just a few feet from my bed. My sleep quality was hit or miss, and I was tired a lot. Since moving into my new cottage, my bedroom has become a sanctuary—not a workspace. My sleep is much deeper, with more dreams, and I'm more awake in the morning.

dimming with the daylight. You need it dark, so wearing sunglasses to lessen light
exposure, going home to a darkened house, and taking a melatonin supplement may
help you get your needed sleep.[74]

THE TAKEAWAY

There are lots of positive ways to deal with stress, but there are just as many negative
ways, such as overeating, drinking too much alcohol, or smoking more than usual.

It's useful, in the long run, to understand how *you* deal with stress. Likewise, how
you love yourself plays an important role in your choices. Do you nurture yourself
with good things, like long walks or making a pot of nourishing vegetable soup? Or
do you just reach for a candy bar or two? Stress is a fact of life. How you deal with it
and manage your responses is up to you—it's within your power to choose what's
good for you. Try some of the stress-reduction techniques we've offered.

Start with whatever technique attracts you the most and practice it for at least a
week. Longer is better: We encourage you to stay with one practice for at minimum
a month. Then explore more ideas. Give yourself time to test-drive several different
methods. Effective stress management goes a long way t oward immune health and
faster recovery from illnesses. Figure out what works best for you. You'll gain a sense
of control and have the power to cope with any challenge.

(continued on page 166)

THE TOP 10 WAYS TO GET A BETTER NIGHT'S SLEEP

Getting a good night's sleep is super-important, but it's not always easy. Here are 10 tips for improving the quality of your shut-eye—or what physicians and researchers call "sleep hygiene."

1. Use your bedroom primarily for sleep and romance—not work—and make sure it's free of disturbing noises or too much light.[57]

2. Reduce or remove electronic devices, including your cell phone, from your sleep area. Plan to dim the lights and turn off screens at least a half hour before turning in.

3. If traffic noises, neighbors, or barking dogs disrupt your sleep, try a white noise machine.

4. Experiment with your thermostat. Most studies show that a temperature between 60 and 67 degrees Fahrenheit is optimal for sleeping, while temperatures above 75 degrees or below 54 degrees are disruptive to sleep.[58]

5. Exercising during the day can improve sleep. However, exercising too close to bedtime might leave you energized. Learn what works for you.[59]

6. Carbohydrates can lead to better sleep than proteins. That's because your brain converts tryptophan—an amino acid found in foods—into a relaxation molecule called serotonin. Eating a high-carb snack like an apple before bed will promote better sleep than eating an egg.[60] Although this sounds confusing, the carb helps the body's tryptophan move into the brain, whereas the protein snack slows down the process.

7. Tryptophan or 5-HTP supplements can promote sleep by directly enhancing serotonin and melatonin in the brain. (Bedtime dosages: 500 to 1,500 mg tryptophan, 50 to 150 mg 5-HTP.) Start with lower amounts and work up. If your issue is wakening in the middle of the night and being unable to fall back to sleep, take the lower amounts of either nutrient if and when you wake between 2:00 and 4:00 a.m.

8. Herbal teas can relax your body and mind to support sleep. (*Note: If you're prone to nighttime trips to the bathroom, you might want to try herbal capsules instead.*) Herbs that are useful for sleep include valerian root, hops, chamomile, passionflower, and lemon balm.[61] Many commercial brands of sleep-enhancing herbal teas or capsules are available.

9. Rub a few drops of lavender oil onto the bottom of your feet. You can massage drops into your temples or rub a few drops on your pillow.[62] For generations, the scent of lavender has been used for inducing relaxation and even sleep. Much of the medical research into lavender has been conducted with hospitalized patients, by either diffusing the scent in the room or having the patients smell the essential oil directly. The nurses observed benefits as well—their patients were sleeping more peacefully! Studies have shown that pure lavender essential oil placed in a jar at night by the bedside of hospitalized patients improved their reported quality of sleep and lowered their blood pressure.[63] In a clinical trial of 64 patients in a hospital critical care unit, the patients who were exposed to 9 hours of lavender aromatherapy for 3 nights reported a much-improved quality of sleep with no need for sleeping pills.[64] One way that inhaling lavender can improve sleep and relaxation is through changing brain waves as measured via an EEG. In studies with healthy adults, inhaling lavender for a few minutes increased the alpha and theta waves—brain waves for deep relaxation.[65]

10. Worries can interfere with quality sleep. Write down any worries on paper in an area other than your bedroom—and leave them there. Then forget about them before you turn in.[66]

When gauging the effects of stress-reduction techniques on your overall immune health, focus on the end result. You're not an experimental subject in a lab where your immune functions are being measured. So look at how these strategies play out in your life. The outcome, over the long run, should be fewer bouts with colds and the flu and better overall health. See what helps you and what you will do regularly. The same goes if you have a painful autoimmune illness or frequent allergy attacks. Lessening your overall stress will likely help you, no matter what other factors are present. You don't need lab tests to observe a change in your health or well-being.

So . . . stress less and relax more to enhance your well-being and physical health. Start by getting to know your mind and body better. When your shoulders are raised up to your ears or your jaw is clenched, ask yourself why your body is preparing to fight or run away. Or—even without asking the question—take a deep breath, lower your shoulders, relax your jaw, and let go of that invisible stressor. What else can you do to change your mind or unwind your body from its tension-producing, energy-reducing reactions? Your health is in your hands and your head.

Next up? Get moving! Exercise is one of the best all-around stress-reduction strategies, and it benefits every other aspect of your health and well-being, too. In Chapter 6, we'll get you and your immune system pumped up and slowed down with exercises you can implement right now to improve your overall health.

CHAPTER 6

Get Moving *for* Better Immunity!

We learned in Chapter 1 that movement is essential to immune health—that's because it accelerates the filtering and cleansing work of your lymphatic system. But that's not all. In this chapter, you'll learn how movement and exercise can help you manage stress, enhance your energy and mood, and improve your sleep[1]—all factors that affect your immune function and overall health. Exercise also lessens inflammation, a factor in unhealthy aging and many chronic illnesses.[2]

In the past, scientists recommended 30 to 60 minutes of uninterrupted exercise every day, and that sounded intimidating to lots of people. If you've got the time and the energy, 60 minutes is great, but if you don't, here's some good news: Research shows that exercising for short time periods multiple times a day is equally beneficial.[3] Just 10 or 15 minutes of physical activity three times daily can provide similar—if not better—benefits in terms of lower blood pressure and better glucose regulation when compared with longer workouts.[4] Dr. Niels Vollaard and colleagues at the University of Bath in England researched the idea of high-intensity interval training (HIT) with 15 healthy sedentary young adults over a 6-week period. The participants had three 10-minute exercise sessions a week. Although they had done less than 10 minutes of hard exercise each time, their cardio fitness and aerobic capacity improved.[5]

An even shorter, more-intense strategy called "burst training" may provide benefits similar to longer programs. Burst training consists of very brief intervals (30 to 60 seconds) of intense exercise repeated a few times a day. Think of sprinting up a steep hill for 1 minute, resting for 30 seconds, then doing it again. Burst training isn't for the couch potato wanting to get fit quick, but once you're in shape (or if you already are), talk to your doctor about exploring the idea.

Just as important, and gaining ground in the world of healthy aging research, is the notion that even the simplest movements are beneficial to your health. Periodically get up from your desk, step away from your screens, walk around your house or office, do some stretches, pull weeds from the garden, visit a neighbor, or pop down to the break room—and take the stairs. Research shows that people who sit many hours each day are more likely to develop chronic illnesses and age poorly,[6] all because of our often discussed nemesis: low-level inflammation.[7]

Your level of daily physical activity even affects your brain. Studies comparing active animals with those that are sedentary have shown that the brains of inactive animals grow more connections to neurons that trigger stress. In one study, rats were given the choice of running on a wheel as much as they wanted. Turned out that those that ran a lot, compared to the less active rats, experienced positive brain changes. And the neurons of the less active rats developed more branches projecting into the stress areas of the brain.[8] Why is this important? Scientists believe that this phenomenon also applies to people. The more you remain sedentary, the stronger stress patterns your brain builds. But when you exercise, your brain develops new neurons that enhance your capacity to learn.[9] In addition, there's a body of research on humans showing that engaging in regular physical activity may keep brains healthy long into the later years.[10] Recent studies show that even if you exercise for 60 minutes every day, but spend the rest of your day sitting, you can still experience unwanted weight gain because the pressure of sitting makes fat cells reproduce.[11] That's more evidence that inactivity increases stress and increases your risk of cardiovascular disease, chronic inflammation, and other long-term conditions.

TRY THIS!

If you're reading this at home, put this book down and go wash dishes, straighten out a cabinet or closet, or head outside and breathe the fresh air and feel the energy of nature. Wherever you are, take a 10-minute walk. How do you feel now? Or write a comment in your journal about how you felt before and after. Now you can go back to reading this book. Try setting a clock or your smartphone to remind you to get up and move around for a few minutes every hour.

The Immune Diaries   Sondra

I recently blogged about research on the importance of getting up from your desk, even though I didn't practice this myself. I could easily sit at the computer all day. When I learned that I could prolong my life and improve my health with this simple shift in my behavior, I started taking regular 10- to 15-minute breaks every hour. I prepare a meal, clean up fallen leaves in the yard, do laundry, or make phone calls while walking around. My surprising discovery: I actually get more done in the day, plus I have more energy. You have nothing to lose by trying!

The big picture: Moving your body moves your mind, molecules, and muscles; gets your immune cells patrolling your body more efficiently; reduces stress; and improves your sleep. It even reduces inflammation.[12] Are you moving your body enough throughout the day? Let's find out!

In this chapter, we'll explore the details of how exercise improves your health and enhances your life, and then we'll look at ways to add more motion to your day. Understanding your current fitness level enables you to make choices that are both beneficial and appropriate for you. Let's take a look at exactly how exercise can keep your immune system healthy and strong.

Exercise Strengthens Your Lymphatic System

Back in Chapter 1, we learned about the lymphatic arm of the immune system—it's a major player in detoxifying and cleansing your body. When the muscles surrounding your lymphatic vessels are flexing and moving, that shifts the intricate lymphatic system into high gear and helps it work more efficiently and effectively. So when you're moving or pumping iron, you're also pumping up the activity of your lymphatics. But if you're sitting around all day, this purifying system becomes sluggish and less effective.

One great way to wake up your lymphatic function is through massage. When you get a massage, your lymph channels receive one, too, because they are "massaged" by the large muscles surrounding them. So besides the pleasure a massage brings, it stimulates

WHAT'S YOUR EXERCISE QUOTIENT (EQ)?

How active are you? Answer the following questions about your lifestyle habits and you might discover areas that need improving.

1 = RARELY OR NEVER   2 = ONCE A WEEK   3 = ALMOST DAILY

I exercise regularly by going to a gym, walking or running, using home equipment, or using exercise or workout videos/DVDs.	1	2	3
I practice yoga, tai chi, qigong, or aikido.	1	2	3
I dance around the house; get out for activities with my partner, friends, or family; or take a movement class.	1	2	3
I walk to the store to pick up small grocery items, park my car at the edge of the parking lot at the mall, or take the stairs instead of the elevator at work.	1	2	3
I clean my house regularly, vacuuming, mopping, dusting, or carrying loads of laundry up and down the stairs.	1	2	3
I get up and move frequently while watching TV or sitting at my desk.	1	2	3
I spend time stretching or doing weight training.	1	2	3
I get a good night's sleep and wake up refreshed and energetic.	1	2	3

Give yourself 1 point for every time you checked box 1, 2 points for every time you checked box 2, and 3 points for every time you checked box 3. Now, add up your EQ points!

1–8 You're a couch potato! Make a conscious effort to get up and move. See the exercises in this chapter and find ways to make movement a regular part of your day.

9–20 You're getting there. Any movement is better than sitting still! Commit to exploring new ways to weave physical activity into your life.

21–24 Congratulations! You know how movement contributes to a healthy life. Keep up the good work—and look for new activities to keep it interesting.

the lymph into removing waste, toxins, and excess fluids. If you can't afford regular massages—or just don't have time for them—don't worry. You can stimulate this movement of the lymph through self-massage, and we'll show you how later in this chapter. Simple self-massage is especially helpful when you feel a cold coming on or during times of acute environmental stimulation, such as allergy season or visits to polluted cities.

Restoring and improving your lymphatic flow are crucial to the health of your immune system. Consider this: When you're sitting still, your lymph flows at a rate of about $1/10$ ounce an hour. But when you're moving, the rate increases 20 times to about 2 ounces an hour. That's important, because a sluggish lymphatic system doesn't propel your filtering lymph, waste, and immune cells fast enough for optimal detoxification. If this system backs up, toxins accumulate and the immune warriors are prevented from finding dangerous invaders. Later in this chapter, you'll learn a variety of ways to stimulate the movement of these protective lymphatic warriors.

Exercise Relieves Your Stress

We've already talked about the effects of chronic stress on your immune system: It throws off the balance of your T cells and heightens inflammation. This puts you at a higher risk of cardiovascular disease, diabetes, depression, Alzheimer's, and even cancer—just to name a few preventable conditions. Moderate and consistent exercise

COPING WITH COLDS

Exercise is important, but there are times when your body needs a break. If you're sick with an upper respiratory infection, severe cold, cough, headache, vomiting, or fever, you should avoid strenuous exercise for the first 2 or 3 days. But if you sense that a cold is just coming on, then working up a good sweat may alleviate your symptoms. Many people claim they can burn through the early onset of a cold with a workout followed by a steam or sauna. So unless you're feeling wiped out, you may do an easy workout during the early stages of a cold. But if you're tired and achy from the flu or other infection, give your body the rest it needs.

can curb the damaging effects caused by chronic stress and keep you healthy[13] by mobilizing your immune cells and lessening inflammation.[14]

Exercise Enhances Your Mood and Promotes Healthy Aging

If you're consistent with your exercise, relaxation, good nutrition, and spending time with good friends, you can remain vital well into your golden years. Evidence among older populations shows that physical exercise improves muscle strength and helps prevent type 2 diabetes, cardiovascular diseases, and osteoporosis. Even short bursts of physical training can lessen inflammation in the elderly. Low-impact activities like yoga, tai chi, and qigong are gaining popularity among older populations and can all improve immune health.[15] Older people who are already highly conditioned have better immune health, perhaps because of exercise and other lifestyle choices they've made.[16]

Exercise keeps you flexible and helps you build strong bones, and that becomes more important with each passing year. When you're fit, you're less likely to lose your balance or fall, so you're better equipped to maintain your independence as you get older. Falls and broken bones are a common downfall as people age.

Exercise Helps You Sleep Better

The relationship between exercise and sleep is complex. As we get older, getting to sleep and staying asleep often become more difficult, especially for women. Most sleep studies involve people over age 50, with or without insomnia. In six different trials, people who engaged in an exercise program reported that they fell asleep faster and relied on far less sleep medication.[17] A large study of 100 adults between ages 60 and 92 who practiced tai chi three times a week for 24 weeks showed improvement in all qualities of sleep—the length of time it took to fall asleep, the amount of uninterrupted sleep, and the duration of sleep. In fact, the tai chi group compared to the low-intensity exercise group averaged almost an hour more sleep each night.[18] Research provides some good indications that exercise will help you sleep better; what works best for you is yet another adventure into discovering more about yourself.

Give the movement plan in this chapter a try. Your immune cells will love you for it—and you will, too, when you get a good night's sleep and wake up feeling refreshed. Research, after all, shows that exercise, performed not too close to bedtime, increases how long someone stays asleep and enhances restorative sleep.[19] What we know for sure: Staying fit and getting a good night's sleep are both important for overall immune health and well-being.

Exercise Keeps Inflammation in Check

Regular exercise clearly reduces blood markers of inflammation. In a 12-week resistance-training program, elderly Japanese women reduced the circulating inflammatory markers in their blood.[20] The program also improved their mobility and strength while lessening pain and fatigue. And as we've said before, regular exercise has been shown to be a factor in lowering cardiovascular disease and type 2 diabetes, conditions linked to inflammation.[21]

It's estimated that about 60 percent of adults in the United States aren't getting regular physical activity, even though the evidence that physical exercise improves heart health is overwhelming. We now know that a key cause of cardiovascular disease is inflammation. In a review of more than 15,000 adults, leisure-time physical

---

MODERATION IN EVERYTHING!

Getting too much exercise isn't a problem for most of us. Competitive athletes and those training for marathons or endurance events, however, need to be proactive with their nutrition and rest to prevent running their immune system into the ground and increasing the risk for more infections. Any strenuous physical exercise creates physiological stress, but the effects of this physiological stress on immune health are short-term and transient. With any exercise program, minimize the risk of injury by not putting too much stress on one particular part of your body. For example, if you do only one repetitive activity, such as playing tennis, you may injure your shoulder or arm; if golf is your only game, your swing may hurt your back. If you're training for a marathon, rest and replenish after the event. Create a balanced program with a good mix of activities.

activity was linked to lower blood levels of CRP (C-reactive protein),[22] a measurement of inflammation. In later studies, physical exercise also decreased proinflammatory cytokines and enhanced the anti-inflammatory cytokines,[23] demonstrating that exercise alters inflammation and blood measurements. The evidence is clear: Moving your body regularly lessens chronic inflammation and balances your immune health.

The verdict is in: Movement is one of your best strategies for a strong, balanced immune system and a long, healthy, happy life. Let's explore the best ways to get started.

YOUR PERFECT PROGRAM: IT'S ALL ABOUT BALANCE

Before choosing a fitness routine, you need to weigh lots of factors, such as your health, age, and gender; your current fitness level; and any past injuries or weak areas in your body. The types of exercises you select, level of intensity, duration, and frequency all depend on your individual needs. Exercises that you enjoy will benefit you the most simply because you'll actually do them!

FIND YOUR FITNESS FIT!

Not sure what exercises to choose? Review these questions, adapted from *The Fitness Instinct*,[24] to help you figure out what activities might be right for you.

Does it seem like fun?

Will I devote time to learning and practicing?

Do I have friends who are involved in this activity?

Do I need special equipment—and if so, can I afford it?

What's my realistic time commitment?

Can I enjoy the activity even as a beginner?

Do I think I can master this activity? Will it help me feel positive about myself?

I've always enjoyed sports and physical activities—I don't feel my best unless I'm exercising regularly. For the past 40 years, I've done some stretching almost every day either at home or at the gym. I have a wide range of physical interests, from tennis, racquetball, baseball, swimming, and Frisbee to tai chi and yoga. Yet like most people, my interests and exercise program have shifted over the years. Right now, my favorite workout is what I call "spin and swim"—an hour-long Spin (biking) class, followed by weight machines, stretching, and 20 minutes of swimming. Then I finish with a short session in the steam room or hot tub.

When I'm at my office seeing patients, I have much more energy, better mental focus, and improved stamina if I take a lunchtime workout break. When I have a lunch meeting and can't get to the gym, my afternoon isn't quite as easy. For me, regular exercise makes all the difference in my energy, mood, and stamina. Of course, my health and well-being are the side benefits.

In addition to finding activities that you truly enjoy and will do consistently, strive for a balanced program that incorporates these five fitness goals:

- Weight training for strength and bone building
- Stretching for flexibility
- Cardio and aerobic activity for endurance and heart fitness
- Deep breathing to lower stress and improve relaxation and overall well-being
- Energy exercises for inner strength and vitality

Explore a few different activities so that you aren't limited by the weather. If you enjoy running or walking but live in a northern climate, join a gym during the winter months or buy workout DVDs to use as backup. Or walk the malls if you live in snow country and need to get out of the house. Create a program that includes the five fitness goals, and develop options that vary with the seasons. Guidelines for older adults have recommended 30 minutes of moderate intensity physical activity at least five times a week, strength training and flexibility twice a week, and balance training.[25]

We've said it before, but it bears repeating: Regular movement leads to good lymphatic flow, better circulation, quality sleep, better moods, and more consistent energy. You'll simply feel better.

The Power of Movement

When it comes to strengthening your immune system, improving your health, and boosting your mood, all exercise in moderation is good. Yet some movement practices are immune-building powerhouses. New research shows that activities like yoga, tai chi, and qigong are super-effective, and it's easy to learn the basics. So these energy-balancing forms are the foundation of your Ultimate Immunity workout. Before we look at the details and the how-tos, though, let's take a look at some of the science behind their effectiveness.

Yoga

Yoga, from a Sanskrit word meaning "union" of body and spirit, is an ancient movement and meditation practice that originated in India thousands of years ago. It emphasizes stretching poses, or postures, called asanas. When practicing these poses, you focus on your breathing, your body, and the subtlety and correctness of your posture. There are many different forms of yoga, including Iyengar, hatha, ashtanga, and Bikram. DVDs abound for you to learn from in the comfort of your living room, but studying with a qualified teacher in person will accelerate your learning and ensure that you're using proper form. An experienced teacher can also offer sensible guidance on how to be aware and present in your body so you can avoid injury or overdoing it. Plus, there's a lot to be said for practicing with a group.

In a review of 81 studies comparing the health benefits of yoga and exercise, yoga was superior to exercise in everything measured except physical fitness.[26] In another study comparing hatha yoga to physical exercise, people with type 2 diabetes who practiced yoga for 6 months showed reduced levels of fasting blood glucose, lipids, and markers of oxidative stress such as superoxide dismutase and oxidized LDL, while those engaging in conventional physical training of mainly aerobic exercise decreased fasting blood glucose without the other beneficial effects.[27] Numerous studies indicate that yoga reduces stress[28] and the release of immune-suppressing cortisol.[29] Most studies of yoga look at its effect on people who've never done it before.

Interestingly, those who practiced yoga most frequently had better health outcomes and health behaviors (they had a better sense of well-being, ate a healthier diet, had a lower body mass index, were less likely to smoke or overuse alcohol, slept better, were less fatigued, had stronger social support, and were more mindful and more active). Their years of practice or class attendance were not a factor in their health outcome— just the frequency with which they practiced.[30] Finally, in a study at Georgia State University of 19 people with heart failure, those who participated in an 8-week regimen of yoga along with their medical treatment improved exercise tolerance and lowered their inflammatory markers.[31]

Tai Chi (or Taiji)

Along with yoga, tai chi and qigong are ancient meditative movement practices. Tai chi, a martial art that originated in China from qigong, emphasizes long, slow, continuous movements along with breathing and meditation. Both tai chi and qigong offer important health benefits, especially for people over age 55.[32] One reason for that finding: Most of the studies are done with an older population, since tai chi and qigong are gentle, low-impact exercises and can be safely practiced by people who've been sedentary for years. Today, especially as it's taught in the United States, tai chi and qigong have become almost interchangeable, having transformed into a stress-management practice that strives to balance mind and body, healing and longevity. As mentioned earlier, tai chi also improved people's quality of sleep. Let's look at tai chi first, since it's more familiar to most Westerners.

As with yoga, there are many different forms of tai chi, and medical research has demonstrated that when people who are 55 years or older practice tai chi, they can improve their balance, mobility, mood, and immune health. In fact, the first studies looked to see what could improve the balance of older people, since falls and broken bones are common problems as we age—and if you're afraid of losing your balance, you'll be less likely to be physically active, which is essential to your immune health. In one study, 22 people ages 68 to 92, who'd undergone knee, hip, or back surgery, were trained in tai chi 5 days a week for 90 minutes for 3 weeks. Results showed that their walking and balance were significantly improved.[33]

As we've noted in earlier chapters, aging impacts your immune strength and response to vaccines. Researchers at UCLA explored how people could boost their immunity to the shingles virus. (If you had chicken pox as a child, the varicella

SUCCESS STORY

Sally Pera, 66

Any way you look at it, Sally Pera is a strong woman. The oldest of seven children—and the mother and stepmother of six—she grew up on a ranch in Colorado, where she learned that even when you don't feel your best, you keep on going and put your best foot forward. She's an entrepreneur who's built up a Silicon Valley business. In her free time, she's a ballroom dancer.

But severe allergies, which plagued her immune system for most of her life, came close to bringing her down. She's allergic to a bunch of things, from strong perfumes and eggs to dust and pollen to cats and dogs. Her reactions ran the gamut: She'd experience skin problems, foggy brain, and lethargy, and three or four times she even went into anaphylactic shock.

Her problems got so severe at one point that she thought she had mono and had to quit grad school. (Strong woman that she is, Sally eventually went back and completed her degree.) But it wasn't until a few years ago, when Dr. Haas put her on the I-PEP diet and the Cool Down anti-inflammation program, that she began to get a handle on her health concerns. "I had to get away from all the conventional common sense," Sally says, "and move into another way of thinking. That's what Dr. Haas's programs did for me." After a battery of tests, Dr. Haas showed her exactly what she was reactive to—and taught her how to get better with the right foods and supplements, plus bio-identical hormones. "Within a month," she says, "I was feeling dramatically better."

At an age where lots of her friends are starting to complain about aches and pains, Sally reports that she's feeling stronger than ever. "I have great energy," she says, "and it all comes from getting a handle on all my health issues that were so debilitating. Tonight, I'm going ballroom dancing with a younger man—I really do have an amazing, fun life."

virus [chicken pox] lies dormant in your nerve cells for your entire life and can rear its ugly head again later on in the form of painful shingles.) In the study, 112 adults ranging in age from 59 to 86 were divided into two groups. One group studied tai chi, while the control group took part in a health education program. After 16 weeks, both groups were given the shingles vaccine, and 2 months later their immunity to shingles was measured. All participants showed increased immunity to shingles, but the tai chi group's immune antibody response was twice that of the control group.[34]

Qigong (or Chi Gung)

Qigong, the 5,000-year-old parent of tai chi, is a series of meditative movements that emphasize the cultivation and balance of qi (chi), or vital energy. In the Chinese system of medicine, everything is energy, with illness resulting from a blockage or imbalance in that energy. First, a little background. According to traditional Chinese medicine, qi flows in meridians or channels throughout and around your body. Your body's qi is focused in three main areas called cauldrons, or dantiens.

The lower dantien is about 2 inches below your navel, deep inside, and is said to store and build energy. The heart center area (the middle dantien) holds another quality of qi, and your head (the third eye) holds "shen," or spiritual qi. But you don't have to believe in this concept to experience qigong's benefits of reducing stress[35] and improving energy and clarity. Although qigong is less well known in the West than tai chi, its popularity is growing fast, since qigong and tai chi are quite similar in their benefits. The advantage of qigong, as it's commonly practiced in the United States, is that you don't need to learn a long sequence of movements to achieve the health benefits—just a few simple movements can do the trick. As with improving the immune response to shingles vaccine, other studies have shown that older adults who practiced tai chi or qigong also have a greater antibody response to the

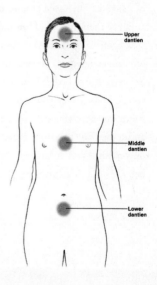

influenza vaccine.[36] Many studies have examined the benefits of qigong, and there is plenty of evidence to convince even the staunchest cynic to try it.

In one Taiwanese study, for example, 37 healthy adults between ages 41 and 55 took part in a 12-week program that included hour-long group tai chi qigong sessions. Participants' mobility and immune functions were tested before and after the study. At the end of 12 weeks, they could walk a 6-minute circuit more quickly and their regulatory T cells increased, which could lessen their risks for misguided immune hyperactivity.[37] And in a study of healthy young women ages 18 to 25, those practicing qigong for 8 weeks showed improved balance.[38]

In addition, a Chinese study showed that people with cancer who practiced qigong improved their DNA repair rate.[39] Remember, it's the DNA repair system that helps your body eliminate cancer cells.

We're mentioning cancer here because people with cancer suffer from some of the same problems we all may face, such as fatigue, depression, and anxiety, along with the additional stress that comes from undergoing treatments and facing an uncertain outcome. This "captive population" is the subject of many mind-body and complementary research studies looking at improving quality of life—and, of course, we can all benefit from that. For those with cancer, practicing qigong for an average of 12 weeks can lessen fatigue, depression, and stress-related cortisol levels as well as enhance their quality of life and immune functions.[40]

Qigong includes slow rhythmic movements, controlled breathing, meditation, and, oftentimes, imagery. The best time to practice qigong is when you first wake up or right before you go to bed. It helps set the tone for your day and awakens your mind. Plus, if you do it first thing, you've already accomplished something important—keeping your commitment to yourself to practice qigong. Practicing outdoors, standing on the earth and connecting to nature, is even better, as long as it's not too windy, raining, too cold, or too hot. Wait at least an hour after eating. You can also use qigong as a warmup before swimming, lifting weights, or going for a walk to help you get in the zone.

The Ultimate Immunity

Since *Ultimate Immunity* integrates the many ways you nourish your body and your mind, including food, movement practices, and meditation, we're providing you with a plan to weave them all into your life. The self-massage practice can be done every day, in the morning when you wake up, at night before you go to bed, or really any time, for as little as 5 minutes or as long as 20. We also encourage you to practice the qigong movements, which take about 10 to 20 minutes, every day for the maximum benefit, or at least every other day. You can add a half-hour walk 5 days a week and do some weight training and stretching to complete the picture. The important thing here is to not stress about it. Just do what you can and notice how it affects your body—and your life.

Here's the plan.

SELF-MASSAGE FOR A HEALTHIER SELF

The benefits of massage and self-massage go beyond skin deep. Massage invigorates your skin—the home of many of your immune cells—and improves circulation, relaxation, and lymphatic movement. Plus, massage provides the benefits of sensual pleasure. Massage therapy is now a bona fide practice of complementary medicine and gaining acceptance as useful for relief of pain and stress[41] and to improve bloodflow and healing. Massage therapy requires an individual trained to administer a session. There are many names or types of massage, such as Swedish, lymphatic, and deep tissue. Of course, these all cost money. Very few studies have examined self-massage, let alone qigong self-massage. In one study out of a wellness center in New Jersey, 40 people with osteoarthritis were divided into two groups. One group was trained in self-massage, the other group was the wait-listed control. The trained group did 20 minutes of supervised self-massage twice a week for 6 weeks. At the end of this period, they reported less pain and stiffness and improved function.[42]

Most people can't get a professional massage daily, but with self-massage, you can experience many of the same benefits every day. Follow the instructions ahead for self-massage to give your immune cells some much-needed soothing therapeutic touch and qi energy.[43] As soon as you wake up, before getting out of bed, begin each day by massaging your arms, face, and neck, plus tapping your head to wake up your brain. You can also do these massages anytime, while fully clothed, or do them in a warm bath or while applying skin lotion. You don't have to do them all—do as many as you'd like, and do each one at least three times. Whenever you practice these massage techniques, imagine you're having some relaxing spa time.

The Immune Diaries — Sondra

More than 20 years ago, as I investigated the nature of healing, I learned that no matter what culture or tradition I looked at, healing always came down to energy. Since the martial arts, such as tai chi and qigong, all focus on managing personal energy, I decided to study qigong. I found a qigong master in San Francisco and studied with him to explore the energy of qi. I've been practicing qigong ever since. In all this time, I've rarely caught a cold or the flu. In this chapter, I share some of my favorite qigong practices.

IN-BED ENERGY MASSAGE SERIES

When you wake, take some good deep
breaths and sit up to perform these few
immune-enhancing exercises. First rub your
hands together to warm them.

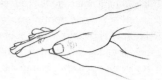

WASH YOUR FACE WITH QI

Say "Good morning, world!" with this simple movement. Bring your warmed
hands up to your face, brushing your hands down the sides and up to your forehead. Some say this movement reduces wrinkles.

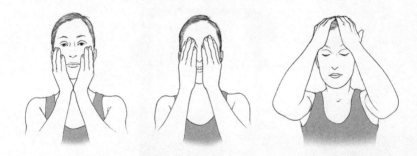

HEAD TAP

Take the time each morning to
awaken your mind as well as your
body. Using your fingertips, tap all
around the top, sides, and back of
your head. Can you feel yourself
waking up?

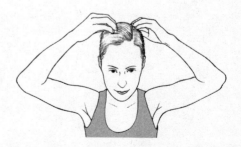

ARM SWEEPS

This soothing massage for your skin also gets the lymphatics moving. Stretch your left arm out in front of you with your palm up and elbow slightly bent. Relax your shoulders. Place your right hand (open palm) on the top of your left shoulder and slowly move your hand down the inside of your left arm. Go across your open left palm to the ends of your fingers. Turn your left palm down and your arm over; move your right hand up the outside of your arm, then up and over your shoulder. Turn your left arm over again and repeat your downward sweep. Repeat three times on each arm or as many times as you'd like.

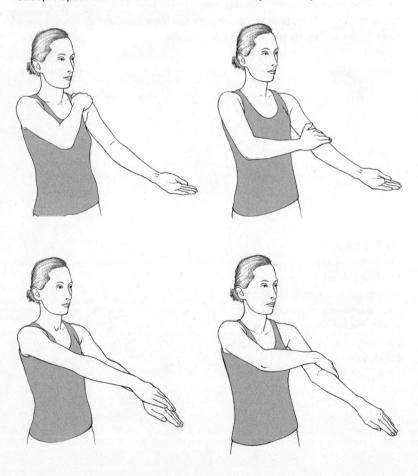

NECK RUB

This massage is particularly helpful if you feel a cold coming on. Rub your hands together again to warm them. Place one open palm on the back of your neck with your other hand over it. Then move them like you are moving a towel back and forth. This, along with the Shoulder Sweep, warms you up and helps stifle that threatening cold.

SHOULDER SWEEP—RUB AND BRUSH

This is another movement that is beneficial if you feel a cold virus knocking on the door. Grasp your left shoulder with your right hand. Press firmly and pull your hand across your shoulder and down, moving diagonally between your breasts. Shake off your hand as if you're flicking off water. Repeat on the other side. Alternate sides three times.

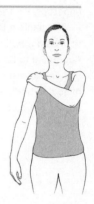

BELLY BOOST

If you're dealing with constipation or diarrhea, this can help. Place one hand, palm down, under your belly button (the lower dantien area). Place your other hand on top. Gently move your hands in a clockwise direction, starting in a small circle, gradually making it larger with your hands. Do this 18 times, and reverse the direction for another 18 times. If you have a tendency to be constipated, move only in a clockwise direction; that's the direction your intestines move their contents. If diarrhea is a problem, move your hands in the opposite or counterclockwise direction.

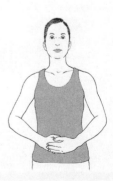

THYMUS PAT AND HUM

The thymus is the orchestrator of the immune network, and this simple step can help strengthen the body's immune regulators (mentioned in Chapter 1). Place your palm over your thymus (beneath your collarbone) and very tenderly circle in a clockwise direction. Then gently pat the area with the palm of your hand or a gentle fist softly and hum deep into your thymus. Another option is to tap the thymus area with your fingertips. Find which way you prefer.

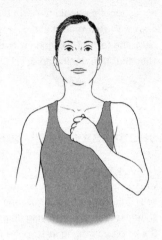

The ancient Greeks believed that the thymus controlled the body's life energy. According to Dr. John Diamond, author of *Life Energy*,[44] the thymus is the link between mind and body because it's one of the first organs affected by mental attitudes and stress.

OUT-OF-BED ENERGY MASSAGE SERIES

Do the following exercises after getting out of bed.

KIDNEY PAT AND HUM

In Chinese medicine, the kidney is important to immune health, and this movement can help you build qi and energy. Place your warmed palms over the kidneys in the small of your back just above your waistline. Rub in a circular motion and warm the area. Then make soft fists and gently tap over your kidneys while making a humming sound.

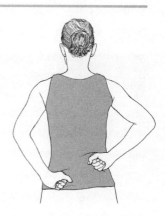

LEG SWEEPS—ENERGY AND LYMPH PULLUP

Similar to Arm Sweeps, Leg Sweeps are good for getting the lymphatics going. Place your hands, palms down, over your hips. Slowly move your hands down the outside of your legs and, bending down, move your hands along the outside edges of your feet, going around your toes. Bring your palms up the insides of your legs, across your groin, up both sides of your belly, and up over your heart and breasts. This helps move the lymph up to where it gets recycled. Repeat at least three times.

WHOLE BODY WAKE-UP TAP

Now it's time to improve the overall circulation of your blood and lymph. Keep your hands open and use your fingertips to gently pat down both sides of your head, shoulders, chest, arms, and legs.

An added benefit of qigong self-massage and movements is that you can do them whenever you need to, not just in the morning. Does your energy slump around 4 p.m.? Try some Wake-Up Taps and notice how you feel afterward. Or try the following Logging On movement series for an energy surge. It's called Logging On because it helps you connect to all your sources of energy—body, mind, earth, and qi.

LOGGING ON: THE QIGONG MOVEMENT SEQUENCE

This simple 10-minute sequence is easy to learn, and your body and mind will love you for it. Ideally, these movements should be performed standing, but they can be adapted for sitting or lying down. Choose a time and place where you won't be disturbed and where the wind is not blowing, and don't do these right after you've eaten. Take off your shoes and loosen any tight clothing. Each movement has imagery associated with it. We'll give you suggestions, but feel free to come up with your own. An online video of this sequence is available at sondrabarrett.com/logging-on.

Do each of the movements at least three times. Your body will tell you if it wants to do more of one or more. Think of yourself as a water creature, soft and curved and floating gracefully. Keep your movements fluid and rounded.

The Immune Diaries   Sondra

During the past 2 decades, I've taught the 10-minute Logging On qigong movement sequence to thousands of people across the United States. After a colleague and I studied with qigong master DaJin Sun, we created a simplified version that beginners could learn without becoming a "master." I came up with the name years later. Following 9/11, I taught this sequence to large groups in areas hit hard by the catastrophe. More than 75 percent of the participants said it helped diminish the energy-draining stress they felt and boosted their mood and perception of energy.

STANDING POSTURE—ANCHOR ON

As with any movement meditation practice, you need to learn the proper posture. With your feet flat on the ground, shoulder-width apart, and parallel to
each other, rock back and forth so that you feel solid on the earth. Imagine that
you have roots growing from the bottoms of your feet, anchoring you solidly
into the earth. Gently bend your knees, tuck in your butt, relax your shoulders,
and, with your chin parallel to the earth, imagine that you have a cord connecting you to the sky or to heaven. The finishing touch for this standing posture is
the Inner Smile. Place the tip of your tongue behind your teeth on your upper
palate. This closes the circuit of qi throughout your body, releases saliva, and
relaxes your face. You can hold this standing posture longer for balancing your
energy. As you decide to explore qi further, you could stand like this, with your
arms forming a circle in front of you, hands down at your waist and palms facing your belly. This posture is often called the Standing Stake. Try standing for a
few minutes if you want. You can also do the Inner Smile anytime, such as when
waiting at a red light or grocery shopping. Or move on to the rest of the movement sequence. You will maintain this same standing posture throughout the
series, all the while imagining that you are connected to both earth and sky
through your body.

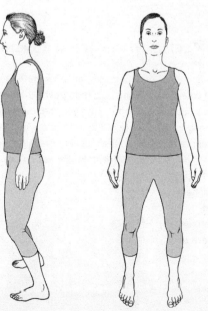

ROOT YOUR ENERGY (ROOTING AND SPIRALING)

Place your hands on your hips with your fingertips pointed toward your spine. Gently make circles with your waist, sort of like belly dancing, keeping your head upright and your shoulders parallel to the earth. Circle clockwise, then counterclockwise. Your belly leads the movement while the rest of your body is upright but not uptight. This loosens the lower back and frees the parasympathetic nerves (those that initiate relaxation) in your lower spine, starting you on this stress-relieving journey.

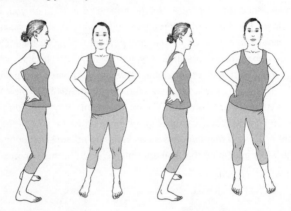

FILL YOUR BELLY WITH ENERGY (OPENING TO BREATH)

Put your hands in front of your lower dantien with the backs of your hands touching and your palms facing out. Then push your hands apart until they are about 6 inches beyond your body. Turn your hands again so that your palms are facing, and bring your hands together in front of your navel. The movement is like pushing curtains open and then closing them. Repeat at least three times. Let your breath guide the movement: Inhale as you push your hands out; exhale as you bring them back. This will help you relax and open your dantien to receive more qi.

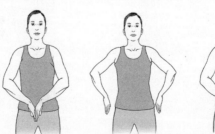

ENERGY WASH

Bring your hands to your sides with your elbows very slightly bent and your palms facing upward. Relax your shoulders. Lift your arms at your sides to above your head. Turn your hands over, with your palms toward the sky to receive more qi. Then turn your hands over, palms down, and imagine golden energy flowing out of your fingers as you lower your hands down in front of your body. Imagine that you're washing away any stress and negative thoughts, and replacing that negativity with fresh light and energy.

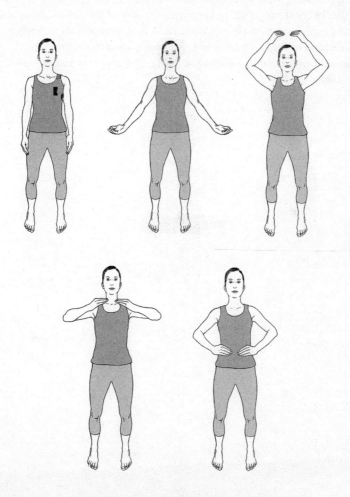

BE A BIRD (WING WAVES)

Bring your arms to your sides, palms facing down, and lift your slightly rounded arms as if there's wind holding them up and you are flying. Lower and repeat.

BE A WAVE (CORE WAVE)

Bring your hands below your lower dantien with palms facing down. Move them toward your sides, keeping them in front of your body. Lift your arms and hands until they're chest high. If you've seen anyone doing tai chi, you will recognize this as a core movement. Lift and lower. Keep your shoulders relaxed and your arms soft and rounded. You may feel your back getting into the motion; go ahead and gently bend your knees and rise up. You are indeed doing wavelike movements.

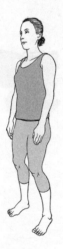
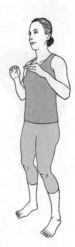
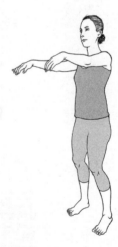

OPEN YOUR HEART AND THYMUS CENTERS

Begin as you did in the Be a Wave movement, and once your arms are chest high, spread them out to your sides with a good stretch. Look over one shoulder and flex your wrists back. Bring your arms back to center, with your palms facing each other. Repeat, looking over the opposite shoulder as you flex your wrists. This movement also opens the thymus area, the home of your T cells and master immune regulator. Chinese medicine holds that this movement opens your thymus-heart area. In Western medicine, we might one day learn that this frees the regulatory T cells. From other traditions, this is also a gesture thought to open your heart.

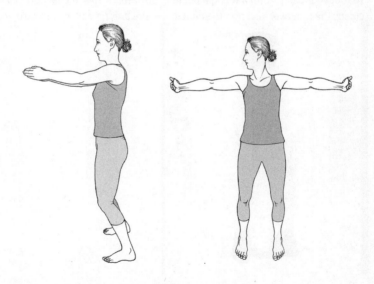

INTEGRATING THE ENERGY

This is the equivalent to alternate nostril breathing in yoga. It balances and integrates the qi and the right and left hemispheres of the brain.

Place one hand, palm down, below your navel and the other hand to your side, palm down, same level.

Now raise both arms until they're over your head with your palms facing each other.

Now the hand that was at your side lowers down your center, and the hand that was originally below your navel goes to the side. Repeat at least three times.

On the fourth time, as your palms are facing each other over your head, bring them together and lower them down the center of your body. Turn your hands so that your palms form a triangle pointing downward. This anchors the qi and closes the practice. Feel free to stand in this posture for as long as you'd like.

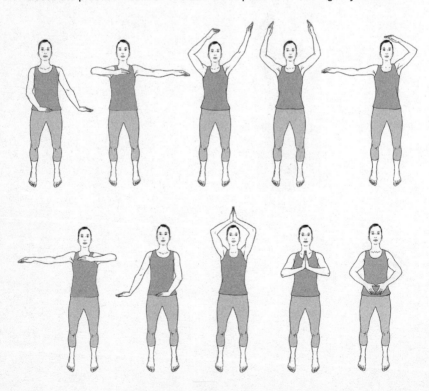

When you finish your qigong practice, you should feel more energy. You can call that qi, vitality, or even power. You will likely feel more centered. This would be an ideal time for some meditation or a nice walk. Or you can simply be quiet and let the qi guide you. When you've been practicing for a while, you may discover that your body wants to move and sway; you may notice that it feels natural and enjoyable to stand with the natural movement of your qi.

THE TAKEAWAY

We hope you'll explore our simple healing energy movements. Research shows many benefits of these approaches, and we've seen the amazing effects they've had on us, our students, and our patients. If you prefer, of course, you can do other activities that you may enjoy more. Remember: The important thing is to keep moving, varying your activities from day to day. Do it! Engaging in a variety of exercise and movement activities will help keep you balanced and healthy. And experiment with using a soundtrack for any of the exercises. Research shows that listening to music helps you maintain your pace and rhythm while enhancing the overall pleasure of the activity.[45]

Your cells are in constant motion, and some scientists say that the movement of cells is proof of their intelligence. To maintain that intelligence, you and your cells must move. Find something you like to do, and find a friend to do it with you. Your intent to enhance your health and well-being will take you to Ultimate Immunity. When you combine healthy movement with healthy eating and a deep sense of mindfulness, it's amazing the changes you'll see in your life. Next, we put the whole program together for you—to balance your immune health and nourish yourself body and mind.

CHAPTER 7

Personalized Programs *for* Immune Imbalances

You picked up this book because you want a stronger, more balanced immune system and a healthier, happier life. We've emphasized all along that lifestyle choices—including what you eat, how you manage stress, and your level of physical activity—have a significant impact on your immune function and overall health. In this chapter, we'll guide you on the first steps of your journey with plans that you can personalize and adapt to suit your specific needs. Our goal is to empower you to make good choices by offering you useful information and new ideas to consider. The rest is up to you.

Now it's time to have a conversation with yourself. What's your biggest health concern or challenge? Have you been thinking of giving up wheat, beer, or sugar to try to ease your stuffy nose, indigestion, or bloat? Is arthritis keeping you from enjoying your walks? Are you tired of itchy eczema? Examine your priorities and ask what you'd like to change first, then consider your options. Make a commitment to do whatever it takes to improve your situation! You're not in this alone. In this chapter, we provide a variety of programs to jump-start your journey toward improved health.

We've talked a lot about what goes on inside your body—all those intricate systems that work together to keep you well. And we've talked about your choices and other factors that can influence the inner workings of your body. In this chapter, we integrate these concepts into a simple program that encompasses nutrition, stress management, and fitness, plus supplements and medications when needed. We'll look in detail at several specific health concerns, but the bottom line is this: The main culprit in almost any illness is too much inflammation and cellular damage caused by oxidative stress (remember those free radicals?). So, much of our advice will focus on ways you can reduce and prevent inflammation and frequent infections and lessen the effects of allergies and autoimmune illnesses.

YOU'RE IN CHARGE!

Let's begin at the beginning: Start with an honest self-assessment of your goals and what health changes you'd like to make first. Having an objective—a measurable outcome—will allow you to gauge your improvement so that you can adjust your program accordingly.

Next, look deeper than your surface symptoms. Can you identify any daily, seasonal, or even yearly health patterns? Some people battle the same illness at the same time every year—bronchitis in the fall, for example, or a sinus infection every spring. In the past, you may have resorted to taking antibiotics once or twice for an infectious illness, and the drug might have eased your congestive cough, but it may not have left you feeling better overall or changed that yearly pattern. Even after you stopped coughing, the effects of the medication or the infection—low energy and poor sleep—may have lingered. Let's look beyond symptom relief to complete recovery. What would it be like to avoid those annual rounds of bronchitis and antibiotics?

Achieving a mind-body state that can prevent your next health threat—or make you better prepared to fight it—is the essence of improved immune health. It's an "inside job," and you're the only one who's qualified to do it.

This proactive attitude is exactly what your body needs. You don't have to battle bronchitis every autumn just because the fallen leaves are moldy. Regular bouts with the same or similar symptoms means that a few layers of imbalance exist in your body, such as a weakened immune system along with the suboptimal performance of another vital function. It's up to you to peel back those layers to get to the problem's core, so begin to pay attention early in the process—before you get sick—and become aware of when and where things start to feel a bit off. Your body speaks to you in many ways; you just need to listen a bit more deeply. When you expand your knowledge and awareness of your body, you can spot patterns in your health. Poor health often mirrors what's going on in your life. Does your autumn bronchitis follow on the heels of a very

THE POWER OF CHANGE

This entire book is about change—changing your mind and health, especially your immune health. But change isn't always easy, since most of the time it involves moving out of your comfort zone.

In the field of health psychology and resilience, experts have identified the principles of "hardiness"[1] that help people stay motivated and make change. Hardiness was originally defined as the three C's (challenge, commitment, and control).[2] We've added a fourth C (community), which goes a long way toward strengthening immune health.

- Make a *commitment.*
- Embrace the *challenge* instead of seeing it as a threat.
- Know that you're in *control.*
- Engage *community* and personal support.

This body of knowledge originated with Dr. Suzanne Kobasa at the University of Chicago. She spent several years following Bell Telephone executives whose lives were undergoing major changes, including losing their jobs or moving to new areas of the country or new positions. Those who stayed well, despite these stressful life changes, exhibited the three C's of commitment, challenge, and control. So put the C's to work for you! Make a commitment to the Ultimate Immunity program and let others know about your decision.

Look at this program as an exciting challenge rather than a punishment. Remember that you're in control of the decisions you make—and your decisions can lead to better health. Connect with others for support and affirmation. Embracing these four C's can make all the difference!

busy summer when you had little rest and poor nourishment? Do you simply expect it and believe there's nothing you can do to prevent it? After all, if you get the same condition every year around the same time, there must be a reason. And you're right! There are probably many reasons, most of which have to do with how you've been taking care of yourself along the way, not just in the days immediately preceding your illness.

You can't overhaul your immune system overnight, so think strategically and begin with what you'd like to change first. Organize your thoughts and your understanding of your body. Can you identify what's out of balance? Are you feeling achy, itchy, irritated, or congested? Are your tissues experiencing the fires of inflammation? You know, if you're honest with yourself, which habits aren't as healthy as they could be.

Make this chapter personal and meaningful for you. Take some time to write down a few realistic goals. Your healing journey is up to you.

BEGINNING YOUR PERSONAL JOURNEY

What do you need for this healing journey? Besides a journal, there are important intangibles, such as patience, commitment, and, ideally, some support from other people in your life. All of these things can boost your initial motivation to change. We'll be your coach, by way of this book, to help you initiate the changes you desire.

We've already talked about setting goals with measurable outcomes. In the back of this book, you'll find tracking tools and journal pages to help you chart your progress. (See pages 298–307.)

SET YOUR GOALS!

Your intentions and goals are powerful motivators. Your intention could be as simple as eating a healthier diet with more fresh vegetables and fruit. Perhaps it's to prevent getting an autoimmune illness that runs in your family. Or it may be to lose weight and lower your risk for diabetes. Write your intentions and goals in your journal. Here are a few examples of strong, clear intentions and measurable goals:

- I will eat at least three servings of greens every day for the next month because that will lessen inflammation in my body.

- I will engage in the Cool Down Inflammation Prevention Program for 1 month to reduce my joint pains.

- I will practice mindfulness meditation daily for 15 minutes for the next 3 weeks; I want to be less stressed and anxious and wish to improve my attitude.

Staying focused on the "why" helps you remain committed if physical results aren't immediately obvious. Use the journal pages starting on page 298, grab a notebook, or download an app to your smartphone. (One great free app is Lose It! For more information, go to loseit.com.)

THE COOL DOWN INFLAMMATION PREVENTION PROGRAM

When it comes to balancing your immune health, the first thing to tackle is inflammation—because inflammation underlies so many health issues, and getting it under control is the foundation for a healthy immune system and a healthy body.[3] To do that, you'll eat a nourishing diet and practice mind-body strategies for managing stress, thus enhancing your energy and engaging in a richer life.

You'll build on—and adapt—the anti-inflammatory plan. We've created specific programs for reducing allergies, preventing infections, and lessening autoimmunity and hyperimmune activity. Each individual program includes food and mind-body stress-managements strategies. Plus, you'll learn about over-the-counter supplements that may help in different situations. Let's get started.

Inflammation is a generalized response of the body to irritation, injury, infection, and immune challenges. It shows up in many ways: the swollen ankle after a fall, the redness around a wound, itchy eyes when allergies strike, the fever from an infection, or the pain from arthritis. Inflammation is a helpful and lifesaving acute response, but when it occurs for a long time and in the wrong place, health problems ensue. Living less inflamed—body and mind—ideally results in less pain, greater flexibility, more energy, healthier relationships, and a more content life.

One key to this program is the healthy eating plan, the I-PEP that you learned about in Chapter 4. And to calm inflammation, it's equally important to calm your body and mind.[4] Remember: Address your stress! Relax. Breathe deeply. Stretch and move your body. When you need to, consider supplemental nutritional and plant products to enhance healing—nature's milder form of pharmaceutical medicine.

If you're currently taking prescription drugs, however, don't stop taking any of them without first discussing it with your health-care provider. As your health improves, you might be able to shift to a lower dosage, or you may even be able to stop taking a drug altogether. But that's an important move to take only after professional consultation. It's possible that pain medications, sleep drugs, hormones, or products used to lower cholesterol, blood pressure, or blood sugar can be tapered off as you live your life differently. Always work with your physician when it comes to adjusting the dosages and frequency of your current medicines.

This book doesn't specifically address common health concerns such as blood sugar, blood pressure, cancer, and high cholesterol, but studies show that when we lessen inflammation through dietary changes, stress reduction, or movement practices, these other conditions—particularly risks for heart disease[5]—also improve.

Let's start out, though, with the Cool Down Program, which has four major components: nutrition, mind-body techniques (including fitness and stress management strategies), healing herbs and supplements, and gut health. These pieces are interconnected—and if you include all the component parts, by the end of the third week of the Cool Down (if not before), you'll discover a happier, healthier, stronger you.

The Nutrition Connection: Defeat Inflammation with Food

For the Cool Down Program, I-PEP will be your anti-inflammation guide, so refer to Chapter 4 often for more food details. I-PEP offers you the best way to soothe inflammation and boost your immune health. Review the plan on pages 127–132. Here are the highlights.

- Eat lots of vegetables, fruits, and quality protein like wild seafood.
- Include colorful produce like greens and berries, plus nuts and seeds, and good oils like olive oil.
- Use healing, anti-inflammatory herbs and spices, such as ginger, turmeric, garlic, and rosemary.
- Drink herbal, green, and/or black teas to keep immune cells cooled down.[6]
- Incorporate plenty of fiber.
- Avoid trans fats and limit processed and packaged foods, especially those with refined flour and sugar.
- Keep your red meat consumption to a minimum and make it lean when you do eat it.
- Be mindful of your intake of substances that are often abused, such as alcohol, caffeine, sugar, marijuana, or prescription narcotics.
- Consider a few supplements, such as a multivitamin/mineral, an omega-3 product, an antioxidant combo, probiotics, and vitamin D. The probiotics and omega-3 oils may offer the best overall immune support. Glucosamine can be helpful to maintain healthy joints as you age.

- Limit chemical exposure in your food, on your body, and in your home. Evaluate your cosmetics, laundry soaps, and cleaning supplies. Whenever possible, choose natural alternatives.

The Mind–Body Connection

Research has shown that many health concerns (including infectious diseases like the flu and other viruses, cardiovascular disease, depression, and even wound healing) are worsened by inflammation and stress.[7] For more than 20 years, scientists have been researching alternative mind-body approaches that reduce stress and inflammation and lead to better health and happiness. As a reminder, here are examples of the science-backed mind-body techniques that we explored earlier.

SINGING MEDITATION (also known as Kirtan Kriya).[8] Researchers at UCLA, working with caregivers of family members suffering from dementia, had participants take part in 12 minutes daily of Kirtan Kriya, or singing meditation, for 8 weeks. Compared to a control group, caregivers using this strategy had lowered expression of inflammation genes as well as improved cognitive skills and better memory.[9]

YOGA. In a study at Ohio State University among small groups of breast cancer survivors, those taking part in a yoga practice for 3 months experienced less inflammation and fatigue and fewer symptoms of depression. Breathing and meditation seemed to be the most important aspects of the yoga practices.[10]

MINDFULNESS MEDITATION. This thoroughly researched practice, taught in many hospitals, health-care settings, and community centers, has been shown to reduce stress. Among the older population, it also reduces loneliness and decreases the production of genes that cause inflammation.[11]

EMOTIONAL DISCLOSURE. Developed by psychologist James Pennebaker,[12] this well-researched strategy that's distinct from journaling offers positive health benefits for people with major stress, asthma, rheumatoid arthritis, arthritis, psoriasis, and cancer.[13]

The Herbal and Supplement Connection

When you take a pharmaceutical drug for a hyperimmune condition, the drug typically lessens or depresses all of your body's immune functions, leaving you more vulnerable

INFLAMMATION-BUSTING HERBS AND SUPPLEMENTS

Numerous supplements—nutrients and herbs—have been shown to reduce inflammation. (Read more about them in Chapter 4.) Our favorites include:

- **Omega-3s with EPA/DHA.** These help to lower irritation from oxidative stress[14] of blood vessels and tissues.

- **Antioxidants.** Choose a general formula with vitamins A, C, and E plus selenium and zinc. NAC (N-acetyl cysteine) is an important building block of glutathione, your cell's most important antioxidant. Antioxidants lessen the damage from infection and inflammation and may prevent gene damage.

- **Vitamin D.** This, the "sunshine vitamin," offers many protective benefits for whole-body health. Besides playing a key role in building strong bones, it helps balance immune health.

- **Probiotics.** These support gut health and immune cell development.

- **Alpha lipoic acid.** This specific antioxidant made by your cells assists the body in detoxifying chemicals and protects the liver.

- **CoQ10.** Another antioxidant your body can produce, CoQ10 is essential for energy production in the cells.

- **Quercetin.** This important bioflavonoid is found in onions, garlic, and citrus and works to lessen allergy and histamine reactions.[15]

- **Bromelain and papain.** Bromelain, an enzyme from pineapple, and papain, an enzyme from papaya, can reduce pain and swelling.[16]

- **Curcumin.** This biologically active component of turmeric is one of the most potent immunomodulators available. Many commercial anti-inflammatory formulations contain both curcumin and ginger, which complement each other.

- **Ginger.** This root helps with circulation, energy, and body warmth.

- **Boswellia.** Derived from tree bark gum resin and often known as Indian frankincense, this herb has been used for centuries in Ayurvedic medicine. Recently, it has been shown to diminish hyperactive inflammatory T cell activity.[17]

to infections. Research is showing that certain powerful anti-inflammatory herbs not only lessen hyperactive reactions but also balance the overall immune response, keeping you healthy. Some herbs are known as *adaptogens*—they can enhance or diminish stress responses, depending on what your body needs. Substances called *immunomodulators* do the same thing for your immune system. Many of the herbs we recommend, like curcumin, are potent immunomodulators.

Begin your program with a probiotic and general antioxidant supplement that contains vitamins C, A, and E as mixed tocopherols, plus zinc and selenium. Later, you can add alpha lipoic acid and vitamin D. Your basic program could also include an anti-inflammatory herbal product that includes curcumin, ginger, and boswellia. Check out the chart below for recommended dosages.

CHOOSE THE RIGHT DOSE!

SUPPLEMENT	DOSAGES	TIMING AND FREQUENCY
Antioxidant blend	Vitamin C (500–1,000 mg) Vitamin A (1,000–2000 IU) Zinc citrate (15–30 mg) Vitamin E as mixed tocopherols (400 IU) Selenium as selenomethionine (200 mcg)	Once or twice daily
Alpha lipoic acid	100–200 mg	Once or twice daily
Vitamin D	1,000–5,000 IU	Once daily
Curcumin (turmeric) Avoid if taking blood thinners	100–200 mg	2–3 times daily before or after meals
Ginger (capsules of ginger-root powder)	500–1,000 mg	2–3 times daily
Probiotics, like lactobacillus and bifidobacteria	1 billion–10 billion per capsule	Once or twice daily
Omega-3 oils with EPA and DHA	300–600 mg capsules	2–6 capsules daily with higher amounts for more inflammation
Quercetin	250–500 mg capsules	1–2 capsules 2–3 times daily
Coenzyme Q10 as ubiquinol or ubiquinone	50–100 mg	2–3 times daily
Boswellia (with at least 60% boswellic acids)	300–500 mg	2–3 times daily

The Gut Connection

Throughout this book, you've read about the busy and bossy little bugs in your belly. We've talked about how important your microbiome is and how those microbes in your gut actually tell the immune cells with which they cohabitate what they're supposed to be doing at any given time. In fact, there's a lot of "conversation" going on between the microbes and your immune cells. But the conversation goes more than two ways: Your emotions, your stress level, and your daily choices and activities contribute their molecular two cents, and that compounds this intestinal chatter.

Your immune system is more complicated than any scientists thought when they first began examining T and B cells in the 1970s. Our mind and stress were not really considered factors in overall health until the late 1990s. Today, the gut, its biome, and epigenetics are recognized as integral parts of the story.

Your belly is really smart: It's packed with cells and neurons that pour out more neurotransmitters than your brain. Immune cells in the gut recognize good microbes, good food, and your own good cells. And the microbes, under those conditions, tell the immune cells to become healthy T regulating (Treg) cells. But when the gut becomes inflamed, miscommunication ensues, and our microbes sound the alarm, telling our T cells that it's time to fight. These aggressive T helper cells trigger imbalance, and that imbalance makes our bodies think that it's time to be more aggressive, hypervigilant, and overreactive. This can result in allergies, autoimmune illnesses, and chronic inflammation, all explosive levels of imbalance that become self-sustaining. How do we break the cycle? We bring the mind and body back into balance by reducing stress, consuming less-inflaming food, and avoiding irritating people. Go with your gut; it's been telling you this all along!

Assessing the microbes living inside the GI tract is a useful practice in integrative medicine. For this evaluation, it's important to work with a practitioner who uses a lab that can offer you a complete microbial picture of what's living in your gut—the healthy probiotic bacteria as well as the potentially pathogenic bacteria, yeasts, or parasites. Once the various species of microbes are properly identified, you and your doctor can choose an appropriate course of treatment, if one is necessary, to improve your immune health. Much of this testing is covered by insurance and Medicare.

Keeping your gut healthy is key when it comes to keeping your immune system strong. In *The Detox Diet*,[18] Dr. Haas offers a "5R" program for healing the gut:

- Remove abnormal microbes.

- Reinnoculate healthy microbes such as probiotics.

- Replace low digestive helpers like enzymes or hydrochloric acid.

- Repair inflamed or damaged gut lining with nutrients and herbs.

- Rebalance your lifestyle with better diet and less stress.

There are many specifics to a program like this, so work with a knowledgeable practitioner who truly understands the importance of gut assessment and healing rebalance.

YOUR PERSONAL COOL DOWN TIME

Ready to get started? Remember, this is an integrative program that asks you to pay attention to your whole lifestyle—to eat well, manage your stress, and engage in strategies that lessen mental and physical inflammation. The mind-body practices we recommend are qigong and meditation. The chart on page 210 and "The Cool Down Plan in Action" (page 208) detail the whole program. In a nutshell:

- Begin every day with brief self-massage followed by the Logging On qigong movement practice (details on pages 183–194).

- What you eat is spelled out in the I-PEP program in Chapter 4.

- At least five times a week, engage in active physical fitness activities—walking, weight training, stretching, or yoga, as you are physically able.

- Also include a 10- to 20-minute meditation practice sometime during the day; this could be simple meditation, the Kirtan, mindfulness, or imagery (explored in Chapter 5). We encourage you to stay with one style of practice for at least a few weeks, since it takes awhile to get yourself cooled and calmed down to experience the benefits of meditation.

- The imagery explorations are an added support for your healing process. Consider the problem you're focusing on, such as an inflamed gut, allergies, or pain; then every night at bedtime, listen to, read about, or remember the imagery for that condition. It's always good to get into a relaxed state before doing the imagery. Don't be surprised if you discover your sleep improves.

IS YOUR HOME AN INFLAMMATION STATION?

Do your skin care products and cleaning supplies inflame, irritate, or worsen your allergies? Are there volatile chemicals outgassing into the air from new paint, from scented candles or air fresheners, or from new products such as carpets and furniture? These, too, can undermine your health. As part of your Cool Down Program, review and reduce your chemical exposure as much as possible. Find great advice and tips at ewg.org/healthyhometips.

On your next day off, plan a trip to a local greenhouse or garden center. Some plants can remove certain chemicals from the air, such as formaldehyde and benzene hydrocarbons. These beneficial plants include aloe vera, spider plants, Gerbera daisies, snake plants, golden pathos, ficus trees, bamboo palms, and peace lilies. Find one you like and bring it home!

You may decide to explore the other suggested mind-body practices, such as emotional disclosure, during a particularly stressful period.

Pay attention to your spiritual life, too, because that's another aspect of healing. Almost every spiritual tradition emphasizes the connection between gratitude and health. Try to express your gratitude in your own way, perhaps by writing in your journal three things you are grateful for, saying a prayer of gratitude, or even telling someone how much you appreciate their friendship. Most of all, be grateful for yourself and let yourself *be*.

COOL FOR YOU: INDIVIDUALIZE YOUR COOL DOWN PROGRAM

Okay, you've learned the basics of the Cool Down Program. Now it's time to customize it. Think about the goals you selected at the beginning of this chapter. What health concerns would you like to address first? Do you have chronic joint pain from arthritis? We'll show you how to kick the NSAID habit and ease your pain naturally. Maybe you're plagued by frequent colds and flu, and you've tried every cold remedy that's out there. We'll show you how to prevent—and relieve—cold symptoms and strengthen your immune system. Or perhaps hay fever season makes you a prisoner

(continued on page 210)

THE COOL DOWN PLAN IN ACTION

It's as easy as 1-2-3! Decide on a start date—be sure to make it soon—and follow the schedule.

Wake Up

Sit up in bed and take a few deep breaths. Rub your hands together to warm them, and do all or some of the self-massage practices on pages 183–188. Do the face wash and Head Tap and the Whole Body Wake-Up Tap. Do Arm Sweeps, Neck Rubs, and the Thymus Pat and Hum.

Take 10 minutes to engage in your morning Logging On qigong movements (pages 189–194).

Take 10 minutes to sit quietly and engage in one of the meditation practices, such as mindfulness. Set your intention for the day.

Breakfast

Drink a cup of water with a squeeze of fresh lemon or lime.

Brew a cup of tea and assemble the ingredients for a smoothie or another morning meal, such as hot steel-cut oatmeal. (See the recipes in Chapter 8.)

Take your supplements after you eat—multivitamin, antioxidant, or omega-3, if you choose, and with your doctor's approval.

Midmorning

Keep your energy level high with a snack of 2 or 3 roasted carrots, an apple, or a few almonds.

If you're incorporating any herbal supplements, this is a good time to take them.

Take a 15-minute stretch or walk break.

Lunchtime

Take a 10-minute walk-and-stretch break before eating.

Eat a big green salad with shredded kale, red leaf lettuce, basil, and shredded carrots. Add a piece of roasted chicken breast or spicy tofu. Or choose a salad from the recipes in Chapter 8.

Afternoon Break

Snack on a handful of almonds or walnuts or a piece or two of fruit.

If you didn't practice qigong in the morning, now is a good time to do so. You can also revive your energy level by doing the Logging On qigong program again.

End of Workday

Unwind with 15 minutes of walking with a friend, or head to the gym for a workout or swim.

Dinner

About 15 to 30 minutes before dinner, drink a glass of water with cucumber slices in it.

Sit down for your meal. No TV, phones, or screens.

Be mindful of what you're eating and who is with you; chew well and savor your food.

Take some supplements after dinner, as appropriate.

Spend the evening relaxing with a movie, a good book, or another enjoyable activity.

Bedtime

About an hour before bedtime, turn off the TV and computers. Dim the lights. Turn on quiet music and take some time to meditate using mindfulness or imagery. (See Chapter 5.)

Do self-massage, this time in a slow and soothing way. (See Chapter 6.) Or massage after a shower while applying moisturizing lotion. (This is a great sleep aid.)

Get into bed, relax, unwind, and have sweet dreams.

THE COOL DOWN PROGRAM

PRACTICE QIGONG DAILY	RELIEVE STRESS: CHOOSE 1 AND STICK WITH IT	
Self-massage Morning or before bed	**Mindfulness** Take a class or learn from a book or online course and practice for 15–30 minutes a day	
Logging On movements Morning, plus any time your energy is lagging	**Kirtan Kriya** 12 minutes, ideally after qigong (6 minutes if you're extra busy)	
	Emotional disclosure writing Do for 15–20 minutes for 4 days only Perhaps wait a few days or a week before adding this to your program	
	Imagery Daily or when needed	

in your own house or makes you drowsy and drippy on allergy medications. Read on! In the pages that follow, you'll learn how to personalize the Cool Down Program to address your own immune health needs.

Ultimate Immunity Approaches for Chronic Pain

Chronic inflammation contributes to many painful conditions, including rheumatoid and osteoarthritis and back pain. Anti-inflammatory medicines (NSAIDs) such as aspirin, acetaminophen, ibuprofen, and naproxen work well because they block the enzymes that trigger both swelling and pain. Problem is, they may come with some unpleasant— and sometimes dangerous—side effects, like abdominal pain and liver damage.

Natural Pain Alternatives

HERBS AND SPICES. Natural alternatives to NSAIDs that offer similar effects include turmeric, green tea, ginger, rosemary, cat's claw, devil's claw, and willow bark. Because some of these supplements work in much the same way as NSAIDs, they do pose some of the same risks, such as stomach upset, irritation, and bleeding; however, the side effects tend to be much less frequent or severe. Most evidence singles out turmeric (as curcumin) as being one of the most effective natural treatments to help ease pain.[19]

TAKE SUPPLEMENTS	MOVE	BE SPIRITUAL
Week 1 Vitamin D Probiotics	Walk at least 15 minutes (30 minutes or more is even better) 5 days a week	Gratitude daily
Week 2 Curcumin Omega-3 fish oils	Stretch 15 minutes 3 times a week	Be present and loving
Week 3 Ginger or another herb like boswellia	Weight train 3 times a week	Try to relax and be present
	Consider yoga as you are able	

FISH OIL can ease inflammation and pain caused by many chronic conditions. The most convincing research tells us to use 2 to 4 g of DHA and EPA or up to 12 g of omega-3 oils daily, often a higher amount than most people take. Gamma-linolenic acid (GLA) from seed oils such as evening primrose at doses between 1,400 and 2,800 mg caused significant improvements in pain in people with rheumatoid arthritis.[20] Beneficial omega-3 fatty acids are available from other sources, but experts agree that fish oil offers the best forms of EPA and DHA.

BODY SCAN EXERCISE

Close your eyes and feel your breath as it comes into your nostrils and leaves. Become aware of the rising and falling of your breath in your chest and belly. Feel where your body touches the chair and your feet touch the floor, and simply breathe with awareness for a few moments. Now pay attention as slowly, with your mind, you scan your body from head to toe. Notice any places that feel tight or painful and breathe relaxation into those places. Continue to move your awareness through your body, relaxing as you do so. And simply note your awareness of your body sensations—where it hurts and where it feels relaxed.

VITAMIN D. Some studies have linked low levels of vitamin D to increased levels of inflammation and chronic pain. Other studies, however, contradict those findings, so the jury's still out. But remember, every cell in your body responds to vitamin D, so if you are low in D, a supplement may diminish any possible risks.

BROMELAIN may also moderate chronic pain. Bromelain is an anti-inflammatory enzyme extracted from pineapple that helps with pain and swelling.

IMAGERY IN ACTION

Imagery exercises can help you relax and enhance your overall healing experience. Early studies of imagery and immune health revealed that people could use their minds to encourage the regression of warts! At Carleton University in Ottawa, researchers looked at whether hypnotic suggestion and imagery would help people lose their warts, a viral condition. Twenty-two people with warts on one or both hands were individually given 5 minutes of relaxation hypnosis and then given directions to spend 2 minutes imagining getting rid of their warts while paying attention to the sensations in their hand: to experience warmth and tingling while imagining that their warts were shrinking and falling off. Following this, they were questioned about the vividness of their images and sensations. Six weeks later, they came back for follow-up; more than 50 percent of the warts were gone in the imagery group and none from the control group. The vividness of the imagery influenced the extent of their positive results. More women benefited from this than men.[21]

An observable physical change helps support the beneficial potential of imagery. We know from athletes that mental rehearsal, another form of imagery, improves performance significantly.[22] One of our clients eliminated her herpes lesions permanently with just one session. We can't guarantee the outcome, but we can promise that imagery soothes the mind, and it may redirect and calm down the immune renegades and accelerate healing in damaged areas of your body. Imagine using your imagination to affect a positive outcome and feel it with all of your senses. Imagery isn't always visual; it can also be kinesthetic—some people feel with their body or sense the imagery, while others may experience a sound or a scent reflecting the imagery. In other words, you can experience the imagery in many different ways.

GUIDED IMAGERY FOR CALMING INFLAMMATION

Imagine you're in a beautiful, secluded grotto, surrounded by lush green plants and serenaded by the gentle calls of birds. This feels like a very welcoming and safe place. Walk around and see what else is there—perhaps moss-covered rocks or a grassy area under a tree that invites you to sit. The sounds of bubbling water entice you to a glistening natural pool with a small waterfall. The air is warm. You're alone, and you feel safe and tranquil. You wade into the clear water and, leaning back, let the cooling water embrace you. As you relax and let the water keep you afloat, release any thoughts of frustration, worry, or anger. Surrender those emotions to the water. Let those feelings disappear. Let the anger and inflaming heat inside you cool down. As you're being held and comforted by this pool, feel that your cells, too, are being embraced and balanced by the water's cooling energy. Picture or sense that all your cells calm down and stop emitting inflammatory chemicals as they come into balance. Let an image come to mind that reminds you of this inner cooling and balance. Or repeat a word or a sound, such as "om." Let yourself be in this peaceful moment for as long as you want. Press your thumb to your first finger to help your body remember this experience. When you're ready, slowly step out of the pool. There's a huge towel waiting for you. Dry yourself, put your clothes back on, and sit on a rock to remember this time. When you're ready, open your eyes and become aware of where you are now. You're feeling relaxed and peaceful and washed free. Take a few minutes to write down this experience; remember and know that you can visit here anytime you need to cool down or soothe your body.

IMAGERY EXERCISE. You can shift your attitude, your mood, and even your behavior with mental imagery and positive expectations. First, relax by meditating or taking a 10-minute walk. Or try a body scan (see page 211), which increases your awareness of your body. Read more about the imagery itself (above). You can record and then play the directions so that you can relax, listen, and simply be guided through the exercise. Images may come to your mind that are different from the ones we describe, and that's okay—it's your own inner wisdom speaking, and you should listen.

Ultimate Immunity Approaches
for Infectious Conditions

Do you frequently experience colds, flus, or other infections? We looked at some common infections in Chapter 2 and their usual mainstream treatments in Chapter 3. So you already know about the troublesome side effects that accompany frequent courses of antibiotics and other medications. Your goal, in improving your immune health, is to live your life free from infectious episodes and antibiotics as much as possible. If frequent colds and the flu are your concern, you can individualize the Cool Down Program to pump up your immune health, keep infections at bay, and accelerate healing if you do happen to catch something.

While there are specific courses of treatment for certain problems (like drinking 100 percent cranberry juice for a bladder infection), our focus is on overall prevention of cyclical colds and flus that notoriously plague people and interfere with quality of life, work, and productivity.

Nobody's "bulletproof"; there's no surefire way to guarantee you'll never get sick. But these science-backed strategies can help you shift the odds in your favor.

Natural Alternatives for Infection Protection

You're surrounded by germs at every turn—every doorknob, every handshake, and every credit card machine may be teeming with microorganisms. That can't be

---

AVOID UNNECESSARY ANTIBIOTICS!

The overuse of antibiotics in the United States costs our health-care system billions of dollars every year. But the problems get much more personal than that. Antibiotics don't know the difference between the good microbes and the pathogenic ones in your GI tract—the medication simply wipes them all out. Altering the intestinal microbiome (flora) affects your digestive, elimination, and immune functions and can potentially lead to food reactions and allergies. Antibiotics themselves can trigger allergic reactions as well as unpleasant side effects (see Chapter 3). In addition, certain antibiotics should not be taken during pregnancy (streptomycin, kanamycin, and tetracycline) because they pose serious risks of birth defects to the fetus.[23]

---

helped. But you can make your body more resistant to those bugs you cannot avoid. Here are some strategies to use in conjunction with the Cool Down Program.

ZINC. This mineral has been shown in some studies to reduce the incidence of all infections, including respiratory and the flu, especially in those over age 60.[24] The highest dose of zinc recommended in the studies was 80 mg a day for older adults; 45 mg is the average needed to restore immune function and prevent infections.

GOOD HYGIENE. It's basic but it works! Wash your hands after touching doorknobs, money, and fixtures in public restrooms. When it's not possible to wash your hands, use a natural hand sanitizer. Avoid touching your face and mouth after being in public until you wash. Keep your own pen handy so you're never tempted to use the "community" pen at a doctor's office or other businesses. Cover your mouth when coughing to lessen the spread of germs. Cough into your bent elbow, not into your hands.

VACCINES. The easiest way to protect yourself against an infection for which a vaccine exists is to simply get the vaccination. You may want the shingles vaccine as you age; the HPV (human papillomavirus) vaccine for the teenager in your life; or basic immunizations for your children. What you do for yourself or your family is still mostly up to you, although the medical establishment pushes all of us to get many vaccinations.

If you travel to places that have endemic infectious issues, such as typhoid, cholera, or malaria, there are specific actions you must take to protect yourself. Although flu shots can help prevent influenza, they're not 100 percent foolproof, and they're not for everyone. (Neither of us has had a flu shot for decades.) The vaccine changes every year because the influenza viruses change. So each shot is only protective for the predicted viruses of that year (the ones that the powers-that-be elect to include), but there are literally hundreds of possible viruses swirling around. Those who should consider receiving a flu shot are those at risk of serious complications from the flu. An annual flu shot is especially important for those over age 60 and those who work with them, people with chronic medical conditions, those on steroids, smokers (who have a higher risk for respiratory conditions), and folks with poor diets who are likely to be nutritionally deficient. People who are immunosuppressed or who have HIV should take only the inactivated flu shot, never the live attenuated virus nasal spray. If you're severely allergic to eggs, never get a flu shot.[25]

REST. Basic, but effective. Getting plenty of sleep protects you from infection, and when you do catch a cold or the flu, rest helps your body heal itself. Your body and its wise immune cells know what to do if you give them time. So make sure you get additional rest the first 72 hours.[26] And stay home—your doctor can't do much to help you, and antibiotics are ineffective against these illnesses, which are caused by a virus. Plus, by staying home, you won't share your germs with friends and co-workers.

Fight Infection with Nutrition

Mother Nature provides a vast array of herbs and plants that may help your body eliminate cold and flu viruses. These common naturopathic remedies can work clinically. Although they've not been fully researched in double-blind, placebo-controlled clinical trials, there are many studies showing the natural antibiotic effects of the following nutrients and herbs. Here's a quick overview.

ECHINACEA is an herbal product that's often considered to have healing qualities. Though it doesn't prevent colds,[27] it may shorten the duration a bit. Echinacea seems to work by activating immune cells, so it's best avoided by people with autoimmune illnesses or even allergies.

VITAMIN A bursts (not beta-carotene supplements)—75,000 to 150,000 IU daily split into three doses for *just a few days* is thought to support immunity and mucous membrane healing. A lower dosage of 20,000 IU is then taken twice daily for a few days, followed by 5,000 to 10,000 IU for 3 to 5 days. This has worked for many practitioners and patients in fighting off early infections. Due to the potential toxicity of vitamin A, use this treatment only under the care of your health practitioner.

VITAMIN D₃. Research indicates that vitamin D_3 is most effective in preventing viral upper respiratory infections, influenza, and TB.[28] The recommended dosage is 5,000 IU daily, especially if you've measured low. Also, some data suggest that 50,000 IU daily for only 3 days may help heal certain infections, such as the herpes viruses (simplex and zoster).[29] Some practitioners believe that 10,000 IU daily during the cold season offers substantial protection.

GLUTATHIONE spray (oral or nasal) may be helpful for respiratory and sinus infections.[30] Taking glutathione as oral tablets or capsules has no apparent benefit, as it gets digested and does not appear to increase blood levels of glutathione.

The Immune Diaries   Elson

I began to have a sore throat and congestion a day after a trip. The day I returned, I also saw patients all day, and some of them were sick with infectious illnesses. The previous week, I had seen many ill patients, and my home office assistant was sick with a cold and cough. People were coughing on the flights up and back from Portland. And while away, my food intake was different than usual. I ate more wheat, breads, and foods that are congestive for me, like cheese; plus, I hadn't slept well. So what triggered my sore throat—all of the above or one thing? I'm exposed to people with colds or flu all the time, so it's not always easy to figure out a specific cause.

Since I was writing a book on immune health, I was inspired to reflect on why this cold and sore throat were attacking me at that moment. I know I was depleted from the busyness and travels. Normally, my body is fairly strong and resistant, and I've been blessed with good health for much of my life. Still, everybody gets sick once in a while. So I jumped into action.

I started with lightening my diet by adding more liquids and veggies and fruits and eating fewer grains as well as some protein. I also did some Master Cleanse lemonade, and, for later in the day, I made vegetable soup with onion, garlic, cabbage, carrot, and zucchini. I pressed a couple of cloves of fresh garlic into my already-served-up hot bowl of soup, since uncooked garlic has more allicin and germ-fighting properties. I began taking extra vitamin A (20,000 to 30,000 IU three times daily), vitamin C (500 to 1,000 mg every hour or two), and an alcohol-based echinacea/goldenseal tincture. I continued this regimen for a couple of days, then lowered the vitamin A. When I felt better, I exercised, took a steam bath, and made sure I got good sleep. All of this lifted my illness within a few days and kept it from going deeper into bronchitis.

GARLIC (*Allium sativa*), and particularly the allicin sulfur compound in garlic,[31] has been considered a natural antibiotic for centuries. Testing shows it inhibits the growth of some bacteria and yeast. It also appears to be helpful in treating parasites.[32]

GRAPEFRUIT SEED EXTRACT (GSE) contains flavonoids and is a natural antioxidant with antibacterial[33] and antiviral properties. It has been shown to kill contaminating viruses on produce and is an effective cleansing agent.[34] GSE can inhibit bacteria and yeast growth on the skin and is a good remedy for athlete's foot.

OREGANO OIL in liquid or capsule form can treat some fungi and bacteria. It's a popular and effective remedy as a natural infection fighter[35] and a potent antiparasitic agent.[36]

GOLDENSEAL[37] (berberine is its known active chemical component) is beneficial for some types of diarrhea and eye infections. It's being actively investigated for its bactericidal activities. In addition, it has been discovered to be an anti-inflammatory agent[38] (in lab tests) as well as a cholesterol-lowering substance.[39]

LICORICE ROOT shows antibacterial effects and contains a sweet-tasting compound called glycyrrhizin, which, if taken in large amounts, can cause high blood pressure.[40] So supplements are available that have removed that compound; they are known as DGL (deglycyrrhized licorice root extract).

OLIVE LEAF EXTRACT has both antimicrobial and antiviral activity and is available in capsules, as a skin cream, or as a mouth rinse. Olive leaf diminishes pain and is anti-inflammatory.[41] As an oral topical elixir, its effects on the size and pain of canker sores are equivalent with the effects of conventional topical steroids.[42] People undergoing intensive chemotherapy and/or radiation for cancer frequently get painful, inflamed mouth sores and swelling called oral mucositis, which affects their quality of life and is often a cause for stopping treatment. In a recent study, patients who used an olive leaf extract mouth rinse, compared to a placebo, showed a much lower incidence and reduced severity of oral mucositis. Another benefit—their markers of inflammation were down.[43]

OSCILLOCOCCINUM is a popular homeopathic treatment for colds and flu. Anecdotally, it works for some people. Research results vary.

Natural Approaches for Specific Infectious Conditions

All the strategies we discussed in the previous pages apply to the conditions we're about to review, but there are certain common illnesses we'll examine more closely to give you more healing options to consider.

Recurrent Infection, in General

If you feel as though you're catching everything that's going around, it means your body is run down and your immune system isn't protecting you from microbes. You need to find out why. Many factors can contribute to this poor body terrain—nutritional deficiencies, exposure to a high volume of microbes, stress, poor sleep, gut imbalance, or yeast overgrowth coupled with a sensitivity or immune antibody reaction to the yeast.

Review the Cool Down Program guidelines and begin to incorporate those mind-body stress management techniques. Work with your practitioner—two heads are better than one! Focus on keeping your cells working optimally with nutrient-rich foods and a multivitamin/mineral supplement as well as omega-3 oils, vitamin D, and probiotics.

Colds and Influenza

There are hundreds of home remedies that people around the world use to treat these common illnesses, from chicken soup to fresh garlic to zinc lozenges and short-term megadoses of vitamins A and C. Most don't pan out in the limited research that's available, but zinc certainly shows promise. Often, the best thing to do is rest, drink lots of fluids to flush your body's impurities, and let your marvelous immune system identify and eradicate those viruses and then produce antibodies to protect you from them in the future.

Ear Infection (Otitis Media)

More common in children, ear infections do occur occasionally in adults. They're generally viral (though often treated with antibiotics) and are caused by the spread of microbes into the middle ear followed by an inflammation reaction. The infection causes fluid to build up, and this creates pressure and pain behind the eardrum. Air travel should be avoided until the ear infection clears, as the increased ear pressure can damage the eardrum.

Allergies and pacifier use in infants are factors that might increase the risk of ear infections. Babies who have been breastfed have a reduced risk, which could be because they've avoided cow's milk longer. Studies indicate that any formula-feeding the first 6 months of life significantly increases the incidence of otitis media.[44] Most ear infections resolve themselves without the use of antibiotics.

A popular product for ear pain and low-grade infections is garlic/mullein flower ear oil. Put several drops into the ear canal several times daily. This old remedy helps lessen ear pain and inflammation. Ear issues often result from colds or sore throats, so it's important to take good preventive care.

Upper Respiratory Infection (Bronchitis, Sinusitis, Pharyngitis, Pneumonia)

All these conditions involve the upper respiratory tract, with inflammation and/or an infection of the nose and sinuses, the throat, or the lungs. Acute bronchitis is often due to a viral or bacterial infection, while chronic bronchitis and chronic obstructive pulmonary disease (COPD) are more often related to smoking and other environmental exposures (not infectious agents) that result in inflamed, irritated, and damaged lung membranes.

Most sinus infections are caused by viruses, some are provoked by fungi, and only a few arise from persistent bacterial infections. Sinusitis can lead to pain around the nose and behind the eyes, where the sinuses are located.

Pneumonia in the elderly has been linked to low zinc levels.[45] Fortunately, restoring zinc levels to normal helps combat pneumonia, can reduce the amount of antibiotics used, and shortens the duration of the illness.[46]

For upper respiratory infections, we generally recommend extra vitamins A and C (often the A burst); N-acetyl cysteine (NAC), which helps generate glutathione and protect respiratory membranes; and an herbal cough medicine with elderberry, wild cherry bark, and/or licorice root. Colloidal silver may also help some people, as can irrigation and cleansing of the nose and sinuses with a hot shower or a neti pot.

Stomach Flu or Food Poisoning

Occasionally, we pick up bothersome infections from spoiled or contaminated food. The people preparing or packaging your food can pass along pathogenic microbes, such as viruses, bacteria, and even parasites. Some people are more vulnerable to these pathogens than others, so that potato salad that sent you running to the bathroom might not bother someone else. Purchase fresh, good quality foods, and wash all produce before serving it to yourself or your family. Wash your hands before you handle

food at home, and use different cutting boards for raw meats or fish. Be especially
diligent with cleanliness in the kitchen!

When traveling or when eating away from home, choose restaurants that are clean
and that select quality foods. When you're traveling out of the country, eat primarily
cooked foods or fruits that you can peel, and choose well-known (and clean) restaurants. Street food may not be a wise idea.

Urinary Tract Infections (UTIs)

Much more common in women than men, UTIs can become a greater problem with
increased sexual activity. It's important to urinate and wash after sexual intercourse
and make sure you wipe yourself from front to back.

Unsweetened, 100 percent cranberry juice and cranberry extracts are natural
remedies that may offer some protection by making the bladder less hospitable to
bacteria.[48] Cranberries contain proanthocyanidins, and studies show that these
compounds help prevent the common bowel bacteria E. coli from sticking to urinary tract walls. Another active ingredient in cranberry (perhaps the key one) is
D-mannose, a natural sugar. D-mannose lessens the adhesiveness of any bacteria in
the bladder, so the germs leave with the urine. Using 50 to 100 mg of D-mannose
two or three times daily can reduce the incidence of bladder infections and the common "honeymoon cystitis."[49]

If you're prone to UTIs, drink plenty of water every day, urinate when you need to (don't hold it in too long), and avoid irritating chemicals (like fragrances) from feminine hygiene products and toilet paper. Probiotics may be helpful and can be taken either orally or used as a douche. Inject a solution of powder (one to two capsules or $^1/_4$ to $^1/_2$ teaspoon, for example, dissolved in purified water) into the vagina.

Herpes (Herpes Simplex)

There are two primary strains of the herpes simplex virus. Type 1 is usually transmitted through infected saliva (think kissing) and causes sores on the lips. Type 2 is sexually transmitted and causes outbreaks of sores near and around the genitals.[50] Common canker sores are not the same as oral herpes. What's the difference? Canker sores are usually inside the mouth and initially painful, but they are not caused by a virus and are not contagious. Canker sores are often related to nutrient deficiencies, acidic foods like tomatoes, or mouth acidity. As mentioned earlier, a mouth rinse containing olive leaf extract can lower the incidence and severity of mouth sores.

On the other hand, herpes type 1 lesions, also known as cold sores or fever blisters, are infectious and contagious. The lesions often start as small, painful patches of blistered skin. In some people, the outbreak of oral herpes is accompanied by a headache or pain at the base of the neck because the herpes virus inflames the nerve roots that supply sensation to the skin. (Similarly, lower-back aches can occur prior to and during genital herpes outbreaks.)

The amino acid lysine appears to be a simple and safe treatment for both oral and genital herpes. For outbreaks, take 500 to 1,500 mg two or three times daily, or take 500 mg once or twice daily as a preventive.[51] Also, don't kiss anyone when you have cold sores.

Topical treatments include manuka honey on the lesions, which may help them heal faster, and zinc oxide cream, which can lessen the severity of a genital herpes outbreak. Other supplements that may ease herpes infections include vitamins A and C, resveratrol, garlic, red algae, lactoferrin, and the herb lemon balm. High doses of vitamin D—50,000 IU daily for 3 days—may speed up the healing process.

Shingles (Herpes Zoster)

Shingles is a painful and often disabling rash caused by the varicella-zoster virus—the same one that causes chicken pox. Once you've had chicken pox, the nasty virus that caused it remains dormant in your nerve cells and may be reactivated years or decades later. When it's reactivated, it takes the form known as shingles. People who are immunized against chicken pox appear to be much less likely to develop shingles.[52] If you've actually had chicken pox, you're at the most risk for shingles.

Shingles occurs primarily in people over age 50 and can last several months—even longer. It's not as contagious as chicken pox, but a person with an active outbreak can transmit the varicella virus to someone who has not had chicken pox or the vaccine, and that person can develop chicken pox.

There are few natural remedies proven to prevent shingles, but several reduce the discomfort and pain. Capsaicin or cayenne ointments may lessen the nerve pain, and cool baths or compresses offer some comfort. The impact of high doses of vitamin D is currently being researched. A shingles vaccine is available for people over 50, and it's estimated to reduce about 50 percent of the cases. However, fewer than 4 percent of older adults have been vaccinated, so there's still not enough research to tell us how effective it is.

Viral Hepatitis

To prevent getting hepatitis in the first place, avoid contact with people who have hepatitis A or B, and don't inject illegal drugs. Unfortunately, lab accidents, such as being stuck by a needle used on someone with hepatitis, can transfer the infectious agent to an innocent bystander. There are vaccines available against hepatitis A and B. Natural remedies that offer some support for healing hepatitis infections include vitamin C (500 to 1,000 mg three times daily), milk thistle (silymarin herb, 60 to 120 mg two or three times daily), lipoic acid (100 to 200 mg three times daily), and selenium (as selenomethionine, 100 to 200 mcg twice a day). Of course, to not additionally stress your liver, avoid alcohol and reduce your exposure to chemicals—in foods, in your home, and on your skin.

More progressive complementary therapies include intravenous vitamin C cocktails and ozone therapy administered into the blood, which disrupts the microbe and may even stimulate immune cells.[53] For chronic hepatitis C, preliminary research indicates that 30 to 60 sessions of ozone therapy administered into the blood and rectum can lessen the symptoms of hepatitis C and appears to eradicate some of the virus.[54] You would need to find a physician who does these types of intravenous and ozone treatments, sometimes referred to as "oxidative therapies."

Ultimate Immunity Approaches for Allergies

Allergic reactions are common in people of all ages, so lessening their symptoms is an important issue for overall immune health. And since the reactions (not the causes) are due to inflammation, following both the I-PEP and the Cool Down Program for a few weeks will help.

General and Seasonal Allergies

If you have seasonal allergies, try implementing the antiallergy approaches on the opposite page in the weeks before the usual onset of your allergy symptoms. For instance, if April is typically your worst month allergy-wise, start using the following strategies by the first of March. These approaches also offer general guidelines for environmental and food allergies, allergic skin rashes like eczema, and asthma.

ORAL ALLERGY SYNDROME

The words "hay fever" technically refer to an allergy to ragweed pollen, but now it's a catchall term for general seasonal allergies. Some people may experience the crossover reactions, normally experienced from ragweed, when they eat bananas, cucumbers, melons, sunflower seeds, or zucchini. This is known as oral allergy syndrome (OAS). Symptoms are caused by similar substances (cross-reacting allergens) in both pollen and raw produce. As seen commonly in practice, a broader definition of OAS also refers to any kind of food immune reaction setting up the body to be generally more reactive to any environmental agents. If you've ever had an itchy mouth after eating fresh salsa, that may be oral allergy syndrome triggered by a reaction to raw tomatoes. The main signs of OAS are swelling of the mouth area, itchy mouth or ears, or scratchy throat. Many of the allergy proteins are on the food's skin, so peeling or cooking can help get rid of the offending allergen. Other OAS partnerships include:

- Allergy to grass pollen may cause reactions to celery, melons, oranges, peaches, and tomatoes.

- Allergy to birch pollen may enhance reactions to apples, almonds, carrots, celery, cherries, hazelnuts, kiwifruit, peaches, pears, and plums.

Uncovering the exact cause of an allergic reaction isn't always easy. Is your itchy, red skin the result of something you ate? Or was it caused by a pollen, a chemical, or your friend's cat? What exactly is making your nose run or causing your latest eczema outbreak? It's time for more detective work!

The eating plans in Chapter 4 begin with the elimination of common food

---

THE FIVE-STEP ANTIALLERGY PLAN

1. **Purify with the 5-Day Elimination, Healing Plan.** (See page 123.) Avoid common allergens (wheat, eggs, dairy, corn, peanuts, and shellfish, for example) and foods you know are issues for you for a few weeks before following up with your physician. Challenge testing entails adding back one food a day and watching for any reactions.

2. **Strengthen.** Consume more anti-inflammatory foods, which can lessen the symptoms of allergic reactions: broccoli, citrus, kale, collards, onions and garlic, elderberries, and parsley.

3. **Balance your belly.** Take probiotics twice daily for at least 2 weeks. If the probiotics seem to lessen your food allergies and reactions, continue taking them.[55] If you have any ongoing digestive issues or have taken antibiotics fairly often in your life, get your gut checked out with a practitioner who is aware of gut con-

nections to immunity and who offers specialized lab testing to look at digestion, microbes, and permeability.

4. **Reduce your stress** and lighten your mood. Research shows that chronic stress can trigger allergy flare-ups.[56]

5. **Supplement.** Include quercetin (250 to 500 mg three times daily) and vitamin C (500 to 1,000 mg three times daily). Add vitamin A (3,000 to 6,000 IU daily) and vitamin D (2,000 to 5,000 IU daily). Try the "honey treatment," starting with ½ teaspoon daily of locally produced honey and working up to 1 tablespoon over 2 to 3 weeks. (The research here is mixed, but many patients report good results, as they do with consuming local bee pollen.) Other herbal treatments include butterbur root (*Petasites hybridus*), stinging nettle (*Urtica dioica*), goldenseal (*Hydrastis canadensis*), and eucalyptus oil as steam.

PROBIOTICS AND ALLERGIES

Over the last 15 years, many studies have examined how and if allergies can be prevented and symptoms lessened.[57] Using probiotics seems like a no-brainer—introducing beneficial microbes into the gut would modulate immune reactions and aid digestion. So far, however, the most convincing evidence comes from introducing probiotics early on in high-risk infants to help prevent or eliminate eczema (allergic dermatitis)—which is often the first sign of allergies. Research is still unclear whether probiotics, in general, affect the incidence of food allergies. But providing your belly with beneficial gut microbes through probiotics balances T cell reactions and still benefits your overall health.

---

allergens, but your doctor can check you for other specific allergies using skin or blood tests. Your personal experience, however, is still what matters most. Lab tests aren't 100 percent foolproof in assessing food reactions.

Environmental Airborne Allergies and Hay Fever

These can be triggered by pollens, weeds, dust, animals, and grasses (not necessarily just hay or ragweed). What you put in your mouth also matters and can affect your overall allergy state. The elimination diet in Chapter 4 can help reduce reactions caused by "oral allergy syndrome" (or pollen-food syndrome). (See "Oral Allergy Syndrome" on page 224) It's worthwhile to try the elimination diet to see if it lowers your environmental reactions, even if there's no clear evidence that certain foods are allergenic for you. In clinical practice, a diet cleanup lowers and often eliminates "hay fever" symptoms.

Here are some vitamins and supplements that are helpful for people with environmental allergies and hay fever:

- **QUERCETIN.** 250 to 500 mg three times daily. Food sources of quercetin, which has antihistamine effects, include red grapes (these also contain resveratrol, a polyphenol with anti-inflammatory and cardioprotective effects), berries, apples, and red onions, so eating these foods may reduce allergies.
- **VITAMIN C.** 500 to 1,000 mg three times daily.

- **VITAMIN D.** 2,000 to 5,000 IU daily.

- **NETTLE LEAF.** Stinging nettle (*Urtica dioica*) has a long history of use with seasonal allergies. Take 150 to 300 mg twice daily.

- **BUTTERBUR** (*Petasites hybridus*), 50 to 75 mg twice daily, may relieve swelling and other inflammatory symptoms of allergic rhinitis (hay fever).[58] Butterbur preparations can contain harmful chemicals called pyrrolizidine alkaloids (PAs), so make sure that any butterbur products you purchase are certified and labeled "PA free."

Other self-care practices may ease hay fever symptoms, allergies, and sinus congestion.

IMAGERY FOR ALLERGIES

As with any imagery exercise, be in a safe, peaceful place where you won't be disturbed for at least 15 minutes. Have your journal handy, plus colored pencils or markers, too, if you'd like.

Begin by relaxing. Humming and singing are easy ways to relax and achieve an inner calm, as is Kirtan Kriya meditation—or even just a quick walk. Then close your eyes, breathe deeply, and feel your body. You can continue singing or humming for a few more minutes if you'd like. Now breathe in and sigh, letting out any tension in your mind and body as you exhale. Imagine your body as a transparent container filled with trillions of glimmering cells and twinkling molecules. To protect this inner space, imagine an invisible cloak or powerful shield wrapped around you. It fits just like your skin, so that whenever your shield is bombarded with pollens, irritating scents, or irritating people, it easily repels that negative energy. Your invisible shield protects you from anything that can cause you harm or put you in danger. Your boundaries are impenetrable. You are safe inside this cocoon. See if you can actually feel or sense your energy emitting this protective layer around you. It's always there, and you can take a few moments every day to check it and reinforce any weak points. Touch your thumbs and first fingers together to hold the shield strong. You can do this a few times a day.

Slowly move your fingers and thumbs apart, feel your breath, and thank your cells and molecules for taking such good care of you. Then go about your day, free from allergies and protected against harmful energies.

- Try saline nasal irrigation with salt and sterile water.

- Wash your bed linens regularly in hot water to remove any dust mites or pet dander that can contribute to household allergies.

- Use a vacuum or an air purifier with a HEPA filter, especially in your bedroom.

Eczema

Eczema is an allergic condition that results in a persistent, itchy, red, and inflamed skin rash, which is exacerbated by dry air, food and environmental allergens, and stress. Gut sensitivity can make eczema worse. Since so many factors can aggravate it, calm your eczema by integrating the programs for allergy, inflammation, and infection protection, and use a quality moisturizer to ease discomfort. The gut health program (see page 205) may also be beneficial, while the elimination diet may assist in unearthing unknown food triggers.

Also, remove bad fats (trans and saturated fats) from your diet. Include only good oils, and take additional omega-3 oils as both fish oil and flaxseed oil if those are tolerated. A higher dosage may be needed to get results, so try two or three capsules two or three times daily. Add vitamins A, C, D, and quercetin. Research shows that a topical licorice gel may prevent and alleviate eczema outbreaks.[59]

Asthma

Asthma is an inflammatory and allergic condition, so both the Cool Down and the general and seasonal allergies programs can help. Typically, people who have asthma also have at least one allergy, so avoid foods and environmental allergens that have caused a reaction. The elimination diet and I-PEP nutrition program can help, too. Respiratory infections will make asthma much worse, so it's important to stay healthy.

When an asthma attack occurs, the airway tightens. Magnesium, butterbur, and perilla seed oil capsules can help relax airway muscles and facilitate better breathing. Vitamin C and quercetin may lower histamine reactions and reduce asthma symptoms.

Butterbur, in particular, shows a lot of promise when taken on a regular basis. Eighty patients with asthma took an extract of butterbur for 2 months, and during that time, the number, duration, and severity of their asthma attacks decreased while lung functions improved. Almost half of the patients were able to reduce their amounts of conventional asthma medications.[60]

You can learn breathing and relaxation exercises to ease the tightening in your throat and calm the body overall. Studies have shown that adding acupuncture and guided imagery with meditation—once weekly, along with weekly group support sessions—to conventional medical management of asthma can result in fewer hospitalized days, fewer emergency room visits, and reduced usage of corticosteroids.[61] And remember that emotional disclosure can help to improve lung function, and yoga may also lessen asthmatic inflammation.[62]

Wheat Allergy, Gluten Sensitivity, and Celiac Disease

The treatment is simple: Avoid wheat and gluten products, which means anything containing wheat, rye, or barley. Those with celiac disease must follow strict gluten-free diets or risk serious complications, whereas people with mild sensitivities may

---

THE ROOT OF THE PROBLEM

Diseases don't exist in bubbles. Many factors feed our illnesses, including the inner workings and imbalances in our bodies. This is especially true for autoimmune illnesses. A sensible approach would be to follow the trails of bread crumbs leading to the primary culprits. Physicians trained in integrative and functional medicine know how to look for these inner imbalances and determine which factors need to be fixed even though they might not know the root or cause of the illness. For autoimmune conditions, it makes sense to explore some of the following potential factors with your practitioner:

- Dietary and nutrient deficiencies
- Gut microbial imbalances and leaky gut syndrome
- Other infectious issues, such as in the teeth or sinuses
- Food immune and allergy reactions, such as to gluten and dairy
- Environmental toxins, including metals like mercury and lead
- Stress
- Hormonal imbalances

Looking closely into these areas, finding the red flags, and correcting these issues can help put you on the road to recovery.

---

still eat small amounts of wheat cautiously. These allergies are a fairly recent phenomenon, a result of the proliferation of processed foods. Food manufacturers pump gluten into virtually everything to add protein and improve texture, so we're consuming a lot more gluten than we should. That's why we encourage you to limit your gluten intake and eat a wider variety of foods that are naturally gluten free. Typically, eating less gluten means consuming less processed food overall.

Be aware that a gluten-free stamp on the package doesn't mean a product is necessarily healthy. There are a lot of processed gluten-free products that contain high-calorie carbohydrate ingredients (other grain flours and sweeteners) to appeal to people as bread substitutes. "Gluten free" has become a multibillion-dollar business.

Ideally, the majority of your diet should be made up of fresh, minimally processed foods. Barring any serious gluten intolerance, feel free to eat your quinoa patty on a whole grain bun once in a while.

Ultimate Immunity Approaches for Autoimmune Disease

If you've been diagnosed with an autoimmune condition, explore the Cool Down Program for at least a few weeks, then see if you notice any improvements. Remember that all hyperactive immune states—including autoimmune disease—are associated with inflammation. This inflammation can be caused by antibodies attaching to some of your own cells and tissues, or it can be caused by chemical signals from rowdy and hyperactive T cells. Regardless of the cells or molecules inflicting the damage, inflammation is still the primary culprit. Cooling it down can certainly improve your well-being, so take advantage of the Cool Down plan.

And check your gut. Do you have belly pain, gas, bloating, constipation, diarrhea, or irregularity? If any of these are common, start improving your gut and immune health with probiotics, and see a practitioner who can help you with more personalized gastrointestinal care. However, be aware that even though probiotics are generally helpful for most of the population, the many microbes within a particular probiotic product could actually stimulate your immune response[63] in a way that is not favorable for an autoimmune disease. A knowledgeable practitioner can direct you to those probiotics that will balance your immune cells in the right direction.

There are more than 100 autoimmune conditions—far too many to discuss here.

But we'll look at some of the more common ones for which we can offer evidence-based solutions. It's not a cure, but following these programs could potentially improve your outcome and make relapses less frequent. Healing is often an individual experience, and what works for one person may not work for another with the same diagnosis.

Autoimmune illnesses tend to be chronic, with cyclic remissions and flare-ups; here you'll find solutions to prolong the duration of your symptom-free remissions. Remember, the goal of healing is balancing the body as well as the mind, mood, and spirit. Lifestyle changes begin with a plan and a firm commitment. Begin with the Cool Down Program for inflammation and take it 1 week at a time. Give the program 3 weeks—at the end of 21 days, you should feel some improvement. If not, or even if you do feel improvement, you might want to try some of the following ideas.

Supplements

These supplements have been shown to help with certain general and/or specific autoimmune issues. They're safe and worth a try.

VITAMIN D is a potent immune regulator. Unfortunately, many people have low laboratory blood levels of vitamin D, which is associated with inflammation and increased risk for autoimmune illnesses. A large study of almost 1,000 adults over age 60 living in Ireland revealed a strong link between low vitamin D status and blood markers of inflammation.[64] A sweeping review of research published from 1973 to 2011 concluded that there is a correlation between low levels of vitamin D and a greater risk for autoimmune illnesses.[65] In addition, individuals who had an autoimmune illness coupled with low vitamin D endured far worse symptoms than people with normal levels. In another study, infants at risk for type 1 diabetes who were given vitamin D supplements were less likely to develop the disease[66] than those who weren't given the supplement. Now numerous studies are being developed on specific autoimmune illnesses and the effects of vitamin D. Taking a simple vitamin D supplement can certainly help lessen autoimmunity.

OMEGA-3 FATTY ACIDS,[67] especially those rich in EPA and DHA (in food or supplements), reduce inflammation. In studies, people with rheumatoid arthritis who took fish oil[68] had less joint pain and morning stiffness and could lower the amount of NSAIDs (pain pills) they were taking. Joint pain caused by other conditions, such as inflammatory bowel disease,[69] was also lessened. *Warning:* Do not take more than 3 grams of fish oil a day.

CURCUMIN is a powerful anti-inflammatory substance with promise as an anti-arthritic. Forty-five patients with active rheumatoid arthritis were randomly selected to receive curcumin (500 mg), conventional drug treatment with diclofenac sodium, or both. The curcumin alone group showed the greatest improvement.[70] Once again, we see evidence that curcumin is not only helpful with arthritis but also may improve any inflammatory condition.

PEONY GLUCOSIDES EXTRACTS from the white peony root have generated a lot of positive research for bringing overactive immune systems back into balance. Peony extracts contain many different molecules, the most predominant of which—paeoniflorin—is thought to be responsible for normalizing out-of-control immune responses.[71] Peony glucosides reduced inflammatory cytokines in lab animals with excessive inflammation like arthritis,[72] and animals that were immunosuppressed (similar to being on steroids) experienced enhanced immune responses. This suggests that people with an autoimmune disease would benefit from both peony's immune-suppressing activity and its enhancing activity.

Most drugs and treatments for autoimmune illnesses suppress immune function; after all, the illness is from too much activity. When immune functions are suppressed, however, you have a greater risk for more infections. If the research holds up to scrutiny, peony glucosides may become a valuable addition to the treatment of autoimmune illnesses.[73] In clinical trials, they have been found to be effective in treating rheumatoid arthritis,[74] lupus, Sjögren's syndrome, and psoriasis.

Mind-Body Practices

Patients diagnosed with a lifelong chronic illness may experience stress, depression, and pessimism.[75] Although you'll find lots of stress-reducing and calming strategies in this book, sometimes it's useful to talk with a professional or join a group of people challenged by similar illnesses. Having support outside your family gives you an opportunity to freely express your fears and discuss your problems. Don't carry the burden alone. Take charge, find additional support, and do the right things for yourself. When you take a proactive stance, your illness may seem to be less of a burden and more like another one of life's challenges. Here are some effective mind-body strategies.

EMOTIONAL DISCLOSURE WRITING. (See Chapter 5 for details.) This practice can lead to improved and more balanced immune health. In studies, it led to improved overall immune health for college students and Holocaust survivors; improved lung function in people with allergic asthma; and lessened joint pain in people with rheumatoid arthritis.[76] People with psoriasis stayed in remission longer after UVB phototherapy when they used emotional disclosure writing.

IMAGERY FOR IMPROVED AUTOIMMUNE HEALTH. Try this exercise: Make yourself comfortable, and know that whatever you imagine will do you no harm and will likely offer you comfort and benefits. Take some deep breaths and feel the gratitude of your whole body come alive. Simply enjoy the inner peace that comes with gratitude. Then close your eyes and journey inside, scanning and feeling all of your body. Now visualize your immune cells, and give them the message and abilities to recognize every part of your body as you. Any immune cell that mistakenly recognizes your cells, tissues, or proteins as alien simply dies, dissolves, and disappears. Watch as these dissolving cells leave your body, and sense their energy leaving your mind.

Take a moment to feel relief, knowing that the damaging, misguided cells are no longer with you. An image or a word may even come to your mind to anchor this moment. Sense and see in your mind that all your damaged tissues are being repaired to their healthy whole states. Visualize yourself doing activities you've been unable to do in the past because of the illness. See yourself whole and fully healed. Take some time to really feel this in your body, anchoring the sensations and memory with the touch of your thumbs to your first fingers. Breathe in, relaxed and peaceful, knowing you can repeat this imagery practice as often as you'd like.

Strategies for Specific Autoimmune Illnesses

You know by now that following the I-PEP eating program, plus the Cool Down Program, is beneficial. Now let's take a closer look at other steps you can take to improve symptoms related to your specific autoimmune condition.

Autoimmune Thyroiditis (Hashimoto's)

In this condition, the thyroid often becomes underactive, so people with the disease benefit from taking a combination of T4 (thyroxine) and T3 (triiodothyronine), the body's primary thyroid hormones. Most physicians prescribe only the T4 component, which your body needs to convert to the more active T3. This process requires selenium and zinc, so adding these nutrients can be helpful in restoring normal thyroid function. In fact, using nutritional treatment in combination with both T3 and T4 hormones can alleviate many hypothyroid symptoms, including fatigue and sluggishness, coldness, dry skin, difficulty losing weight, and depression.

Psoriasis

If you're plagued with psoriasis, think oils, oils, and more oils. Include in your diet healthy omega-3 oils from fish and flaxseed oil and omega-9 from olive oil. You can even add omega-7 oil, which comes from the sea buckthorn plant. Taking a combination of these oils is a great place to start. Vitamins D and A can also support skin healing.

In some cases, psoriasis may have microbial (bacteria and yeast) triggers, so some people benefit from antifungal medicines. Other factors that set off psoriasis outbreaks include stress, cold weather, alcohol, smoking, and some medications, including lithium, beta-blockers, and antimalarial drugs. In addition, some people with psoriasis are very sensitive to chemicals and may have allergies to anything that contacts their skin, like laundry detergents, soaps, perfumes, and metals; they may also experience foods allergies. Gut health, as usual, is another factor to consider.

Light therapy, particularly UVB light,[77] may be useful. In one study, people with psoriasis who did the emotional disclosure writing exercise immediately after light therapy stayed in remission longer.[78] Creams containing vitamins D and A, such as calcipotriene and tretinoin (Retin-A), may also be useful. Other natural approaches include supplementing vitamins A and D (5,000 to 10,000 IU each daily) and fish or mixed oils with EPA and DHA (two capsules three times daily, not to exceed 3,000 mg daily). Of course, include healthy oils in your diet from fatty fish like salmon, sardines, and mackerel.

Inflammatory Bowel Disease (IBD)

Inflammatory bowel disease is a group of conditions affecting the colon and small intestine. The two primary conditions are ulcerative colitis and Crohn's disease. Both can cause pain, diarrhea, and bloody stools. Inflammation is the key, so the Cool Down Program is your first step. Pathogenic gut microbes from bacteria, yeasts, and parasites can cause an underlying infection. Food reactions may play a part, so an elimination diet is an excellent starting point. Learning to manage stress is especially important for people with IBD. As possibly a related issue, many people also suffer from IBS (irritable bowel syndrome, which is often a diagnosis of exclusion—that's what happens when the doctor didn't find an exact cause of digestive complaints of cramps and pains, constipation, or diarrhea). It's likely that food reactions and abnormal gut microbes play a role in both IBD and IBS. People diagnosed with IBS find that their symptoms are lessened with mindfulness meditation.[79] We suggest that this process of stress reduction also helps the symptoms of IBD.

Boswellia extract has been shown to reduce inflammatory molecules, which appear to play a role in IBD attacks. In two separate studies, IBD patients taking 300 to 350 mg of boswellia three times daily had as good or better improvement compared to those taking common sulfa drugs.[80]

Type 1 Diabetes

Young people diagnosed with type 1 diabetes who use insulin must pay close and constant attention to their blood sugar levels and care for their health impeccably to manage their disease. They must be acutely aware of their diet and how exercise affects their blood sugar levels, and they must know how to manage their stress. One lapse in judgment for people with type 1 diabetes can cause their health to go downhill quickly and may even lead to hospitalization. On the other hand, those who engage in attentive self-care often do quite well over their lifetimes—the length of which is often determined by their behaviors.

The Cool Down Program outlines many healthy lifestyle behaviors. Anyone with diabetes, even the more common type 2, can add years and better health to their lives if they add the Cool Down plan to their diabetes program. Living with a chronic lifelong illness is certainly stressful, so dealing with their stress and emotions is essential for those with diabetes.

Arthritis

Rheumatoid arthritis (RA) is a chronic autoimmune disease characterized by inflammation of the joints. It often leads to significant pain and disability. The commonly used drug therapies are not always effective and have significant side effects, especially when used long term. The most common form of arthritis, osteoarthritis (OA), may also be an autoimmune illness, at least in part.[81] Studies have shown that taking

1,500 mg of glucosamine sulfate daily for 12 weeks significantly reduced pain, improved functioning, and lessened the need for painkillers in patients with OA of the knee. We can add glucosamine sulfate[82] to our list of supplements that likely offer some benefit to people with RA or OA.

Studies show that psychological-based interventions can be helpful for the treatment of RA.[83] Both cognitive- and disclosure-based therapies resulted in less pain, better moods, and better coping for RA patients. We use the rationale and findings from these studies on RA to suggest that psychological-based interventions be included as part of an integrative healing program for anyone with an autoimmune condition.

Also, if you have any form of arthritis, consider supplements containing curcumin and boswellia to decrease pain and swelling while increasing your mobility.[84]

Multiple Sclerosis (MS)

MS is a chronic, neurological autoimmune disorder with emotional, cognitive, and physical consequences.[85] Patients can experience a wide range of symptoms, including impaired mobility, sensory disturbances, chronic pain, fatigue, bladder and bowel dysfunction, depression, and cognitive impairment. Patients also report high levels of stress. In a survey of more than 1,000 MS patients, one-third had used mind-body modalities and reported a highly perceived benefit.[86] Self-reporting is a common assessment technique in mind-body clinical studies: It asks people to indicate if they felt better, if they perceived or sensed that their symptoms improved, with less pain or other complaints—all subjective experiences.

If you have MS, lower your stress; keep a positive attitude; eat a nourishing, well-balanced diet; and do simple energy exercises like tai chi, qigong, and yoga. A review of 11 mind-body studies of patients with MS revealed four helpful modalities: yoga, mindfulness, relaxation, and biofeedback.[87] While research regarding any of these immune illnesses is still limited, we do know that mind-body programs alleviate stress and can be a useful part of home self-care.

Many people with MS also report improvement with a vegetarian or vegan diet that includes quality oils and supplementation with omega-3s and evening primrose oil, which contains linolenic acid. Cannabis (marijuana) treatment often helps with spasticity and relaxation.

Connective Tissue Disorders (Lupus, Scleroderma, Sjögren's Syndrome, and Polyarteritis Nodosa)

These complicated multisystem diseases can involve the skin, kidneys, and blood vessels as well as other organs. Recent clinical trials indicate that supplements of vitamin D, omega-3 fatty acids, N-acetyl cysteine, and turmeric show promise for reducing lupus activity. In addition, mind-body approaches, such as cognitive behavioral therapy and counseling, may improve mood and quality of life for those with lupus.[88] All connective tissue disorders make the skin especially sensitive to sun exposure, so wear a hat and use natural sunblock when staying outside.

Note: Today, women with lupus can safely have children, but it's important to consult with your doctor before getting pregnant to discuss your medications as well as potential risks and complications.

THE TAKEAWAY

You've come a long way on your journey to make healthy changes to your body, mind, and life. Like every journey, it's one step at a time. We've provided you with ideas that are based in science and proven in practice, but we don't expect you to try them all. All we ask is that you choose a few that sound appealing and make a commitment to yourself. Select the ideas that make the most sense and feel the best to you. Then stick with them.

See this as an adventure in discovery that will take you to a good life and a healthier balanced immune system where you can enjoy Ultimate Immunity.

CHAPTER 8

Recipes *for* Ultimate Immunity

Many or all of these dishes could be enjoyed at any mealtime. They are especially good for starting the day. Also, some of these recipes are for only one or two people, since that's a more common arrangement for breakfast. Getting a good breakfast is a healthy way to start your day.

HEARTY OATMEAL

PREP TIME: 5 MINUTES ▓ TOTAL TIME: 35 MINUTES ▓ MAKES 2 SERVINGS

$1/2$ cup steel-cut oats (not instant or quick)

$1^1/2$ cups almond or oat milk or water, or a mixture

Dash of sea salt

$1/2$ teaspoon ground cinnamon

$1/4$–$1/2$ teaspoon fresh ginger, peeled and grated

$1/2$ cup fresh or frozen blueberries

$1/4$ cup walnuts

1 tablespoon sweetener—honey, pure maple syrup, blackstrap molasses, or firmly packed brown sugar

In a small saucepan, combine the oats, milk or water, salt, and cinnamon. Bring to a boil, then reduce the heat to medium-low. Cook, stirring occasionally, for 25 to 30 minutes, or until the oats are soft and have absorbed the liquid.

Remove the saucepan from the heat and stir in the ginger, blueberries, nuts, and sweetener.

VARIATIONS:

- **Vary the fruit.** Add 1 sliced banana, 1 chopped apple, or $1/2$ cup dried cranberries or chopped dried apricots, or other fresh fruit in season.
- **Go nutty.** Add $1/4$ cup sunflower seeds or chopped almonds or 2 tablespoons peanut butter or almond butter.

NUTRITION INFORMATION (PER SERVING)
322 calories, 9 g protein, 49 g carbohydrates, 13 g total fat, 1 g saturated fat, 7 g fiber, 163 mg sodium

NICE RICE

PREP TIME: 5 MINUTES ■ TOTAL TIME: 10 MINUTES ■ MAKES 4 SERVINGS

$^3/_4$ cup apple juice or water

$^1/_2$ cup raisins

1 tablespoon grated lemon peel

1 cinnamon stick or $^1/_4$ teaspoon ground cinnamon

2–2$^1/_2$ cups cooked rice or oatmeal

$^1/_4$ cup lightly toasted and coarsely chopped walnuts or almonds

In a medium saucepan, bring the apple juice or water, raisins, lemon peel, and cinnamon to a boil. Reduce the heat and simmer for 3 minutes, or until the raisins are plump. Add the rice and simmer for 2 minutes.

Remove the saucepan from the heat and add the nuts. Remove the cinnamon stick (if used) before serving.

NUTRITION INFORMATION (PER SERVING)
234 calories, 4 g protein, 44 g carbohydrates, 6 g total fat, 0.5 g saturated fat, 3 g fiber, 5 mg sodium

PROBOWL

PREP TIME: 5 MINUTES ■ TOTAL TIME: 5 MINUTES ■ MAKES 1 SERVING

$^1/_2$–1 cup 0% Greek yogurt with live cultures

$^1/_2$ cup blueberries

2 tablespoons ground flaxseeds (fresh or refrigerated)

$^1/_4$ cup walnuts or pumpkin seeds

In a bowl, mix the yogurt, blueberries, flaxseeds, and walnuts or pumpkin seeds. Stir well and enjoy.

VARIATIONS:

- Add grated ginger or ground cinnamon for heat and flavor.
- Add your choice of seasonal fruits.
- Make a smoothie: Combine the ingredients in a blender or food processor with $^1/_2$ cup almond milk (or other nondairy milk, such as rice, oat, hazelnut, or hemp).

NUTRITION INFORMATION (PER SERVING)
353 calories, 17 g protein, 23 g carbohydrates, 23 g total fat, 2 g saturated fat, 8 g fiber, 47 mg sodium

SCRAMBLED TOFU WITH TURMERIC

PREP TIME: 15 MINUTES ■ TOTAL TIME: 30 MINUTES ■ MAKES 4 SERVINGS

Lighter than eggs and with less fat.

14 ounces extra-firm tofu

1 tablespoon light miso

2 tablespoons toasted sesame oil, divided

1 cup sliced mushrooms

2 scallions, including the greens, thinly sliced

¼ cup finely chopped black olives

2 medium tomatoes, seeded and chopped

2 teaspoons ground turmeric

¼ teaspoon cayenne pepper

Sea salt, soy sauce, or Bragg Liquid Amino

¼ cup fresh parsley or cilantro, finely chopped

In a medium bowl, combine the tofu, miso, and 1 tablespoon of the oil. Mash together thoroughly.

Heat the remaining 1 tablespoon oil in a large skillet over medium-high heat. Add the mushrooms and cook for 2 minutes. Add the scallions and cook for 3 minutes, or until the whites of the scallions are translucent and limp and the mushrooms begin to brown.

Add the tofu mixture, olives, tomatoes, and turmeric. Stir together well, cover, and simmer over low heat for 5 minutes. Season to taste with the cayenne pepper and sea salt, soy sauce, or liquid aminos. Add the parsley or cilantro and serve.

VARIATIONS:

- Add or substitute onion and garlic, carrot (finely chopped or grated), and celery slices.
- Change flavorings and spices with nutritional yeast, thyme or rosemary, and/ or dill.
- For a spicy, more egg-colored scrambled tofu, add ½ teaspoon curry powder or salsa as desired after cooking.
- Mix and mash the tofu with 2 hard-cooked eggs for even better nourishment from both. Or scramble the eggs with the tofu.

NUTRITION INFORMATION (PER SERVING)
166 calories, 12 g protein, 8 g carbohydrates, 10 g total fat, 1.5 g saturated fat, 3 g fiber, 282 mg sodium

VEGGIE FRITTATA

2 tablespoons salted or unsalted butter or olive oil

1 onion, diced

2–3 cloves garlic, chopped or minced

1 cup sliced mixed mushrooms

$1/_2$ cup chopped broccoli

2 zucchini, sliced

8 eggs, beaten and mixed with 3 tablespoons water

$1/_4$ teaspoon sea salt

1 teaspoon chopped fresh rosemary or $1/_2$ teaspoon ground dry

Heat the butter or oil in a large skillet. Add the onion and garlic and cook for 4 minutes, or until translucent. Add the mushrooms and cook for 2 minutes, then add the broccoli and gently cook until the vegetables are soft. Add the zucchini and cook for a minute or so.

In a medium bowl, combine the eggs and water with the salt and rosemary. Pour over the veggie mixture.

Cover the skillet. Reduce the heat to medium-low and cook on the stove top until the eggs are set. Alternatively, place the skillet in a preheated 350°F oven and bake for 10 to 15 minutes.

VARIATIONS:

- Top with $1/_2$ cup shredded Cheddar cheese or feta cheese.
- Add 1 cup chopped tomatoes.
- Spice it up with cayenne pepper or salsa.
- Make this scramble by stir-frying the vegetables, then adding the eggs and stirring regularly until done.
- Add smoked salmon with the eggs for a protein-rich frittata or scramble.

NUTRITION INFORMATION (PER SERVING)

230 calories, 15 g protein, 8 g carbohydrates, 16 g total fat, 7 g saturated fat, 2 g fiber, 304 mg sodium

TOASTED OAT MUESLI

PREP TIME: 5 MINUTES ▇ TOTAL TIME: 55 MINUTES
▇ MAKES 22 (¹/₂ CUP) SERVINGS

Top a serving of this delicious breakfast with soy milk or with coconut or soy yogurt and ground flaxseeds.

- 1¹/₄ cups unsalted, raw, sliced natural almonds
- 6 cups old-fashioned oats, preferably thick cut
- 1 package (7 ounces) dried fruit bits

- 1 cup toasted wheat germ
- ¹/₂ cup unsalted raw pumpkin seeds
- ¹/₂ cup unsalted raw sunflower seeds

Preheat the oven to 325°F.

Spread the almonds in a small baking pan. Spread the oats on a jelly roll pan or large baking sheet. Bake, stirring often, until the almonds are toasted (20 to 25 minutes) and the oats are lightly browned (30 to 35 minutes). Transfer the oats and almonds to a large bowl and cool completely.

Add the fruit bits, wheat germ, and seeds. Toss to combine. Store in an airtight container.

NUTRITION INFORMATION (PER SERVING)
233 calories, 8 g protein, 26 g carbohydrates, 11 g total fat, 1 g saturated fat, 5 g fiber, 11 mg sodium

It's always nice to have some simple recipes to start a meal or add to your main course, to perk up your appetite or fill you up. Try a tasty dip with cut-up vegetables like celery, carrots, or cucumbers or spread on rice crackers.

ZUCCHINI AND SWEET POTATO ROUNDS

PREP TIME: 5 MINUTES ■ TOTAL TIME: 30 MINUTES ■ MAKES 4 SERVINGS

2 medium zucchini, sliced into $1/4$" rounds

2 sweet potatoes, sliced into $1/4$" rounds

2 tablespoons extra virgin olive oil

$1/4$ teaspoon sea salt

$1/2$ cup freshly grated Parmesan cheese or Asiago cheese (optional)

Preheat the oven to 400°F. Coat a baking sheet with oil or cooking spray.

In a medium bowl, toss the zucchini and potatoes with the oil. Add the salt. Stir in the cheese, if using, making sure each piece of vegetable is covered.

Spread the vegetables in a single layer on the baking sheet. Bake for 25 to 35 minutes, or until tender-crisp.

NUTRITION INFORMATION (PER SERVING)
130 calories, 2 g protein, 15 g carbohydrates, 7 g total fat, 1 g saturated fat, 3 g fiber, 141 mg sodium

GUACAMOLE

PREP TIME: 10 MINUTES ▦ TOTAL TIME: 10 MINUTES ▦ MAKES 4 SERVINGS

2–4 cloves garlic (more or less
    as you like)

$^1/_2$ teaspoon sea salt

2 medium avocados

1 small red onion, finely chopped

$^1/_4$ cup chopped cilantro

2–3 tablespoons fresh lemon juice

$^1/_2$ teaspoon chili powder

$^1/_8$ teaspoon cayenne pepper (more
    or less as you like)

Mince the garlic and sprinkle with the salt, then transfer to a bowl. Add the avocados and mash with a fork to the desired consistency. Add the onion, cilantro, lemon juice, chili powder, and cayenne pepper and mix to combine.

Serve with fresh veggies or corn chips.

NUTRITION INFORMATION (PER SERVING)
126 calories, 2 g protein, 9 g carbohydrates, 11 g total fat, 1.5 g saturated fat, 5 g fiber, 204 mg sodium

HUMMUS SPREAD OR DIP

PREP TIME: 5 MINUTES ▦ TOTAL TIME: 10 MINUTES ▦ MAKES 8 SERVINGS

1–2 cloves garlic (more or less
    as you like)

1 can (15 ounces) organic
    chickpeas, rinsed and drained

$^1/_3$–$^1/_2$ cup tahini

$^1/_2$ cup water

$^1/_4$ cup fresh lemon juice or lime
    juice

1 teaspoon sea salt

$^1/_2$–1 teaspoon ground cumin

3 tablespoons extra virgin olive oil

In a food processor or blender, pulse the garlic until chopped. Add the chickpeas and tahini and combine. Then add the water, lemon or lime juice, salt, cumin, and oil and process or blend until smooth. You may need to add more water, juice, or oil to reach the desired consistency and taste.

Serve with carrot and celery sticks, blue corn tortilla chips, or small rice crackers.

NUTRITION INFORMATION (PER SERVING)
140 calories, 4 g protein, 8 g carbohydrates, 11 g total fat, 1.5 g saturated fat, 2 g fiber, 297 mg sodium

TOMATO SALSA

PREP TIME: 10 MINUTES ■ **TOTAL TIME: 10 MINUTES** ■ **MAKES 3–4 CUPS (AS A DIP) OR 8 SERVINGS**

3 cups chopped ripe tomatoes

1 small yellow or red onion, chopped

1 small jalapeño or other chile pepper, seeded and finely chopped (wear plastic gloves when handling), or $1/4$–$1/2$ cup chopped bell pepper (for a milder salsa)

2 cloves garlic (more if you like), minced

$1/2$ teaspoon chili powder or $1/4$ teaspoon cayenne pepper

2 teaspoons fresh lemon juice or lime juice

$1/4$ teaspoon sea salt

2 tablespoons chopped cilantro (optional)

$1/4$–$1/2$ teaspoon ground cumin (optional)

1–2 sprigs fresh oregano, chopped, or $1/2$ teaspoon dried (optional)

In a large bowl, mix the tomatoes, onion, chile or bell pepper, garlic, chili powder or cayenne pepper, lemon or lime juice, and salt. Add the cilantro, cumin, and oregano, if using. For a creamier salsa, put the mixture in a blender or food processor and pulse.

Serve with corn chips, other chips, or veggie strips.

NUTRITION INFORMATION (PER SERVING)
14 calories, 1 g protein, 3 g carbohydrates, 0 g total fat, 0 g saturated fat, 1 g fiber, 62 mg sodium

BRUSCHETTA TOPPINGS

PREP TIME: 10 MINUTES ■ TOTAL TIME: 10 MINUTES ■ MAKES 12 SERVINGS

Bruschetta is thinly sliced, grilled or toasted bread rubbed with olive oil and garlic, then topped with one of the spreads. For a gluten-free version, use gluten-free bread, thin rice crackers, or corn tortillas for the base.

OLIVE HERB SPREAD

1 cup chopped, pitted black or green olives

1 cup chopped, pitted kalamata olives

2 tablespoons chopped cilantro

2 cloves garlic

3 tablespoons chopped fresh mint

2 tablespoons balsamic vinegar or red wine vinegar

1 tablespoon rinsed capers

5 tablespoons extra virgin olive oil

In a food processor, combine the olives, cilantro, garlic, mint, vinegar, and capers and process, slowly adding the oil until you have a finely chopped or chunky paste. Spoon onto the bruschetta. The spread will keep for a few weeks refrigerated.

NUTRITION INFORMATION (PER SERVING)
109 calories, 0 g protein, 2 g carbohydrates, 11 g total fat, 1 g saturated fat, 0 g fiber, 347 mg sodium

TOMATO, BASIL, AND MOZZARELLA STACKS

2 large Roma tomatoes, sliced

12 ounces fresh mozzarella, sliced

1 cup fresh basil leaves

Place 1 tomato slice, 1 cheese slice, and 1 or 2 leaves of basil on each piece of bruschetta.

NUTRITION INFORMATION (PER SERVING)
78 calories, 5 g protein, 1 g carbohydrates, 6 g total fat, 4 g saturated fat, 0 g fiber, 87 mg sodium

Salads are a high priority for a healthy diet and especially for I-PEP. Fresh greens in particular can be eaten two or three times daily for the good fiber and nutrients they contain. Salads keep us going inside and out, providing some bulk without many calories—especially important if you want to keep your weight down and energy up. Create some meals with a salad as the main course, like a big mixed green salad with vegetables and some avocado, seeds, and/or legumes, all wrapped in a nice warm organic corn tortilla with a bit of dressing or salsa or the Avocado Dressing on page 282. Try growing some of your own greens and fresh herbs.

QUINOA TABBOULEH

PREP TIME: 15 MINUTES ■ TOTAL TIME: 20 MINUTES ■ MAKES 4 SERVINGS

$1/2$ cup quinoa, rinsed well

$1/2$ teaspoon salt, divided

3 cups water, chicken stock, or vegetable stock

2 cloves garlic, minced

$1/2$ cup fresh lemon juice

$1/2$ cup olive oil

2 Persian cucumbers, finely chopped

$1/2$ pint cherry tomatoes, halved

$2/3$ cup chopped fresh flat-leaf parsley

$2/3$ cup chopped fresh mint

Ground black pepper

In a medium saucepan, bring the quinoa, $1/4$ teaspoon of the salt, and the water or stock to a boil. Reduce the heat to medium-low, cover, and simmer for 10 minutes. Turn off the heat and let sit, covered, for another 5 minutes. When the quinoa is done, each grain displays a little thread. Drain and fluff.

In a small bowl, whisk together the garlic, lemon juice, oil, and the remaining $1/4$ teaspoon salt. Pour the dressing over the hot or cooled quinoa.

Let cool, then mix in the cucumbers, tomatoes, parsley, and mint. Season with black pepper and more salt, if desired.

VARIATION:

Use bulgur in place of the quinoa.

NUTRITION INFORMATION (PER SERVING)
212 calories, 6 g protein, 24 g carbohydrates, 11 g total fat, 1.5 g saturated fat, 4 g fiber, 177 mg sodium

MIXED GREENS SALAD

PREP TIME: 10 MINUTES ■ **TOTAL TIME: 10 MINUTES** ■ **MAKES 4 SERVINGS**

Serve this with our simple dressing or use a salad dressing of your choice.

SALAD

- 3 cups mixed lettuces, such as red or green leaf, romaine, or butter, washed and dried
- 1 cup shredded red, green, or savoy cabbage, washed and dried
- 1 cup baby spinach leaves, stems removed
- $1/2$ cup diced yellow, green, or red bell pepper
- 3 carrots, sliced or grated
- $1/2$ cup wiped and sliced button mushrooms
- 3 scallions, sliced (optional)
- 1 avocado, sliced
- $1/4$ cup alfalfa sprouts
- $1/2$ cup bean sprouts (such as mung), green peas, chickpeas, azuki beans, or microgreens
- $1/2$ cup sunflower seeds

SIMPLE DRESSING

- 3 tablespoons fresh lemon juice or lime juice
- $1/2$ cup olive oil
- $1/4$ teaspoon sea salt
- 1–2 cloves garlic, minced
- $1/4$ teaspoon ground black pepper (optional)

To make the salad: In a large bowl, combine the lettuces, cabbage, spinach, bell pepper, carrots, mushrooms, scallions, avocado, sprouts, and seeds.

To make the simple dressing: In a small bowl, combine the lemon or lime juice, oil, salt, garlic, and pepper, if using. Drizzle over the salad.

VARIATIONS:

- Add 1–2 roasted chicken breasts, sliced.
- Add 1–2 cans wild sardines, sliced or chopped.
- Add 1 can water-packed tuna, drained.
- Add 2 sliced hard-cooked eggs.

NUTRITION INFORMATION (PER SERVING)
374 calories, 5 g protein, 13 g carbohydrates, 36 g total fat, 5 g saturated fat, 4 g fiber, 201 mg sodium

ASIAN GINGER SLAW

PREP TIME: 15 MINUTES ■ TOTAL TIME: 15 MINUTES + MARINATING TIME ■ MAKES 4 SERVINGS

DRESSING

- 1/2 cup soy sauce
- 1/4 cup sugar
- 1/4 cup mirin (sweet rice wine) or dry sherry
- 1/4 cup rice vinegar
- 1/4 cup peanut oil or olive oil
- 1 tablespoon sesame oil
- 3–4 cloves garlic, minced
- 2" piece fresh ginger, peeled and grated
- 1 tablespoon fresh lime juice
- 3 good shakes of hot sauce (optional)

SLAW

- 1 cup finely shredded green cabbage
- 1 cup finely shredded red cabbage
- 1 cup grated carrots
- Toasted sesame seeds, chopped roasted peanuts, or sliced almonds (optional)

To make the dressing: Whisk together the soy sauce, sugar, mirin or sherry, vinegar, oils, garlic, ginger, lime juice, and hot sauce, if using. Mix well.

To make the slaw: In a large bowl, combine the cabbages and carrots. Pour about 1/2 cup of the dressing over the slaw. Marinate in the refrigerator for at least 20 minutes and up to 4 hours.

Serve topped with a sprinkling of the sesame seeds or nuts, if using. Leftover dressing can be stored indefinitely.

VARIATIONS:

- For a main course, toss the slaw with shredded roasted chicken.
- Marinate the vegetables in the dressing overnight.

NUTRITION INFORMATION (PER SERVING)
114 calories, 2 g protein, 13 g carbohydrates, 6 g total fat, 1 g saturated fat, 2 g fiber, 720 mg sodium

WARM RED CABBAGE SALAD

PREP TIME: 5 MINUTES ▦ TOTAL TIME: 20 MINUTES ▦ MAKES 4 SERVINGS

1 small head red cabbage

1 small onion, sliced

5 tablespoons olive oil

$1/2$ cup sweet peas or snow pea pods

3 tablespoons rice vinegar

$1/2$ cup toasted walnuts

$1/4$–$1/2$ cup feta cheese or chèvre or sheep's milk cheese, crumbled (optional)

Cut the cabbage lengthwise into 4 pieces, then slice into $1/4$" strips. In a large skillet, steam with $1/4$ cup water for 5 minutes, or until soft. Remove and set aside.

In the same skillet, lightly cook the onion in 1 tablespoon of the oil for 3 to 5 minutes, or until transparent. Add the cabbage and peas.

In a small bowl, combine the remaining oil and vinegar. Pour over the cabbage mixture and toss. Top with the walnuts and the cheese, if using. Serve warm.

NUTRITION INFORMATION (PER SERVING)
231 calories, 3 g protein, 18 g carbohydrates, 18 g total fat, 2.5 g saturated fat, 4 g fiber, 220 mg sodium

SIMPLE KALE SALAD

PREP TIME: 5 MINUTES ▪ TOTAL TIME: 10 MINUTES ▪ MAKES 4 SERVINGS

Many kinds of kale are available, including dinosaur or lacinato (dark green bumpy leaves) and curly kale (frilly leaves). Baby kale is more tender. Our favorite is dinosaur or lacinato. Kale, with both antioxidant and anti-inflammatory properties, is rich in fiber and alpha-linolenic acids (ALA), one of the building blocks of the omega-3 fatty acids—100 calories' worth of kale provides 7 grams of fiber and 350 mg of ALA. Make sure you buy organic kale, as conventionally grown kale may contain lots of pesticides, as can any leafy greens.

1 bunch kale

1–2 tablespoons olive oil

1 teaspoon Himalayan pink salt

Wash and dry the kale and slice into thin ribbons across the width of the leaf. If the center stems are tough, slice vertically and discard the stems or save them for soup.

Place the kale in a large bowl and sprinkle with the oil and salt. Then massage the leaves with your hands for about 5 minutes, squishing the leaves almost like you are kneading dough. This tenderizes the kale (and your hands as well!).

VARIATIONS:

Add one of the following ingredients:
- Sliced avocado
- Cherry tomatoes
- Chickpeas
- Roasted walnuts or sunflower seeds
- Black or kalamata olives
- Feta cheese

NUTRITION INFORMATION (PER SERVING)
46 calories, 1 g protein, 3 g carbohydrates, 4 g total fat, 0.5 g saturated fat, 1 g fiber, 207 mg sodium

ZESTY TOFU "EGG" SALAD

PREP TIME: 20 MINUTES ■ TOTAL TIME: 20 MINUTES ■ MAKES 4 SERVINGS

1 package (12 ounces drained weight) extra-firm tofu

1 tablespoon olive oil

3 tablespoons 0% plain Greek yogurt

2 tablespoons prepared mango chutney

2 teaspoons curry powder

$1/4$ teaspoon salt

2 scallions, chopped

1 carrot, shredded

1 rib celery, finely chopped

$1/4$ cup raisins

2 cups mixed greens

Remove the tofu from the package and place in a colander in the sink to drain. Place a flat plate on top of the tofu and a heavy can of vegetables on the plate for 15 minutes.

Meanwhile, whisk together the oil, yogurt, chutney, curry powder, and salt. Stir in the scallions, carrot, celery, and raisins. Crumble the tofu and add to the bowl. Toss gently to coat.

To serve, top $1/2$ cup of the greens with one-quarter of the tofu mixture.

NUTRITION INFORMATION (PER SERVING)
144 calories, 8 g protein, 19 g carbohydrates, 4 g total fat, 1 g saturated fat, 2 g fiber, 321 mg sodium

CITRUS-GRILLED SALMON SALAD

PREP TIME: 5 MINUTES ■ TOTAL TIME: 1 HOUR ■ MAKES 4 SERVINGS

3 tablespoons frozen orange juice concentrate

2 tablespoons lime juice

$^3/_4$ teaspoon salt, divided

$^3/_4$ teaspoon hot-pepper sauce

$^1/_2$ teaspoon ground cumin

$1^1/_4$ pounds wild salmon fillet

1 red onion, cut into thick rounds

2 red bell peppers, cut lengthwise into 4 pieces

1 green bell pepper, cut lengthwise into 4 pieces

1 large tomato, cut into wedges

1 tablespoon olive oil

In a medium bowl, combine the orange juice, lime juice, $^1/_4$ teaspoon of the salt, the hot-pepper sauce, and cumin. Add the salmon and onion, turning to coat. Set aside to marinate for 30 minutes at room temperature.

Preheat the grill to medium. Oil a grill rack (and a perforated grill topper, if possible).

Reserving the marinade, place the fish on the rack, cover, and grill for 20 minutes, or until the fish is opaque. Remove from the grill and set aside. Place the onion and bell peppers, skin side down, on the grill topper or rack. Cover and grill, turning and basting the vegetables with some of the reserved marinade, for 7 minutes, or until the peppers are charred and the onion is tender-crisp.

When cool enough to handle, peel the peppers and cut into $^1/_2$"-wide strips. Break the salmon into bite-size pieces.

In a medium bowl, gently combine the salmon, peppers, onion, tomato wedges, oil, and the remaining $^1/_2$ teaspoon salt.

NUTRITION INFORMATION (PER SERVING)
301 calories, 30 g protein, 15 g carbohydrates,13 g total fat, 2 g saturated fat, 3 g fiber, 537 mg sodium

Soups are an excellent way to get nourishment and warmth, especially during the colder months. Also, they are a great way to eat more vegetables. You can even boil up vegetable trimmings from preparing other recipes to make a simple broth. Any soup can be put in a blender to make a creamier version. Enjoy soups year-round, even for breakfast! A simple nutritious meal can be a bowl of soup and a salad—think green and lean.

CARROT-GINGER SOUP

PREP TIME: 10 MINUTES ■ TOTAL TIME: 40 MINUTES ■ MAKES 4–6 SERVINGS

5 cups water

2 pounds carrots, peeled and cut into thirds

1" piece fresh ginger, peeled and sliced

$1/2$ teaspoon sea salt

Bring the water to a boil in a medium saucepan. Add the carrots, ginger, and salt. Reduce the heat to medium-low, cover, and simmer for 25 to 30 minutes, or until the carrots are tender.

Carefully transfer the soup to a blender or food processor, or use an immersion blender, and puree until smooth.

VARIATIONS:

- Spicy version. Chop and add $1/2$ onion, 2 cloves garlic, and $1/2$ rib celery. Top with $1/4$ teaspoon sesame seed–salt blend and $1/2$ teaspoon turmeric (optional).
- Roasted version. Instead of boiling the carrots and ginger, roast them at 350°F for 30 minutes. Proceed as for the rest of the recipe. Roasted vegetables tend to have richer flavors.
- Heartier version. Cook 1–2 peeled parsnips along with the carrots.

NUTRITION INFORMATION (PER SERVING)
50 calories, 1 g protein, 12 g carbohydrates, 0.5 g total fat, 0 g saturated fat, 3 g fiber, 223 mg sodium

RICH VEGETABLE SOUP

PREP TIME: 15 MINUTES ■ TOTAL TIME: 50 MINUTES ■ MAKES 4 SERVINGS

4–5 cups water (more if needed)

1–2 pounds small or medium unpeeled potatoes, or cauliflower pieces

1/2 teaspoon dried basil

1/2 teaspoon ground cumin

2–4 cloves garlic, chopped (optional)

3 tablespoons sesame oil or olive oil

1/2–1 teaspoon sea salt

1/4 teaspoon cayenne pepper (optional)

1 small or medium onion, chopped

1 small tomato, diced

1/2 cup each chopped carrots, celery, zucchini, broccoli, and cauliflower

1/2 cup chopped green bell pepper or beets, for pink soup (optional)

1 cup chopped kale

1/2 cup chopped scallions (optional)

Bring the water to a boil in a large saucepan. Add the potatoes or cauliflower and parboil for 15 minutes. Allow to cool a bit, then transfer the vegetables and water to a blender or food processor, or use an immersion blender. Add the basil, cumin, garlic, oil, salt, and cayenne pepper (to taste), if using, and puree until smooth.

Return the mixture to the saucepan. Add the onion, tomato, carrots, celery, zucchini, broccoli, cauliflower, and bell pepper or beets, if using. Cover and cook over low heat for 5 to 10 minutes. Add the kale and cook for 5 to 10 minutes.

Top with the scallions, if using, and serve.

VARIATIONS:

- For a cream soup, use milk (preferably 1% or 2%), yogurt, or buttermilk.
- For a dairy-free "cream" soup, blend in 1 cup well-cooked, moist oatmeal or a milk alternative like oat milk, rice milk, almond milk, or even coconut milk.

NUTRITION INFORMATION (PER SERVING)
216 calories, 4 g protein, 28 g carbohydrates, 11 g total fat, 1.5 g saturated fat, 5 g fiber, 252 mg sodium

CHICKEN-LIME SOUP

PREP TIME: 30 MINUTES ■ TOTAL TIME: 2 HOURS 40 MINUTES
■ MAKES 6 SERVINGS

2 bone-in chicken breasts halves, with skin

2 carrots, roughly chopped

1 onion, quartered

2 parsnips, roughly chopped

2 ribs celery, preferably with leaves, roughly chopped

4 cloves garlic, lightly smashed

1 tablespoon kosher salt

2–2$\frac{1}{2}$ quarts water (enough to cover the chicken and vegetables)

$\frac{1}{2}$ pound fine egg noodles (optional)

2 avocados, sliced

$\frac{1}{2}$ cup cilantro, roughly chopped

2–4 tablespoons fresh lime juice

Lime wedges, for garnish

Tortilla chips, for garnish (optional)

Place the chicken in a large soup pot. Add the carrots, onion, parsnips, celery, garlic, salt, and water. Bring to a boil over medium-high heat, then reduce the heat and simmer, uncovered, for 2 hours, periodically skimming off any foam and debris that rise to the surface.

Remove the chicken to a plate and strain the stock, discarding the vegetables. As the stock sits, drops of fat will begin to collect on the surface. While the chicken cools, gently skim off the fat from the stock.

When the chicken is cool enough to handle, remove the skin and take the meat off the bones. Shred or chop as desired. Prepare the noodles according to package directions, if using.

Into each of 6 bowls, place some shredded chicken, a few avocado slices, and a sprinkling of cilantro. Stir the lime juice into the broth, then ladle the broth into the bowls. Add the noodles, if using. Garnish with lime wedges and tortilla chips, if using.

NUTRITION INFORMATION (PER SERVING)
298 calories, 31 g protein, 15 g carbohydrates, 13 g total fat, 2.5 g saturated fat, 3 g fiber, 454 mg sodium

DR. SUN'S SEASONAL SAVORY SOUP

PREP TIME: 15 MINUTES ▪ TOTAL TIME: 25 MINUTES ▪ MAKES 4 SERVINGS

Choose your favorite veggies currently in season.

2 carrots, sliced

2 green or yellow zucchini, sliced

1 red bell pepper, sliced

4–6 mushrooms, sliced

1 onion, chopped

4–6 cloves garlic, chopped

1 cup each of these additional veggie options (choose all or some you like): eggplant, chopped green cabbage, broccoli pieces

2–3 cups water

1 can (13.5 ounces) light coconut milk

1 teaspoon curry powder

$1/4$ teaspoon cayenne pepper

In a large saucepan, place the carrots, zucchini, bell pepper, mushrooms, onion, garlic, and additional veggies. Add just enough of the water to cover the veggies. Bring to a boil, then reduce the heat and simmer for 5 minutes, or until the vegetables are starting to soften.

Add the coconut milk, curry powder, and cayenne pepper (to taste) and simmer for a couple minutes, stirring occasionally, until the veggies are tender.

NUTRITION INFORMATION (PER SERVING)
122 calories, 3 g protein, 17 g carbohydrates, 6 g total fat, 4 g saturated fat, 4 g fiber, 69 mg sodium

SPLIT PEA SOUP

PREP TIME: 5 MINUTES ▪ TOTAL TIME: 1 HOUR 10 MINUTES
▪ MAKES 4 SERVINGS

2 cups dry green split peas

1 onion, chopped

1 large or 2 medium carrots, sliced

2–3 cloves garlic, minced or pressed,
divided

1 tablespoon safflower or peanut
oil (optional)

8 cups water

$\frac{1}{4}$ teaspoon sea salt

Ground black or cayenne pepper
(optional)

Ground cumin or curry powder
(optional)

1 tablespoon miso (optional)

2 tablespoons parsley, chopped

Rinse the peas and drain.

In a large soup pot, lightly cook the onion, carrots, and 1 clove of the garlic in the oil,
if using. Add the water and peas. Bring to a boil, reduce the heat to low, and simmer
for 30 minutes. Add the remaining garlic and the salt. Season to taste with the pepper,
and cumin or curry powder, if using. Simmer for 30 minutes, or until the peas are soft.

Dissolve the miso, if using, in a small amount of water and stir into the soup. Serve
with the parsley and any additional seasonings to taste.

VARIATIONS:

- For a more complete meal, add 2 cups cooked rice to the pot midway (about
  30 minutes) through the cooking time.
- If you eat gluten, add croutons made from whole grain bread: Cube several
  slices and bake at 350°F for 15 to 20 minutes.
- If you like food spicy, add $\frac{1}{2}$ teaspoon cayenne pepper or 1 teaspoon
  smoked paprika.
- For another whole-meal option, serve the soup with a large salad.

NUTRITION INFORMATION (PER SERVING)
362 calories, 25 g protein, 65 g carbohydrates, 1 g total fat, 0 g saturated fat, 26 g fiber,
155 mg sodium

BUTTERNUT SQUASH–TORTILLA SOUP

PREP TIME: 5 MINUTES ■ TOTAL TIME: 1 HOUR 10 MINUTES
■ MAKES 4 SERVINGS

1 medium (2–3 pounds) butternut squash, peeled, seeds removed, and cut into 1" cubes

1 tablespoon olive oil

1 medium onion, chopped

2 cloves garlic, minced

1 tablespoon chili powder

1 large tomato, chopped (optional)

$1/4$ teaspoon ground cumin (optional)

5 cups water or chicken or vegetable broth

$1/2$ teaspoon sea salt

3 corn tortillas (6" diameter), sliced into strips, or tortilla chips

4 kale leaves, sliced into thin strips

$1/2$ cup chopped toasted almonds (optional)

Preheat the oven to 350°F.

Place the squash cubes on a baking sheet and roast in the oven for 40 minutes. Remove from the oven and set aside.

In a large soup pot, heat the oil and cook the onion and garlic for 5 minutes, or until translucent. Add the chili powder and the tomato and cumin, if using. Heat for 1 minute. Add the squash, water or broth, and salt. Bring to a boil and simmer, covered, for 30 to 45 minutes, or until the squash is fork-tender.

Meanwhile, spread the tortilla strips on a baking sheet, coat with cooking spray or rub lightly with olive oil, and bake for 10 minutes, or until golden and crisp. (If you use tortilla chips, omit this step.)

Puree the soup in a blender or food processor, adjust the seasoning, and garnish with the tortilla strips or chips, kale, and almonds, if using.

VARIATION:

Garnish with 1 cup or more of organic blue corn tortilla chips, instead of the tortilla strips, as a nice color contrast.

NUTRITION INFORMATION (PER SERVING)
185 calories, 4 g protein, 37 g carbohydrates, 4 g total fat, 0.5 g saturated fat, 6 g fiber, 232 mg sodium

TUSCAN MINESTRONE

PREP TIME: 30 MINUTES ■ TOTAL TIME: 1 HOUR 10 MINUTES
■ MAKES 6 SERVINGS

2–3 tablespoons olive oil, divided

1 red onion, finely chopped

2 ribs celery, finely chopped

3 carrots, peeled and finely chopped

1 tablespoon fennel seeds

1/4 cup shredded savoy cabbage

2 medium Yukon Gold potatoes, cubed

3 zucchini, cubed

1 can (28 ounces) crushed tomatoes

2 cloves garlic, sliced and smashed

4–5 cups water or meat or vegetable stock

1/2 teaspoon salt

1 can (15 ounces) cannellini, great Northern, or navy beans, rinsed and drained

1 teaspoon chopped fresh sage, or to taste

1 teaspoon chopped fresh thyme, or to taste

1–3 cups lacinato kale, torn, or fresh spinach, stems removed

2 ounces Asiago cheese, shaved or grated, for garnish (optional)

In a large soup pot over medium heat, heat 2 tablespoons of the oil, the onion, celery, and carrots. (This is called a *soffrito* or mirepoix and is a great starter for any soup.) Cook, stirring frequently, for 15 minutes, or until golden brown. Add the remaining 1 tablespoon oil as the vegetables are cooking, if necessary.

Add the fennel seeds, stir, and cook for 1 minute. Add the cabbage, potatoes, zucchini, tomatoes, and garlic. Add enough of the water or stock to reach just below the vegetables. Add the salt, bring to a boil, and stir. Reduce the heat and simmer for 20 minutes, or until the vegetables are tender. Add the beans and another cup of water if the mixture is too thick and simmer for 3 to 4 minutes. Add the sage, thyme, and kale or spinach and cook for another few minutes. The vegetables should be tender but not overcooked.

Serve garnished with the Asiago, if using.

VARIATION:

Add 1/2 cup cooked pasta—rotini, radiatore, ziti, orzo, or macaroni.

NUTRITION INFORMATION (PER SERVING)
336 calories, 13 g protein, 58 g carbohydrates, 9 g total fat, 1 g saturated fat, 16 g fiber, 663 mg sodium

Here are some delicious main dish recipes, including vegetarian choices. Be sure to focus on getting lots of veggies along with some protein. These protein sources focus on legumes, fish, and poultry—there's no beef or pork since one of our goals is to reduce red meat intake. These recipes are relatively simple to prepare and are especially tasty jump-starts for your immune-healthy food adventure.

SPICY TOFU

PREP TIME: 15 MINUTES ■ TOTAL TIME: 25 MINUTES ■ MAKES 4 SERVINGS

2 tablespoons peanut or olive oil

4 cloves garlic, crushed

1–2 slices (1" each) fresh ginger, peeled and finely chopped

1 small onion, sliced into $3/4$" pieces

1 block extra-firm tofu (16 ounces), sliced into $3/4$" pieces

2 tablespoons soy sauce

$1/2$ teaspoon honey

$1/2$ teaspoon hot-pepper sauce or cayenne pepper

Heat the oil in a 10" skillet or wok over medium-high heat. Add the garlic, ginger, and onion and cook for 4 minutes, or until golden. Add the tofu and cook until lightly browned. Flip the pieces to brown the other side, about 6 minutes total. Add the soy sauce, honey, and hot-pepper sauce or cayenne pepper.

VARIATIONS:

- Add other vegetables like broccoli, mushrooms, or chard.
- Baked option: Preheat the oven to 350°F and oil a baking dish. Mix together the tofu and the sautéed garlic, ginger, and onion. Spread in the baking dish and bake for 15 minutes. In a small bowl, mix the soy sauce, honey, and hot pepper. Brush the sauce on the tofu mixture and return the dish to the oven. Bake for 15 to 20 minutes.
- Serve the dish immediately over Coconut Rice (page 264).

NUTRITION INFORMATION (PER SERVING)
163 calories, 10 g protein, 6 g carbohydrates, 11 g total fat, 1.5 g saturated fat, 1 g fiber, 480 mg sodium

ROASTED VEGETABLES DELUXE

PREP TIME: 15 MINUTES ▪ TOTAL TIME: 1 HOUR 5 MINUTES ▪ MAKES 4 SERVINGS

Your veggie choices for this dish can be seasonally based. Add pieces of cooked chicken, salmon, or tofu to the roasted vegetables to make this a one-dish warm meal. Or serve with Veggie Tomato Sauce (page 283).

4 carrots

4 red-skinned potatoes, quartered

$1/2$ pound Brussels sprouts, halved

1 winter squash, such as butternut, acorn, hubbard, or delicata, peeled, seeds removed and cubed

$1/2$ pound mushrooms

3 cloves garlic

3 zucchini, cut into chunks

1 green or red bell pepper, seeds removed and sliced

2 tablespoons olive oil

2 tablespoons balsamic vinegar

2 tablespoons Bragg Liquid Aminos

Preheat the oven to 350°F.

To roast the vegetables: On a large baking sheet, place the carrots, potatoes, Brussels sprouts, and winter squash. Bake for 10 to 15 minutes. Stir and add the mushrooms and garlic and bake for another 10 to 15 minutes. Stir in the zucchini and peppers and bake for another 15 to 20 minutes.

Put the roasted vegetables into a serving bowl and lightly season with the oil, vinegar, and liquid aminos. Stir to coat the pieces and serve.

VARIATIONS:

- Spring: garlic, mushrooms, greens, asparagus, peas, spring onions
- Summer: zucchini, corn, tomato, fennel, peppers
- Autumn: potatoes, carrots, garlic, cauliflower, hard squash
- Winter: cabbage, Brussels sprouts, kale, arugula, acorn and other hard squash
- For a complete meal, roast chicken, fish, or tofu with the vegetables.

NUTRITION INFORMATION (PER SERVING)
357 calories, 11 g protein, 65 g carbohydrates, 8 g total fat, 1 g saturated fat, 11 g fiber, 426 mg sodium

CHICKEN-SHIITAKE LETTUCE WRAPS

PREP TIME: 5 MINUTES ▪ TOTAL TIME: 20 MINUTES ▪ MAKES 4 SERVINGS

3 tablespoons peanut oil

1 teaspoon minced garlic

1 pound ground chicken or turkey

½ pound shiitake mushrooms, stemmed and sliced

1 teaspoon grated fresh ginger

1 teaspoon Chinese five-spice powder

8 largest leaves from 1 head butter lettuce, washed

3 tablespoons bottled hoison sauce

Heat the oil in a large skillet over medium heat. Add the garlic and cook for 1 minute. Add the chicken or turkey, increasing the heat a bit. After 5 minutes, add the mushrooms, ginger, and five-spice powder. Cook for 10 minutes, or until the meat is no longer pink.

Into each lettuce leaf, brush 1 teaspoon of the hoison, add some of the meat mixture, and roll up like a burrito. Serve with coconut rice (recipe below).

NUTRITION INFORMATION (PER SERVING)
302 calories, 22 g protein, 10 g carbohydrates, 20 g total fat, 4.5 g saturated fat, 2 g fiber, 247 mg sodium

COCONUT RICE

PREP TIME: 5 MINUTES ▪ TOTAL TIME: 35 MINUTES ▪ MAKES 8 SERVINGS

2 cups jasmine, basmati, or brown rice

2 cups light coconut milk

1¾ cups water

½ teaspoon sea salt

In a large saucepan, combine the rice, coconut milk, water, and salt. Heat on medium-high, stirring occasionally to prevent the rice from sticking or burning. When the liquid begins to gently bubble, reduce the heat to low. Cover tightly. Simmer for 15 to 20 minutes, or until the liquid has been absorbed by the rice. Turn off the heat and let the pan sit, covered, for 5 to 10 minutes, or until you're ready to eat.

Before serving, fluff the rice with a fork or chopsticks.

NUTRITION INFORMATION (PER SERVING)
193 calories, 3 g protein, 38 g carbohydrates, 3 g total fat, 2 g saturated fat, 0 g fiber, 119 mg sodium

POLENTA WITH TOMATO-LENTIL SAUCE

PREP TIME: 10 MINUTES ▪ TOTAL TIME: 50 MINUTES ▪ MAKES 4 SERVINGS

1 small onion, chopped finely

1 carrot, chopped finely

1 rib celery, chopped finely

1 clove garlic, minced

2 tablespoons olive oil

1 pound fresh tomatoes, peeled, or 1 can (15 ounces) whole or crushed tomatoes

1 cup lentils

1 cup sliced mushrooms

$1/4$ teaspoon sea salt

$1/4$ teaspoon ground black pepper (optional)

1 cup polenta

4–5 cups water

In a large saucepan, cook the onion, carrot, celery, and garlic in the oil for 5 minutes, or until the onion is limp and transparent. Add the tomatoes with their juice and lentils and simmer for 30 to 40 minutes with the lid ajar. Add the mushrooms and cook for 5 minutes. Season to taste with the salt and pepper, if using.

Meanwhile, place the polenta in a medium saucepan. Slowly stir in the water, adding a small amount to first make a paste, then continue to add the water, at least 4 cups. Turn on the heat to medium and bring to a boil while stirring. Reduce the heat and continue to stir. Cook for 20 to 30 minutes, stirring occasionally.

Transfer the polenta to a large serving bowl and pour the sauce over it.

VARIATIONS:

- Serve the veggies over rice instead of polenta.
- Sprinkle grated Asiago cheese over the whole dish or mix the cheese with the polenta before adding the vegetables.

NUTRITION INFORMATION (PER SERVING)
432 calories, 18 g protein, 73 g carbohydrates, 8 g total fat, 1 g saturated fat, 17 g fiber, 358 mg sodium

TURKEY CHILI

PREP TIME: 5 MINUTES ■ TOTAL TIME: 1 HOUR 15 MINUTES
■ MAKES 4 SERVINGS

For those who can eat gluten, serve this chili with garlic bread or cornbread. Add a big green salad and you have a complete meal.

2 tablespoons olive oil

1 onion, chopped

4 cloves garlic, sliced

1 pound ground turkey or chicken

1 can (15 ounces) kidney beans, rinsed and drained

1 can (15 ounces) Great Northern beans, rinsed and drained

1 can (28 ounces) crushed tomatoes

1–2 teaspoons ground cumin

1–2 tablespoons chili powder

$^1/_2$ teaspoon cayenne pepper

$^1/_2$ teaspoon sea salt

$^1/_2$ teaspoon ground black pepper (optional)

$^1/_2$ cup shredded sharp Cheddar cheese (optional)

Heat the oil in a large skillet over medium heat. Add the onion and garlic and cook for 5 minutes, or until translucent. Add the turkey or chicken and cook for 10 minutes, or until no longer pink. Drain off any fat. Add the beans, tomatoes with their juice, cumin, chili powder, cayenne pepper (to taste), salt, and black pepper, if using. Mix well and simmer, covered, over low heat for 30 to 45 minutes. Turn off the heat and let sit in the pan for 10 minutes.

Divide into 4 bowls and sprinkle some cheese over each, if desired.

VARIATION:

Try different rice possibilities—Jasmine, basmati, forbidden black rice—for wonderful variations.

NUTRITION INFORMATION (PER SERVING)
386 calories, 32 g protein, 29 g carbohydrates, 17 g total fat, 3.5 g saturated fat, 8 g fiber, 483 mg sodium

RAINBOW VEGGIE RICE

PREP TIME: 5 MINUTES ▪ TOTAL TIME: 50 MINUTES ▪ MAKES 8 SERVINGS

This dish is tasty served with a tofu or Miso/Tahini Dressing (see page 284). This is a good cold salad as well.

2 cups brown rice

2 tablespoons sunflower oil, sesame oil, olive oil, or canola oil

1 small onion, finely chopped

1 red bell pepper, finely chopped

3 carrots, finely chopped

1 yellow squash, finely chopped

1 zucchini, finely chopped

1/4 purple (red) cabbage, shredded

4 scallions, thinly sliced

1/2 cup water

2 teaspoons soy sauce, or to taste

Cayenne pepper (optional)

1–2 cups cut-up cooked chicken or tofu cubes (optional, for more protein and to make a complete meal)

1 cup stemmed and chopped fresh parsley

Prepare the rice according to package directions.

In a large skillet, heat the oil and cook the vegetables in the oil in this order, adding the next one every 3 minutes or so: onion, bell pepper, carrots, yellow squash, zucchini, cabbage, and scallions, stirring frequently. Stir in the water and soy sauce and season to taste with the cayenne pepper, if using. Add the cooked rice in clumps, stir, and heat gently for 5 minutes. Add the chicken or tofu, if using.

Leave covered and serve warm. Add the parsley before serving.

NUTRITION INFORMATION (PER SERVING)
230 calories, 5 g protein, 42 g carbohydrates, 5 g total fat, 0.5 g saturated fat, 5 g fiber, 110 mg sodium

BASMATI RICE WITH ROASTED BUTTERNUT SQUASH

PREP TIME: 10 MINUTES ■ TOTAL TIME: 50 MINUTES ■ MAKES 8 SERVINGS

2 cups brown basmati rice

3³/₄ cups water

1 teaspoon ground turmeric

¹/₂ teaspoon salt

2 tablespoons vegetable oil

20 ounces precut butternut squash

2" cinnamon stick

4 whole cloves

¹/₄ teaspoon ground cardamom

In a large saucepan, bring the rice, water, turmeric, and salt to a boil. Reduce the heat to medium-low and simmer, covered, for 35 to 45 minutes, or until the rice is tender.

Meanwhile, preheat the oven to 400°F.

Heat the oil in a large heavy skillet over low heat. Add the squash, cinnamon, and cloves and stir to coat. Cook for 5 minutes, stirring occasionally, taking care not to burn the spices.

Spread the squash on a large baking sheet. Bake for 15 to 20 minutes, turning once or twice. Remove from the oven and discard the cloves and cinnamon stick.

Fluff the rice with a fork and stir in the cardamom. Toss gently with the roasted squash.

NUTRITION INFORMATION (PER SERVING)
203 calories, 4 g protein, 40 g carbohydrates, 5 g total fat, 0.5 g saturated fat, 3 g fiber, 148 mg sodium

CITRUS SHRIMP AND GARLIC

PREP TIME: 15 MINUTES ■ TOTAL TIME: 20 MINUTES ■ MAKES 6 SERVINGS

$\frac{1}{4}$ cup olive oil

4 cloves garlic, minced

1 cup finely chopped scallions

2 pounds medium shrimp, peeled and deveined

$\frac{1}{4}$ cup fresh lime juice or lemon juice

$\frac{1}{4}$ cup chopped fresh parsley

Pinch of ground black pepper (optional)

Tabasco or other hot sauce (optional)

Warm the oil over medium heat in a large skillet. Add the garlic and scallions and cook for 1 to 2 minutes, or until the scallions turn bright green. Add the shrimp and lime or lemon juice. Maintain the heat at medium-high and cook for 3 to 4 minutes, or until the shrimp curls and turns opaque. Stir in the parsley and pepper and hot sauce (to taste), if using.

Serve over rice, if desired.

VARIATION:

More vegetables can be included in this dish, such as sliced carrots, zucchini, peppers, and mushrooms.

NUTRITION INFORMATION (PER SERVING)
186 calories, 19 g protein, 4 g carbohydrates, 11 g total fat, 1.5 g saturated fat, 1 g fiber, 753 mg sodium

VEGGIE BURGERS

PREP TIME: 5 MINUTES ▦ TOTAL TIME: 30 MINUTES ▦ MAKES 4 SERVINGS

$^2/_3$ cup millet or 16 ounces extra-firm
  tofu, mashed

2 tablespoons sesame oil, divided

1 carrot, grated

1 onion, diced

1 clove garlic, minced

1 scallion, finely chopped

$^1/_2$ cup chopped fresh parsley or
  spinach (optional)

1 tablespoon tamari

1–2 eggs or $^1/_4$–$^1/_2$ cup water, divided

$^1/_2$ cup whole grain bread crumbs

2 tablespoons chopped almonds,
  peanuts, or roasted sesame
  seeds

$^1/_2$ teaspoon dried thyme

$^1/_2$ teaspoon sea salt

If using the millet, in a small saucepan, combine the millet with 1$^1/_3$ cups water. Bring to a boil, reduce the heat, cover, and simmer for 15 minutes. Remove the saucepan from the heat and let stand, covered, for 10 minutes. Fluff with a fork.

Meanwhile, heat 1 tablespoon of the oil in a skillet. Lightly cook the carrot, onion, garlic, scallion, and parsley or spinach (if using) for 5 minutes, or until soft. Transfer to a bowl. Add the millet or mashed tofu, tamari, 1 beaten egg or $^1/_4$ cup of the water, the bread crumbs, nuts or seeds, thyme, and salt to the bowl. Mix with a wooden spoon to a pasty burger consistency, adding the remaining beaten egg or $^1/_4$ cup water if necessary.

Form into 4 patties and cook in the same skillet in the remaining 1 tablespoon oil for 3 minutes per side, or until browned on both sides. Alternatively, preheat the oven to 350°F and bake the patties on a baking sheet for 20 minutes, or until golden brown. Or preheat the oven to 375°F, form the mixture into a loaf, and bake for 40 minutes, or until browned on top.

VARIATIONS:

- Melt your cheese of choice on the burgers and serve with your choice of trimmings, such as buns or toast, corn tortillas, sliced tomatoes, lettuce or alfalfa sprouts, ketchup, mustard, and relish.
- Combine with salad, steamed vegetables, corn on the cob, or, for a classically American treat, some baked fries: Preheat the oven to 350°F. Cut potatoes into long strips (or use a food processor to make chips). Bake until golden brown. Salt lightly and serve with homemade ketchup.

NUTRITION INFORMATION (PER SERVING)
318 calories, 9 g protein, 30 g carbohydrates, 12 g total fat, 2 g saturated fat, 6 g fiber, 567 mg sodium

VEGGIE-TURKEY MEAT LOAF

**PREP TIME: 15 MINUTES ■ TOTAL TIME: 1 HOUR 5 MINUTES
■ MAKES 6 SERVINGS**

1 tablespoon olive oil

2 pounds ground turkey

1 cup rolled oats

2 eggs

1 tablespoon olive oil

1 cup tomato sauce

6 cloves garlic, chopped

1 cup each of the following
chopped vegetables: carrot,
zucchini, onion, mushroom

$1/2$ teaspoon sea salt

Preheat the oven to 350°F. Coat a loaf pan with the oil.

In a large wooden bowl, combine the turkey, oats, and eggs. Mash together well, then add the tomato sauce, garlic, and your choice of veggies. Mix again.

Bake in the loaf pan for 40 to 50 minutes, or until a thermometer inserted in the center registers 165°F and the meat is no longer pink.

VARIATION:

For an Italian twist, add 1 teaspoon dried oregano, 1 teaspoon dried basil, and $1/2$ teaspoon rosemary to the ground turkey.

NUTRITION INFORMATION (PER SERVING)
348 calories, 15 g protein, 16 g carbohydrates, 17 g total fat, 4 g saturated fat, 3 g fiber, 592 mg sodium

STIR-FRIED VEGETABLES WITH TEMPEH OR TOFU

PREP TIME: 10 MINUTES ■ TOTAL TIME: 25 MINUTES ■ MAKES 4 SERVINGS

1 large onion

3 tablespoons toasted sesame oil, divided

1 cup vegetable stock, divided

3 ounces shiitake mushrooms, stemmed and sliced

2 carrots, thinly sliced on the diagonal

8 ounces extra-firm tofu or tempeh, cut into bite-size cubes

1 cup broccoli florets

1 can (15 ounces) sliced water chestnuts

1 cup bean sprouts

1 clove garlic, minced

2 tablespoons grated fresh ginger

1 tablespoon tamari or soy sauce

$1/8$ teaspoon cayenne pepper

Cut the onion into windowpanes: Cut in half lengthwise, then cut each half into 3 or 4 sections lengthwise, depending on the size of the onion. Slice each section cross-wise into $1/4$" pieces.

In a wok or large skillet over medium heat, cook the onion in 1 tablespoon of the oil until it starts putting out its juice. Add $1/2$ cup of the stock and bring to a rapid boil over high heat. Add the mushrooms, cover, reduce the heat, and simmer for 5 minutes. Add the carrots and cook for a few minutes, adding more stock if necessary. Then add the tofu or tempeh, broccoli, water chestnuts, bean sprouts, and garlic, in that order. Cook for a few more minutes, until the broccoli is bright green.

Squeeze the ginger through cheesecloth and add the solids to the vegetables. Stir and cook for 1 minute. Remove from the heat and stir in the remaining 2 tablespoons oil. Season to taste with the tamari or soy sauce and cayenne pepper.

NUTRITION INFORMATION (PER SERVING)
222 calories, 9 g protein, 18 g carbohydrates, 14 g total fat, 2 g saturated fat, 5 g fiber, 355 mg sodium

CHICKEN YUCATAN-STYLE

**PREP TIME: 10 MINUTES ■ TOTAL TIME: 40 MINUTES + MARINATING TIME
■ MAKES 4 SERVINGS**

2 tablespoons ground annatto/
achiote seed

2 teaspoons fresh oregano

1 teaspoon ground cumin

1/4 teaspoon ground cloves

1 teaspoon sea salt

1 tablespoon olive oil

3 tablespoons fresh lemon juice

1 pound boneless, skinless chicken
breasts (or 8 boneless, skinless
chicken thighs)

8 tortillas (6" diameter), warmed

2 avocados, sliced

1/2 cup cilantro, chopped

In a small bowl, stir together the annatto/achiote seed, oregano, cumin, cloves, salt, oil, and lemon juice until they form a paste, adding a bit of water if necessary.

Place the chicken in a baking dish and spread the paste over the chicken. Marinate in the refrigerator for 4 hours or overnight.

Preheat the oven to 350°F.

Bake the chicken for 20 to 30 minutes, or until a thermometer inserted in the thickest portion registers 165°F and the juices run clear.

Thinly slice or shred the chicken. Place in the tortillas and top with the avocado and cilantro.

NUTRITION INFORMATION (PER SERVING)
395 calories, 29 g protein, 31 g carbohydrates, 19 g total fat, 3 g saturated fat, 9 g fiber, 555 mg sodium

BAKED DILL SALMON

1 tablespoon soy sauce

1–2 tablespoons fresh lemon juice

4 wild salmon fillets (4–6 ounces each)

4 lemon slices

4 tomato slices

4 sprigs fresh dill

Preheat the oven to 375°F.

In a small bowl or dish, mix together the soy sauce and lemon juice. Dip the salmon in the mixture to coat both sides. Place the fillets in a large baking dish. Place a lemon slice, a tomato slice, and a sprig of dill on top of each fillet. Cover the dish with its lid or foil. Bake for 15 to 20 minutes, or until the fish is opaque and flakes easily.

NUTRITION INFORMATION (PER SERVING)
270 calories, 38 g protein, 3 g carbohydrates, 12 g total fat, 1.5 g saturated fat, 1 g fiber, 334 mg sodium

RISOTTO WITH MUSHROOMS, ASPARAGUS, MANCHEGO, AND THYME

PREP TIME: 10 MINUTES ▦ TOTAL TIME: 45 MINUTES ▦ MAKES 6 SERVINGS

1 tablespoon + 1 teaspoon olive oil

$3^{1}/_{2}$ ounces fresh shiitake mushrooms, stemmed and halved or quartered

8 ounces cremini mushrooms, stemmed and sliced

6 ounces portobello mushroom caps, stemmed and sliced

10 spears asparagus, cut into 1" pieces

1 quart chicken stock

2 tablespoons salted butter or 1 tablespoon olive oil

1 onion, diced

1 cup arborio rice

3 teaspoons fresh thyme, chopped + more for garnish

1 clove garlic, minced

$^{1}/_{4}$ teaspoon sea salt

$^{1}/_{4}$ teaspoon ground black pepper (optional)

$^{1}/_{2}$ cup white wine or sherry

$^{1}/_{2}$ cup grated Manchego cheese

Heat 1 tablespoon of the oil in a medium skillet over medium-high heat. Cook the mushrooms, working in batches so as not to crowd the pan, until browned and soft. Remove from the heat and cut the portobello slices into bite-size pieces. Transfer all the mushrooms to a bowl and set aside.

Lightly sauté the asparagus in the remaining 1 teaspoon oil in a small saucepan over low heat. Transfer to a dish and set aside. Add the stock to the saucepan and warm over low to medium heat.

Melt the butter or warm the oil in a large, deep skillet over medium heat. Add the onion and cook, stirring occasionally, for 3 to 5 minutes, or until softened. Add the rice, stirring for 1 minute. Pour in the warm stock, 1 cup at a time, stirring until the rice has absorbed the liquid before adding another cup. Stir in the thyme and garlic, cooking for an additional minute. Add the salt and pepper, if using, then the wine or sherry. Stir and let the liquid bubble away.

When the rice is al dente, stir in the reserved mushrooms and asparagus. Add the cheese and serve.

NUTRITION INFORMATION (PER SERVING)
277 calories, 11 g protein, 33 g carbohydrates, 11 g total fat, 5 g saturated fat, 3 g fiber, 541 mg sodium

SNACKS AND SIDE DISHES

Everyone likes a snack now and then, so here are some healthy ones to enjoy. The bars are good travel foods or can be enjoyed after a workout at the gym or during a hike.

KALE CHIPS

PREP TIME: 10 MINUTES ▪ TOTAL TIME: 25 MINUTES ▪ MAKES 4 SERVINGS

1 bunch kale, preferably dinosaur kale

2 tablespoons extra virgin olive oil— just enough to coat each leaf

1–2 sprinkles of sea salt

Preheat the oven to 275°F.

Wash and thoroughly dry the kale. Remove the thick stems and tear the leaves into bite-size pieces.

In a large bowl, combine the oil and salt. Add the kale and massage with the oil. Spread the pieces on a baking sheet or pizza pan without too much overlap. (You may need to use 2 baking sheets or bake the chips in 2 batches.) Bake for 10 to 15 minutes, or until the edges are crisp.

Serve immediately. Store leftovers in an airtight container (such as a snap-top container). The chips often lose their crispness with storage.

VARIATIONS:

- Try different kinds of salt, such as garlic salt or truffle salt.
- Try with some Parmesan cheese or, even better, nutritional yeast, which gives the chips a cheesy flavor.
- Before baking, sprinkle with different spices—such as ground turmeric, chili powder, fennel powder, or chipotle powder.

NUTRITION INFORMATION (PER SERVING)
79 calories, 1 g protein, 3 g carbohydrates, 7 g total fat, 1 g saturated fat, 1 g fiber, 209 mg sodium

FIG AND ALMOND ENERGY BITES

PREP TIME: 35 MINUTES ■ TOTAL TIME: 1 HOUR 5 MINUTES ■ MAKES 24 SERVINGS

1 cup rolled oats

$^1/_2$ cup unsweetened shredded coconut

$^3/_4$ cup chopped dried figs

$^1/_2$ cup dark chocolate chips

$^1/_2$ cup ground flaxseeds

1 teaspoon ground cinnamon

1 teaspoon ground ginger

Pinch of sea salt

$^1/_2$ cup almond butter

$^1/_4$ cup honey

1 teaspoon almond extract

In a large bowl, combine the oats, coconut, figs, chocolate chips, flaxseed, cinnamon, ginger, and salt. Stir in the almond butter, honey, and almond extract. Mix well and refrigerate for about 30 minutes.

Roll into 24 balls, using about 2 tablespoons mixture per ball, and set on a plate or baking sheet. If the mixture becomes too sticky, return it to the fridge for a couple minutes, or lightly grease your hands with cooking spray.

Store the bites in the refrigerator.

NUTRITION INFORMATION (PER SERVING)
117 calories, 3 g protein, 13 g carbohydrates, 7 g total fat, 2.5 g saturated fat, 3 g fiber, 46 mg sodium

TRIPLE-GINGER CRANBERRY BARS

PREP TIME: 10 MINUTES + OVERNIGHT SOAK FOR THE CRANBERRIES
■ **TOTAL TIME: 40 MINUTES + COOLING TIME** ■ **MAKES 24 SERVINGS**

1 cup dried cranberries

$^1/_2$ cup brandy or orange liqueur or ginger liqueur

2 cups firmly packed light brown sugar

8 tablespoons (1 stick) unsalted butter, room temperature

$1^1/_2$ teaspoons sea salt

2 eggs

$2^3/_4$ cups almond flour

1 tablespoon grated fresh ginger

1 teaspoon ground ginger

$^1/_2$ cup chopped crystallized ginger

$^1/_2$ cup slivered almonds or chopped walnuts

In a small bowl or glass, combine the cranberries and brandy or liqueur. Cover and let soak overnight.

When ready to cook, preheat the oven to 350°F. Coat a 13" x 9" baking pan with butter or coconut oil, then line with parchment paper.

In a medium bowl, beat together the sugar, butter, and salt until light and fluffy. Add the eggs, one at a time, scraping the bowl between each addition. Stir in the almond flour, fresh ginger, ground ginger, and the soaked cranberries (they should have completely absorbed the liquid).

Spread the mixture in the baking pan. Sprinkle the top with the crystallized ginger and nuts. Bake for 25 to 30 minutes, or until light golden brown and slightly firm to the touch. Let cool completely in the pan, then cut into 24 bars. Store in an airtight container at room temperature.

VARIATION:

Substitute dried cut apricots or dried blueberries for the cranberries.

NUTRITION INFORMATION (PER SERVING)
237 calories, 4 g protein, 29 g carbohydrates, 12 g total fat, 3 g saturated fat, 2 g fiber, 115 mg sodium

PUMPKIN-CARROT SNACK BARS

PREP TIME: 15 MINUTES ▪ TOTAL TIME: 40 MINUTES ▪ MAKES 16 SERVINGS

1 cup canned solid-pack pumpkin

1 cup shredded carrots

$\frac{1}{2}$ cup sugar

$\frac{1}{3}$ cup raisins, chopped

$\frac{1}{4}$ cup peanut, grapeseed, or
   sunflower oil

2 large eggs

1 cup whole grain pastry flour

1 teaspoon baking powder

1 teaspoon ground cinnamon

$\frac{1}{2}$ teaspoon baking soda

$\frac{1}{4}$ teaspoon salt

$\frac{1}{4}$ cup shelled pumpkin seeds or
   chopped walnuts

Preheat the oven to 350°F. Coat a 13" x 9" x 2" baking pan with cooking spray.

In a large bowl, combine the pumpkin, carrots, sugar, raisins, oil, and eggs. Stir until well blended. Add the flour, baking powder, cinnamon, baking soda, and salt. Mix until blended.

Pour the batter into the prepared pan and spread evenly. Sprinkle with the seeds or nuts. Bake for 22 to 25 minutes, or until the top springs back when pressed lightly. Cool completely in the pan on a rack.

NUTRITION INFORMATION (PER SERVING)
114 calories, 2 g protein, 16 g carbohydrates, 5 g total fat, 1 g saturated fat, 2 g fiber, 81 mg sodium

GREEN BEANS WITH ALMOND PESTO

PREP TIME: 10 MINUTES ■ TOTAL TIME: 20 MINUTES ■ MAKES 8 SERVINGS

$^1/_2$ cup coarsely chopped fresh basil

$^1/_2$ cup coarsely chopped fresh parsley

$^1/_2$ cup sliced almonds, toasted + additional for garnish

1 large clove garlic

$^1/_3$ cup extra virgin olive oil

Sallt

Ground black pepper

1 pound fresh green beans, trimmed

In a food processor, combine the basil, parsley, almonds, garlic, and oil. Pulse until finely chopped to make pesto. Season to taste with salt and black pepper.

In a large saucepan of boiling water, or in a steamer basket in a large pot with 2" of boiling water, blanch the green beans for 4 minutes, or until just tender.

Drain the beans and top with the pesto and garnish with almonds just before serving.

NUTRITION INFORMATION (PER SERVING)
135 calories, 1 g protein, 5 g carbohydrates, 12 g total fat, 2 g saturated fat, 2 g fiber, 5 mg sodium

THYME-ROASTED CARROTS

PREP TIME: 10 MINUTES ■ TOTAL TIME: 40 MINUTES ■ MAKES 4 SERVINGS

1 pound young carrots, sliced

1 tablespoon olive oil

$^1/_2$ teaspoon sugar

$^1/_4$ teaspoon thyme

$^1/_4$ teaspoon coarse salt

Preheat the oven to 425°F. Lightly oil a rimmed baking sheet.

Arrange the carrots on the baking sheet. Drizzle with the oil and sprinkle with the sugar, thyme, and salt. Toss to mix.

Roast the carrots, stirring three or four times, for 30 minutes, or until tender and lightly browned.

NUTRITION INFORMATION (PER SERVING)
85 calories, 1 g protein, 13 g carbohydrates, 3 g total fat, 0 g saturated fat, 3 g fiber, 180 mg sodium

NORI ROLLS

3 cups water

1 cup short-grain brown rice

$1/4$ teaspoon salt

$1/4$ cup seasoned rice vinegar

4 sheets nori

1 cup grated carrots

1 cup grated cucumber

1 cup grated baked tofu

$1/4$ medium avocado, sliced thin

$1/4$ cup pickled ginger

In a medium saucepan over medium heat, place the water, rice, and salt. Cover and bring to a boil. Reduce the heat to low and simmer for 1 hour, or until the rice is very tender and all the water has been absorbed. Cool. Stir in the vinegar. Set aside.

To assemble the rolls, place a sheet of nori on a bamboo sushi mat. Spread about 1 cup rice in a thin, even layer on the sheet, leaving a 1" band uncovered along the top of the sheet.

Arrange about $1/4$ cup each of the carrot, cucumber, and tofu across the center of the rice, from edge to edge of the roll. Top with slices of the avocado and ginger.

To form the roll, hold the filling in place with your fingertips and use your thumbs to lift the bottom edge of the mat so that the nori edge nearest you is lifted over to meet the top edge of the rice. Use the uncovered portion of the nori as a flap to seal the roll. Use your hands to gently shape the roll, then let it sit on its seam to seal. If bite-size pieces are desired, use a sharp, wet knife to cut the roll crosswise; clean the knife between cuts.

Repeat with the remaining 3 sheets of nori.

NUTRITION INFORMATION (PER SERVING)
414 calories, 20 g protein, 61 g carbohydrates, 11 g total fat, 1 g saturated fat, 7 g fiber, 318 mg sodium

Nothing dresses up a simple food more than seasonings or a sauce. You can use these on salads, omelets, rice, or roasted veggies. Exercise your creativity and explore new, healthful ways to enhance your food.

AVOCADO DRESSING

PREP TIME: 5 MINUTES ▨ TOTAL TIME: 5 MINUTES ▨ MAKES 6–8 SERVINGS

2 medium avocados

3 tablespoons fresh lemon juice

$^3/_4$ teaspoon sea salt or tamari

$^3/_4$ cup water

$^1/_8$–$^1/_4$ teaspoon cayenne pepper

1 clove garlic

In a blender, combine the avocados, lemon juice, salt or tamari (to taste), water, cayenne pepper (or to taste), and garlic. Blend well. Add more water, a tablespoon at a time, to make the dressing thinner, if desired. Toss with your salad.

NUTRITION INFORMATION (2 TABLESPOONS)
39 calories, 0 g protein, 2 g carbohydrates, 4 g total fat, 0.5 g saturated fat, 2 g fiber, 101 mg sodium

VEGGIE TOMATO SAUCE

PREP TIME: 5 MINUTES ■ TOTAL TIME: 30 MINUTES ■ MAKES 8 SERVINGS

Serve this over chicken breasts or pasta.

1 tablespoon olive oil

1 clove garlic, minced

1 chile pepper, finely chopped
(wear plastic gloves when
handling)

1 can (28 ounces) peeled tomatoes,
chopped, or 2 pounds fresh
tomatoes, peeled and chopped

$\frac{1}{4}$ cup chopped black olives

2 tablespoons capers

$\frac{1}{8}$ teaspoon sea salt

Heat the oil in a medium saucepan over medium heat. Add the garlic and chile pepper and cook for 1 minute, or until slightly golden. Remove the chile pepper and add the tomatoes with their juice. Bring to a simmer, then reduce the heat, and simmer with the lid ajar for 20 minutes.

Add the olives and capers and simmer for 5 minutes. Season to taste with the salt.

NUTRITION INFORMATION (PER SERVING)
43 calories, 1 g protein, 5 g carbohydrates, 2 g total fat, 0.5 g saturated fat, 1 g fiber,
320 mg sodium

MISO/TAHINI DRESSING

PREP TIME: 5 MINUTES ■ TOTAL TIME: 5 MINUTES ■ MAKES 4 SERVINGS

This dressing can be used on salad, but it's even better on rice and veggie dishes.

1 tablespoon light miso

3 tablespoons toasted sesame tahini

1 tablespoon brown rice vinegar

$\frac{1}{4}$ teaspoon rice malt syrup or honey

3 tablespoons water

In a small bowl, or using a blender or food processor, combine the miso, tahini, vinegar, malt syrup or honey, and water. If a thinner consistency is desired, add more water.

Adjust the miso/tahini ratio to taste. More miso will make the dressing saltier; less miso will reduce the salt content.

NUTRITION INFORMATION (PER SERVING)
82 calories, 3 g protein, 4 g carbohydrates, 7 g total fat, 1 g saturated fat, 0 g fiber, 214 mg sodium

WALNUT MISO SAUCE

PREP TIME: 5 MINUTES ■ TOTAL TIME: 5 MINUTES ■ MAKES 4 SERVINGS

This sauce can be used over rice and veggies.

1 cup toasted (or raw) walnut pieces

1 tablespoon light miso

1 tablespoon rice vinegar

$\frac{1}{2}$ tablespoon stone-ground mustard

$\frac{1}{4}$ cup water

$\frac{1}{2}$ teaspoon pure maple syrup or honey

In a blender or food processor, combine the walnuts, miso (to taste), vinegar, mustard, water, and maple syrup or honey until smooth.

NUTRITION INFORMATION (PER SERVING)
165 calories, 4 g protein, 6 g carbohydrates, 15 g total fat, 1.5 g saturated fat, 2 g fiber, 270 mg sodium

DAIRY-FREE PESTO SAUCE

PREP TIME: 5 MINUTES ■ TOTAL TIME: 5 MINUTES ■ MAKES 4 SERVINGS

Serve this sauce as a garnish on soup. Of course, this nondairy pesto can also be used with pastas or grain vegetable dishes, if you wish.

1 cup packed fresh basil or spinach, stems removed

1 tablespoon light miso

1 or 2 cloves garlic (more if you like)

½ cup pine nuts and/or walnuts

¼ cup olive oil

In a blender or food processor, puree the basil or spinach, miso, garlic, nuts, and oil. If the dressing is too thick, dilute with a little water.

VARIATIONS:

- A more traditional (and fattening) pesto sauce will include grated Romano cheese.
- Some fresh parsley can be added to the blender or food processor.
- Omit the miso and replace with ½ teaspoon salt and 1 more clove garlic, minced, plus a bit more olive oil.

NUTRITION INFORMATION (PER SERVING)
243 calories, 3 g protein, 3 g carbohydrates, 26 g total fat, 3 g saturated fat, 1 g fiber, 186 mg sodium

LIME AND OLIVE OIL DRESSING

PREP TIME: 5 MINUTES ▥ TOTAL TIME: 5 MINUTES ▥ MAKES 2 SERVINGS

1–2 tablespoons fresh lime juice

3–4 tablespoons extra virgin olive oil

$\frac{1}{2}$ teaspoon salt (Himalayan pink is delicious)

In a small bowl, combine the lime juice, oil, and salt or dukkah. Adjust the seasonings to taste.

VARIATION:

Use lemon juice or 1–1$\frac{1}{2}$ tablespoons balsamic vinegar or apple cider vinegar instead of the lime juice.

NUTRITION INFORMATION (PER SERVING)
191 calories, 0 g protein, 1 g carbohydrates, 21 g total fat, 3 g saturated fat, 0 g fiber, 393 mg sodium

CREAMY DILL DRESSING

PREP TIME: 5 MINUTES ▥ TOTAL TIME: 5 MINUTES ▥ MAKES 12 SERVINGS

1 package (10$\frac{1}{2}$ ounces) firm silken tofu

1 teaspoon minced garlic

2 teaspoons chopped dill

$\frac{1}{2}$ teaspoon salt

2 tablespoons water

1$\frac{1}{2}$ tablespoons lemon juice

1 tablespoon seasoned rice vinegar

In a food processor or blender, combine the tofu, garlic, dill, salt, water, lemon juice, and vinegar. Blend until completely smooth. Store in an airtight container in the refrigerator.

NUTRITION INFORMATION (2 TABLESPOONS)
13 calories, 2 g protein, 1 g carbohydrates, 0 g total fat, 0 g saturated fat, 0 g fiber, 153 mg sodium

Who doesn't like a good homemade—and healthy—dessert? Think fresh fruit! Since most of us are attempting to lower our added sugar intake, most of the desserts here contain no or little natural added sweeteners. You can also lower the sugar content in any of these recipes by substituting cinnamon for some of the sugar.

BAKED APPLES

PREP TIME: 10 MINUTES ▪ TOTAL TIME: 55 MINUTES ▪ MAKES 4 SERVINGS

4 medium to large apples, a crisp variety like Fuji or Granny Smith

$1/4$ cup honey, pure maple syrup, firmly packed light brown sugar, or agave syrup

$1/4$ cup chopped walnuts

$1/4$ cup raisins

$1/2$ teaspoon vanilla extract

$1/4$–$1/2$ teaspoon ground cinnamon

$4^1/2$ teaspoons unsalted butter

Preheat the oven to 350°F. Butter a baking dish or pie plate.

Core the apples, without going all the way through to the bottom, and place in the dish or pie plate.

In a small bowl, mix the honey, maple syrup, sugar, or agave with the nuts, raisins, vanilla, and cinnamon. Place about 1 tablespoon of the mixture inside each cored apple. Top with a dab of butter.

Bake for 45 minutes, or until soft.

NUTRITION INFORMATION (PER SERVING)
273 calories, 2 g protein, 51 g carbohydrates, 9 g total fat, 3 g saturated fat, 5 g fiber, 42 mg sodium

FRUIT FREEZES

PREP TIME: 5 MINUTES ■ TOTAL TIME: 10 MINUTES + FREEZING TIME

Many fruits will work well for these frozen yogurt treats. Either hand-mash or puree the fruit in a blender with a little honey or pure maple syrup and water or lemon juice for a tangy taste. Combine with whole-milk, low-fat, or fat-free plain yogurt. Of course, you can make these freezes without yogurt, just fruit, for a dairy-free version. Add chopped walnuts or almonds, coconut flakes, carob or cacao powder, or natural flavorings for variation. Pour the mixture into freezable cups or scoop into ice-pop containers. The nutrient information is calculated for whole-milk yogurt. If you use low-fat or fat-free yogurt, the fat content and calories go down. Here are some sample fruit freezes.

BANANA-COCOA YOGURT FREEZE
2 SERVINGS

Mash or puree 1 ripe banana with $1/2$ teaspoon honey. Mix in 1 cup plain yogurt and 1 tablespoon unsweetened cocoa or carob powder. Freeze in cups or ice-pop containers.

NUTRITION INFORMATION (PER SERVING)
143 calories, 5 g protein, 22 g carbohydrates, 5 g total fat, 2.5 g saturated fat, 2 g fiber, 57 mg sodium

BANANA-MANGO FREEZE
1 SERVING

Mash or puree 1 medium banana with $1/2$ fresh mango and $1/2$ teaspoon fresh lime juice. Mix in 1 cup plain yogurt. Freeze in cups or ice-pop containers.

NUTRITION INFORMATION (PER SERVING)
178 calories, 6 g protein, 32 g carbohydrates, 5 g total fat, 2.5 g saturated fat, 3 g fiber, 58 mg sodium

PEAR-MAPLE FREEZE
1 SERVING

Puree 1 cup diced pear with 2 teaspoons pure maple syrup, a pinch of ground cardamom, and 1 cup plain yogurt. (May substitute diced apple or 1 cup applesauce for the pear.) Freeze in cups or ice-pop containers.

NUTRITION INFORMATION (PER SERVING)
134 calories, 5 g protein, 21 g carbohydrates, 4 g total fat, 2.5 g saturated fat, 2 g fiber, 58 mg sodium

CREAMY BERRY FREEZE
1 SERVING

Puree 1½ cups organic raspberries, blueberries, strawberries, or blackberries with 1 tablespoon honey, ½ teaspoon fresh lemon juice, and a splash of water. If using frozen, thawed berries, do not add water. Mix in 1 cup plain yogurt. Freeze in cups or ice-pop containers.

NUTRITION INFORMATION (PER SERVING)
155 calories, 5 g protein, 25 g carbohydrates, 5 g total fat, 2.5 g saturated fat, 6 g fiber, 58 mg sodium

VARIATION:

Other berries or fruits, such as peaches or nectarines, can be used. Blend 1–2 cups fresh or fresh frozen fruits with 1 tablespoon honey. Add 1 cup plain yogurt for a creamier version. Freeze in cups or ice pop containers.

NUTRITION INFORMATION (PER SERVING)
273 calories, 10 g protein, 43 g carbohydrates, 8 g total fat, 5 g saturated fat, 2 g fiber, 114 mg sodium

CHOCOLATE-TOFU MOUSSE

PREP TIME: 5 MINUTES ■ TOTAL TIME: 15 MINUTES ■ MAKES 4 SERVINGS

16 ounces soft tofu

2 tablespoons almond butter

3 tablespoons pure maple syrup

1 tablespoon vanilla extract

¼ cup water

3 tablespoons instant grain coffee (such as Pero, Postum, Cafix) or instant real coffee

6 tablespoons dark organic unsweetened cocoa powder

In a medium bowl, beat the tofu, almond butter, maple syrup, and vanilla until creamy.

Bring the water to a boil in a small saucepan. Remove from the heat and stir in the coffee and cocoa to make 3 tablespoons of liquid. It should have the consistency of cream. Add to the tofu mixture and blend again until very smooth.

Serve in individual parfait glasses.

NUTRITION INFORMATION (PER SERVING)
220 calories, 12 g protein, 25 g carbohydrates, 9 g total fat, 0.5 g saturated fat, 4 g fiber, 118 mg sodium

BLACKBERRY-GINGER-APPLE CRISP

PREP TIME: 15 MINUTES ■ TOTAL TIME: 1 HOUR 15 MINUTES
■ MAKES 8 SERVINGS

4–5 organic apples, a crisp variety like Fuji, Gala, or Rome, washed, seeded, and sliced (no need to peel)

6–12 ounces blackberries

3" piece fresh ginger, peeled and grated

1 teaspoon ground cinnamon

1/4 cup firmly packed light brown sugar, more if the berries are tart (optional)

TOPPING

1/3 cup whole wheat or nongluten flour

1/2 cup rolled oats (not steel cut)

1/4–1/2 cup granulated sugar

1/4 cup chopped pecans or other nuts

Pinch of cinnamon (optional)

1/4 cup salted or unsalted butter or cold coconut oil, cut into small pieces

Preheat the oven to 350°F. Coat an 8" x 8" baking dish with coconut oil or butter.

In a large bowl, combine the apples, blackberries, and ginger. Add the cinnamon and brown sugar, if using. Mix well. Transfer to the prepared baking dish.

To make the topping: In a medium bowl, mix the flour, oats, granulated sugar, nuts, and cinnamon, if using. With your fingers, work the butter or oil into the dry ingredients until well blended. Crumble over the top of the fruit mixture.

Bake for 1 hour, or until the fruit mixture bubbles and the topping is golden brown.

VARIATIONS:

- Use a mixture of berries in season.
- This dish can be made without sugar or ginger, and it's still good and sweet. Or you can substitute agave syrup or honey for the sugar in the fruit mixture.
- For a juicy breakfast, mix about a cup of the "crisp" with 1 cup plain yogurt and a sprinkling of ground flaxseeds.
- For another breakfast option, mix about a cup of the crisp with your morning bowl of oatmeal.

NUTRITION INFORMATION (PER SERVING)
222 calories, 2 g protein, 36 g carbohydrates, 9 g total fat, 4 g saturated fat, 5 g fiber, 54 mg sodium

MOYA'S FLOURLESS CHOCOLATE TORTE

PREP TIME: 15 MINUTES ■ TOTAL TIME: 30 MINUTES ■ MAKES 12 SERVINGS

2$\frac{1}{2}$ cups almond flour

$\frac{1}{4}$ cup sugar or sweetener of your choice (or 1 tablespoon agave syrup or honey added to the wet ingredients)

$\frac{1}{4}$ teaspoon sea salt

1 egg yolk

$\frac{1}{4}$ cup grapeseed oil, walnut oil, or melted unsalted butter

1 tablespoon vanilla extract or $\frac{1}{2}$ teaspoon almond extract

FILLING

16 ounces dark chocolate, melted over a double boiler

$\frac{1}{2}$ cup whole-milk plain yogurt

Preheat the oven to 350°F.

In a large bowl, mix together the almond flour, sugar or sweetener, and salt.

In a separate bowl, whisk together the egg yolk, oil or butter, and vanilla or almond extract. Add to the flour mixture and combine. Press into a 10" torte pan or cake pan. Prick the bottom and bake for 15 minutes, or until lightly toasted.

To make the filling: Let the chocolate cool slightly so as not to kill the live cultures in the yogurt. Then blend the yogurt into the chocolate and pour onto the nut crust. Cool completely to set.

NUTRITION INFORMATION (PER SERVING)
415 calories, 7 g protein, 32 g carbohydrates, 30 g total fat, 9 g saturated fat, 5 g fiber, 54 mg sodium

TROPICAL FRUIT SALAD

PREP TIME: 5 MINUTES ■ TOTAL TIME: 10 MINUTES ■ MAKES 4 SERVINGS

$1^1/_2$ cups papaya cubes

$1^1/_2$ cups mango pieces (cubes or balls)

2 bananas, sliced

1 cup fresh pineapple chunks

$^1/_4$ cup fresh lime juice or orange juice

1 cup pumpkin seeds or sliced almonds

In a large bowl, toss the papaya, bananas, mango, and pineapple with the lime or orange juice. Add the seeds or nuts and stir to combine.

VARIATIONS:

- Combine the ingredients in a blender or food processor for a tropical smoothie.
- To the smoothie, add 1–2 cups almond milk for a refreshing tropical drink.
- For those who enjoy a bit of alcohol, add 1 cup dark rum to the smoothie.

NUTRITION INFORMATION (PER SERVING)
279 calories, 10 g protein, 33 g carbohydrates, 15 g total fat, 2.5 g saturated fat, 6 g fiber, 82 mg sodium

There's always a need for nourishing drinks. The nut milks can be used as a base for a smoothie or blended drink. Since increasing your fluid intake supports your health (and lessens wrinkles), experiment with some of these recipes for building your healthy drink repertoire.

NUT MILKS—ALMOND, CASHEW, COCONUT

PREP TIME: 10 MINUTES ■ TOTAL TIME: 10 MINUTES ■ MAKES 2 SERVINGS

Dairy-free, nutrient-rich beverage treats can be made in a blender with a variety of nuts, water, and a touch of sugar or maple syrup and sea salt. Almonds, Brazil nuts, cashews, or coconut can be used.

½–1 cup nuts, preferably unsalted, raw, whole organic nuts; or chopped, broken, or shredded fresh coconut

1–2 cups purified water

1–2 teaspoons sugar or pure maple syrup

1–2 pinches of sea salt

Put the nuts or coconut in a blender, then cover with twice the level of water. Blend for about 30 seconds, adding half of the sugar or maple syrup and salt. Strain the nut milk into a bowl and transfer the liquid to a storage jar. Return the nut solids to the blender and repeat the process with the remaining water, sugar or maple syrup, and salt, again straining out the liquid "nut milk."

Refrigerate and serve as a drink or on cereal. The milk lasts several days refrigerated. The remaining nut "mash" can be used in cooking, such as in grain or vegetable dishes, or in baking, such as in cookies.

NUTRITION INFORMATION (PER SERVING)
357 calories, 14 g protein, 18 g carbohydrates, 30 g total fat, 2 g saturated fat, 8 g fiber, 109 mg sodium

BEET-ORANGE BLISS

PREP TIME: 5 MINUTES ■ TOTAL TIME: 5 MINUTES ■ MAKES 2 SERVINGS

$1/2$ cup chilled unsweetened brewed green tea

$1/3$ cup chilled carrot juice

$3/4$ cup chopped cooked beets

$1/2$ cup frozen or fresh chopped kale

2 oranges, cut into segments

In a blender, combine the tea, carrot juice, beets, kale, and oranges. Process for 30 seconds, or until smooth.

NUTRITION INFORMATION (PER SERVING)
133 calories, 3 g protein, 32 g carbohydrates, 1 g total fat, 0 g saturated fat, 6 g fiber, 80 mg sodium

MANGO-STRAWBERRY POWER-UP

PREP TIME: 5 MINUTES ■ TOTAL TIME: 5 MINUTES ■ MAKES 2 SERVINGS

$3/4$ cup coconut water

$1/2$ cup Greek yogurt

$1^1/4$ cups frozen mango chunks

$1/4$ cup frozen strawberries

2 tablespoons almond meal (ground almonds)

1 tablespoon fresh lemon juice

In a high-powered blender, combine the coconut water, yogurt, mango, strawberries, almond meal, and lemon juice. Puree until smooth. Divide between 2 glasses.

NUTRITION INFORMATION (PER SERVING)
181 calories, 8 g protein, 30 g carbohydrates, 5 g total fat, 1 g saturated fat, 4 g fiber, 26 mg sodium

TROPICAL FRUIT SMOOTHIE

PREP TIME: 5 MINUTES ■ TOTAL TIME: 5 MINUTES ■ MAKES 4 SERVINGS

1 ripe mango, peeled, pitted, and cubed (about 1/2 cup)

1/2 cup coconut milk

1/2 ripe papaya, peeled, seeded, and coarsely chopped (about 3/4 cup)

1 ripe banana, sliced

6 strawberries, stemmed and halved (about 1 1/2 cups)

1 tablespoon fresh lime juice

6 ice cubes, coarsely crushed

In a blender, combine the mango and coconut milk. Puree until completely liquefied. Add the papaya, banana, strawberries, lime juice, and ice. Blend for 2 to 3 minutes, or until smooth and very thick. Pour into chilled glasses.

NUTRITION INFORMATION (PER SERVING)
156 calories, 2 g protein, 26 g carbohydrates, 7 g total fat, 5 g saturated fat, 3 g fiber, 8 mg sodium

MORNING ENERGY DRINK

PREP TIME: 5 MINUTES ■ TOTAL TIME: 5 MINUTES ■ MAKES 2 SERVINGS

1 1/2 cups fat-free vanilla soy milk

1 banana, sliced and frozen

1/4 cup frozen loose-pack blueberries

2 tablespoons almond or cashew butter

1 tablespoon wheat germ

1 tablespoon ground flaxseeds

In a blender, combine the milk, banana, blueberries, nut butter, wheat germ, and flaxseeds. Blend for 30 seconds, or until smooth.

NUTRITION INFORMATION (PER SERVING)
231 calories, 10 g protein, 28 g carbohydrates, 10 g total fat, 2 g saturated fat, 5 g fiber, 127 mg sodium

WATER VARIATIONS

We all know that we're supposed to drink at least 8 glasses of water every day; it helps maintain our energy level, weight, and fluid level. And it's best if what you add to your water is organic. If you want to oomph up your *agua*, try one of these options, which may boost your metabolism.

- Add citrus—lemon, orange, or lime—to your water to help your cells produce more energy with a shot of vitamin C. Add about 3 thin slices to a glass of water and sip.

- Try something different: cucumber. This beverage is served at one of our favorite restaurants and spas and is a real treat to sip at home, too. To a quart pitcher of water, add 8 to 10 slices of cucumber for a wonderfully refreshing way to increase your water intake.

- Add a packet of flavored nutrients, such as the popular Emergen-C, or add a tablespoon or two of a juice like orange or apple.

- Some folks suggest that adding cayenne pepper to your water can boost metabolism, so this is a bit like drinking a variation of the Master Cleanse. You can start slow with $1/8$ teaspoon of cayenne pepper to a glass of water that you've sweetened with a handful of squashed berries, 1 teaspoon of honey, or 1 tablespoon of chopped mango or watermelon.

- Other favorite tasty infusions to prepare with water are watermelon, mint, or pineapple. Place a piece of the chopped fruit or whole fresh mint leaves in a glass of water. When you find a combination that you like, fill a pitcher with water and add a cup of the fruit or a few sprigs of mint. Experiment with other herbs, such as rose geranium or basil.

Before beginning the program, take a few minutes to evaluate yourself and answer the questions below. Take some time and think deeply about your physical, mental, and emotional health and what you would like to change. There are no wrong answers; this exercise simply reviews where you are now. When you have finished the program, or your first round of it, you will have a chance to revisit these questions to see what has changed. Please visit us on Facebook at wwww.facebook.com/UltimateImmunitythebook/info.

WHAT IS YOUR MOST BOTHERSOME SYMPTOM OR PROBLEM THAT YOU'D LIKE TO ADDRESS? _____

How severe was that problem in the last week?

None		1	2	3	4	5	6	7	8	9	10	Severe

In the last 24 hours?

None		1	2	3	4	5	6	7	8	9	10	Severe

My stress level in the last week was:

None		1	2	3	4	5	6	7	8	9	10	Severe

My sleep in the last week was:

Excellent		1	2	3	4	5	6	7	8	9	10	Poor

My exercise regimen is:

Excellent		1	2	3	4	5	6	7	8	9	10	Poor

My stress management strategies are:

Excellent		1	2	3	4	5	6	7	8	9	10	Poor

My eating habits are:

Excellent		1	2	3	4	5	6	7	8	9	10	Poor

My energy level is:

Excellent		1	2	3	4	5	6	7	8	9	10	Poor

My mood is:

Excellent		1	2	3	4	5	6	7	8	9	10	Poor

My ability to focus is:

Excellent		1	2	3	4	5	6	7	8	9	10	Poor

My digestive function and bowel movements are:

Excellent		1	2	3	4	5	6	7	8	9	10	Poor

My level of body pain is:

None		1	2	3	4	5	6	7	8	9	10	Severe

After completing the above questions, look back at your answers. The more circles on the left, the better you are feeling now. Circles closer to the right indicate challenges to address throughout the program. Add up your scores and write the sum of your answers here:

By the end of the program, it's likely that you will have many more circles on the left and a significantly lower total number. Now it's time to begin!

MY STARTING STATS

Weight:	Waist circumference:
BMI:	Blood pressure:

IF YOU KNOW THE FOLLOWING NUMBERS, INCLUDE THEM HERE:

Total cholesterol:	Triglycerides:
HDL:	Blood glucose:
LDL:	TSH (thyroid):

MY ULTIMATE IMMUNITY JOURNAL

DATE:_____

Here's a simple review chart for your transitional elimination diet. List the foods you eat and when you eat them, and be aware of how you feel before and after. Notice your energy level and how you feel as you progress. You may experience some early negative effects as you begin this process, but these should lessen or even disappear by day 3. Pay attention to your overall attitude, mood, energy level, digestion, and any allergy symptoms. Let's see how you improve.

MEAL TYPE	FOOD EATEN	MOOD/ENERGY BEFORE	MOOD/ENERGY AFTER
BREAKFAST One or two 6-oz portions of fruit and grain			
OPTIONAL **MORNING SNACK** 1 small handful of nuts/seeds			
LUNCH Large bowl of salad Optional protein: 3–4 oz beans or 3–4 oz fish or poultry			
OPTIONAL **AFTERNOON SNACK** 1 or 2 pieces of fruit			
DINNER Steamed or roasted veggies Optional protein or optional one or two 6–8 oz servings of a simple vegetable soup			

Don't forget to begin each day with 1 or 2 glasses of water with a squeeze of fresh lemon and follow this up with 1 or 2 glasses of water 30 minutes before lunch and dinner, as well as other times throughout the day!

Check a box for every glass of water consumed throughout the day:

☐ Lemon water in the morning

☐ Before lunch

☐ Before dinner

☐ Additional glasses of water

MIND-BODY CHECKLIST

ACTIVITY	TIME OF DAY	DURATION	MOOD/ENERGY BEFORE	MOOD/ENERGY AFTER
Self-massage				
Logging On				
Stretching				
Weights				
Aerobics				
Walking				
Meditation				
Social interactions				
Outdoor time				

5-DAY ELIMINATION SYMPTOM CHECKLIST:

Headaches
None   1   2   3   4   5   6   7   8   9   10   Severe

Digestion
None   1   2   3   4   5   6   7   8   9   10   Severe

Allergy symptoms
None   1   2   3   4   5   6   7   8   9   10   Severe

Bowel movements
Excellent   1   2   3   4   5   6   7   8   9   10   Poor

Body pain
None   1   2   3   4   5   6   7   8   9   10   Severe

Mood
Excellent   1   2   3   4   5   6   7   8   9   10   Poor

Focus
Excellent   1   2   3   4   5   6   7   8   9   10   Poor

Stress
None   1   2   3   4   5   6   7   8   9   10   Severe

Sleep
Excellent   1   2   3   4   5   6   7   8   9   10   Poor

Once again, add up your score and compare it to your earlier score. How does it compare? Do you feel different from how you felt at the beginning of the program?

REFLECTIONS/CHALLENGES/OBSERVATIONS:

_____

_____

_____

_____

_____

_____

_____

_____

_____

_____

_____

_____

_____

_____

_____

_____

BASIC MASTER CLEANSE RECIPE
Adapted from Stanley Burrough's original recipe

Mix the following ingredients. Adjust the cayenne to your taste.

    2 tablespoons fresh lemon juice

    1 tablespoon pure maple syrup

    $\frac{1}{10}$ teaspoon cayenne (ground red) pepper

    8 ounces water

NOTE:

- You can drink one to two glasses of the juice at a time.
- Rinse your mouth with water after each glass so as not to damage your tooth enamel.
- Don't carry the Master Cleanse in plastic or metal.
- Feel free to also drink herbal tea throughout the day and add a separate drink of fresh vegetable juices that include greens like kale plus celery, cucumber, and carrots.

Glasses of juice consumed

| 1 | 2 | 3 | 4 | 5 | 6 | 7 | 8 | 9 | 10 |

Glasses of water or herbal tea consumed

| 1 | 2 | 3 | 4 | 5 | 6 |

Number of times bowels moved

| 1 | 2 | 3 | 4 |

Number of times urinated throughout the day

| 1 | 2 | 3 | 4 | 5 | 6 | 7 | 8 | 9 | 10 | more |

Energy level

| Excellent | 1 | 2 | 3 | 4 | 5 | 6 | 7 | 8 | 9 | 10 | Poor |

Mood

| Excellent | 1 | 2 | 3 | 4 | 5 | 6 | 7 | 8 | 9 | 10 | Poor |

Here's your chart for tracking your I-PEP (Immune-Power Eating Plan) to help you make good food choices and monitor how you are feeling. Pay attention to how the foods you eat affect your mood and energy.

MEAL TYPE	FOOD EATEN	MOOD/ENERGY BEFORE	MOOD/ENERGY AFTER
BREAKFAST Grain with fruit (choose less reactive grains like quinoa, millet, rice, and oatmeal) Small handful of nuts/seeds (can be added to grain if you desire more food or want to add more protein/oils to breakfast)			
***OPTIONAL* MORNING SNACK** Small handful of nuts/seeds (like almonds, walnuts or sunflower seeds) or another piece of fruit			
LUNCH Salad or vegetable stir-fry with protein like fish, poultry, or legumes			
***OPTIONAL* AFTERNOON SNACK** Veggies (like celery, carrots, or cucumber with hummus) or rice cake with nut butter and sliced organic apple or banana (1 piece of fruit)			
DINNER Protein Veggies Optional rice/quinoa			
***OPTIONAL* EVENING SNACK** 1–2 pieces fruit			

Don't forget to begin each day with 1 to 2 glasses of water with a squeeze of fresh lemon and follow this up with 1 to 2 glasses of water 30 minutes before lunch and dinner, as well as other times throughout the day!

Check a box for every glass of water consumed throughout the day:

☐ Lemon water in the morning

☐ Before lunch

☐ Before dinner

☐ Additional glasses of water

MIND-BODY CHECKLIST

ACTIVITY	TIME OF DAY	DURATION	MOOD/ENERGY BEFORE	MOOD/ENERGY AFTER
Self-massage				
Logging On				
Stretching				
Weights				
Aerobics				
Walking				
Meditation				
Social interactions				
Outdoor time				

I-PEP SYMPTOM CHECKLIST

Headaches
None 1 2 3 4 5 6 7 8 9 10 Severe

Digestion
None 1 2 3 4 5 6 7 8 9 10 Severe

Allergy symptoms
None 1 2 3 4 5 6 7 8 9 10 Severe

Bowel movements
Excellent 1 2 3 4 5 6 7 8 9 10 Poor

Body pain
None 1 2 3 4 5 6 7 8 9 10 Severe

Mood
Excellent 1 2 3 4 5 6 7 8 9 10 Poor

Focus
Excellent 1 2 3 4 5 6 7 8 9 10 Poor

Stress
None 1 2 3 4 5 6 7 8 9 10 Severe

Sleep
Excellent 1 2 3 4 5 6 7 8 9 10 Poor

Once again, add up your score and compare it to your earlier score. How does it compare? Do you feel different from how you felt at the beginning of the program?

MY ULTIMATE IMMUNITY JOURNAL

WHAT WAS YOUR MOST BOTHERSOME SYMPTOM OR PROBLEM BEFORE BEGINNING THE PROGRAM? _____

How severe was that problem in the last week?

None   1   2   3   4   5   6   7   8   9   10   Severe

In the last 24 hours?

None   1   2   3   4   5   6   7   8   9   10   Severe

My stress level in the last week was:

None   1   2   3   4   5   6   7   8   9   10   Severe

My sleep in the last week was:

Excellent   1   2   3   4   5   6   7   8   9   10   Poor

My exercise regimen is:

Excellent   1   2   3   4   5   6   7   8   9   10   Poor

My stress management strategies are:

Excellent   1   2   3   4   5   6   7   8   9   10   Poor

My eating habits are:

Excellent   1   2   3   4   5   6   7   8   9   10   Poor

My energy level is:

Excellent   1   2   3   4   5   6   7   8   9   10   Poor

My mood is:

Excellent   1   2   3   4   5   6   7   8   9   10   Poor

My ability to focus is:

Excellent   1   2   3   4   5   6   7   8   9   10   Poor

My digestive function and bowel movements are:

Excellent   1   2   3   4   5   6   7   8   9   10   Poor

My level of body pain is:

None   1   2   3   4   5   6   7   8   9   10   Severe

Now add up your score. How does it compare to your original score and your score after the 5-Day Elimination, Healing Plan?

Throughout the program, which symptoms improved the most?

_____

Which symptoms still need to be addressed?

_____

How long did you stay with the program?

_____

When did you begin to notice improvements or changes?

_____

What were the biggest changes and challenges for you?

_____

Overall, how do you feel now compared to how you felt before the program?

_____

MY POSTPROGRAM STATS:

Weight:	Waist circumference:
BMI:	Blood pressure:

IF YOU KNOW THE FOLLOWING NUMBERS, INCLUDE THEM HERE:

Total cholesterol:	Triglycerides:
HDL:	Blood glucose:
LDL:	TSH (thyroid):

GLOSSARY

acquired immunity or adaptive immune response: The second immune response that is mounted by lymphocytes to specific antigens, which results in activated immune cells, antibody production, and memory cells.

adaptogens: Substances or herbs that help regulate physiology and homeostasis, or balance.

allergens: Innocuous environmental antigens that give rise to hypersensitivity or allergic reactions.

allergies or allergic reaction: An immune response to an allergen (antigen) due to an antibody, most commonly IgE. The binding of the allergen to IgE on mast cells causes symptoms of allergies through the release of inflammatory molecules, such as histamine.

anaphylaxis: A whole-body or severe localized reaction to an allergen that causes closing of the airways and other potentially life-threatening reactions.

antibody: A protein that recognizes a specific antigen. Antibodies are also known as immunoglobulins, abbreviated as Ig. They help in the elimination of the invader or antigen. The main types of antibodies are IgA, IgG, IgM, and IgE.

antigen-presenting cells (APC): Highly specialized cells that can break a microbe or protein into smaller pieces, called antigens, and carry them to specific T cells able to recognize the antigen. This process activates the T cell to do its part in the immune process. APCs include dendritic cells, monocytes, and macrophages.

antigens: Substances that stimulate an immune response, recognized as "nonself," and results in the production of antibodies and activated T cells to eliminate them. Antigens can be pollens, plants, animal dander, microorganisms, chemicals, or altered cells.

anti-inflammatory: A substance that helps reduce, stop, or prevent inflammation.

antioxidant: A substance that protects the cells from damage caused by free radicals (oxidative stress). Antioxidants are also known as free radical quenchers or balancers.

apoptosis: Programmed cell death due to a normal genetic program that initiates the process. This is a natural process, considered "gentle" to the cell, unlike cell death caused by external events like toxicity or poisoning.

atopic dermatitis: See eczema.

autoantibodies: Antibodies made against one's own cells or tissues that recognize "self" as antigens.

autoimmune disease: An immune attack on your own cells, tissues, or proteins. It is a case of mistaken identity, a misguided attack against something inside of you. It happens when your immune system doesn't recognize part of your own body as *you*.

B lymphocytes (B cells): One of the two major types of lymphocytes; upon activation and further development, they will become plasma cells that produce antibodies.

bacteria: Microscopic single-celled microorganisms that can live anywhere in or outside the human body. Those that are pathogenic can cause a wide variety of infectious diseases. The human body is also home to billions of beneficial bacteria, especially in the gut.

biome or microbiome or microflora: Those microbes that live peacefully in your gut and throughout your body and support immunity and other digestive functions.

bowels: The small and large intestines.

cancer: A disease in which abnormal cells reproduce out of control. The DNA of regulator genes becomes damaged; this mutation contributes to cells growing out of control. Cancer is not one disease; it's many different diseases, depending on the cell type where the abnormal cell originated and the way the genes are regulated and expressed.

capsaicin: A chemical component of chile and cayenne peppers, it causes a burning sensation on tissues and is responsible for the "heat" in certain foods. It helps block pain by interacting with the same receptor sites as endorphins, the body's painkilling substances.

carotenoids: Substances found in yellow and orange vegetables and fruits and dark green vegetables that act as antioxidants. They are one of many phytonutrients that cells use.

celiac disease: An autoimmune condition in which the smallest amounts of gluten can't be tolerated. Autoantibodies are produced against one of the proteins in the intestines (transglutaminase enzyme), leading to intestinal inflammation and damage, worsened significantly by the presence of gluten.

cells: The basic units of life and the sites for all of the body's functions.

chronic inflammation: A result of tissue damaged or when inflammatory activity persists over time.

corticosteroids: A class of drugs related to naturally produced steroids made in the adrenal gland such as cortisol.

cortisol: The major steroid produced by the adrenal cortex.

CRP (C-reactive protein): A protein made during an acute phase of infection and inflammation. It has become a useful molecular marker in the blood for any kind of inflammation. High levels in the blood are considered an indicator of risk for coronary artery disease.

cytokines: Proteins produced primarily by immune cells that affect the behavior of other cells. Cytokines of the immune system are involved in signaling between cells and regulating various aspects of the immune response. Some cytokines can cause a rise in the body's temperature or induce sleep. Others can trigger inflammation (proinflammatory cytokines), while others can stop it.

dendritic cells: Potent stimulators of T cell responses and are also antigen-producing cells (APC). They help process microbes, and they prepare and present the antigens to the lymphocytes so they can remove them more readily through specific immune responses.

DNA (deoxyribonucleic acid): The core molecule that carries genetic information. The genetic code of DNA holds the instructions or blueprints for all the proteins in your body. There are switches surrounding the DNA that turn genes on and off. The switches outside the molecule are called epigenetic, and they can change the expression of a gene without changing the code.

eczema: An inflammatory and allergic condition of the skin; it is also known as atopic dermatitis.

edema: Swelling due to buildup of fluid in the tissues.

enzymes: Protein catalysts that lower the energy necessary for a metabolic reaction, facilitating the speed of reactions.

eosinophils: White blood cells that are increased in allergic reactions and are thought to be important in the defense against parasitic infections.

epigenetic: Refers to the external and environmental switches influencing gene expression. Epigenetic changes, in comparison with genetic mutation, tend to be reversible.

estrogen: A female sex hormone.

flare or flare-up: An acute, sudden worsening of symptoms after a period of remission or relatively mild and stable condition.

free radicals: Highly reactive unstable oxygen compounds that can damage cells and molecules in cells. Also known as oxidants, they are electrically out of balance.

gene: A segment of DNA that carries the coded information for the production of a specific protein.

glutathione: The cell's primary antioxidant, it works with vitamin E, alpha lipoic acid, and vitamin C to keep cells healthy and to limit free radicals.

gluten: A protein in wheat, barley, and rye. (Gliadin is another wheat protein.)

histamine: An inflammatory molecule stored in mast cells and released by allergenic antigens binding to IgE on mast cells. It is also released when tissue cells are damaged.

human leukocyte antigens (HLA): The major histocompatibility antigens that indicate cell identity and immune responsiveness. They mark which cells are compatible with others, meaning the cells and tissues that have similar genes and immunological expression. Some HLA subtypes are indicative of risk for allergies or autoimmune disease and are used in tissue typing for organ transplantation.

hyperactive immune states: An overactive immune response, including allergies, autoimmune illnesses, and chronic inflammation, that can lead to irritation, organ damage or destruction, and chronic illness.

immune response: The response made by the immune cells to defend against a pathogen. An immune response can be triggered by damage to the tissue initiating inflammation. A microbe being engulfed by a phagocyte is an immune response. Other immune responses include the production of antibodies or T killer cells.

immunity: The ability to resist infection and protect the body.

immunization: The deliberate stimulation of the adaptive immune response by introducing into the body an antigen to specific microbes.

immunoglobulin: Another name for antibody or Ig.

immunomodulator: A substance that affects immune responses. Examples are cytokines as well as certain drugs that weaken, regulate, or normalize immune functions.

immunosuppression: A state in which the ability of the body's immune system to respond is decreased. This condition may be present at birth or caused by certain infections, drugs, radiation, or stress.

immunosuppressive: Suppression of the natural immune responses.

infection: An invasion of the tissues by disease-causing microbes.

inflammation: The general response of the cells and tissues to irritation, injury, infection or localized immune response. Acute inflammation refers to an early, quick, and temporary event; chronic inflammation is long lasting from infection, allergies, or autoimmune diseases. Inflammation is an innate nonspecific immune response handled by neutrophils, monocytes, macrophages, and tissue mast cells. The physical signs of inflammation are redness, heat, swelling, and pain.

innate immune response/innate immunity: The early phase of the immune response against pathogens. It is inborn, present at all times, immediate, and does not change with repeated exposures. It is not specific toward any particular organism. Cells involved in this phase include neutrophils, monocytes, and macrophages.

interleukins: A group of peptides or proteins that are chemical signals between immune and other cells of the body. They are cytokines.

leaky gut syndrome: Increased intestinal permeability. Symptoms include bloating, gas, cramps, food sensitivities, and general aches and pains.

lectin: A specific type of protein that binds to certain carbohydrates triggering immune responses. Lectins are pattern-recognizing proteins and are present on the surface of immune cells, plant foods, and microbes.

leukotrienes: Molecules that can prolong or turn off inflammatory responses.

lycopene: A carotenoid phytochemical found in ripe fruits, especially tomatoes.

lymph: The clear, thin fluid of the lymphatic system carrying cells and wastes away through the lymphatic vessels to be recycled back into the blood.

lymphatic system: A system of channels and tissues that drain the fluid that leaks outside of the cells. This part of the immune system includes the lymph fluid, lymph vessels, lymphocytes, and lymph nodes, whose overall function is filtration and immune responses.

lymphedema: A disorder in which lymph accumulates in the soft tissues, resulting in swelling. It refers to swelling in an arm or leg that is commonly caused by removal of lymph nodes as part of cancer treatment, mainly surgery. Lymphedema may be caused by inflammation, obstruction, or removal of the nodes.

lymphocytes: Part of the adaptive immune system, these are white blood cells that fight infection and disease. They are born with the ability to recognize only one specific antigen. There are NK, T, and B lymphocytes.

lymphoid organs: Tissues with high numbers of lymphocytes and include the bone marrow, thymus, lymph nodes, spleen, and GALT, comprising the intestine, the appendix, and Peyer's patches.

macrophages: Monocytic phagocytes that have become activated and are important in innate immunity and immune regulation.

mast cells: Immune cells that live at the body's vulnerable borders, including the skin and the GI and respiratory tracts, and that contain packets of molecules, particularly histamine, which signal inflammation to begin.

melatonin: A hormone produced by the pineal gland in response to light and dark cycles. It induces sleep, influences immune cells, and affects mood.

metabolism: The process by which the body converts food to energy and then gets rid of waste products.

microbiome: The collection of microbes that normally occupy your entire body and is as unique to you as your fingerprints.

molecule: A chemical made of atoms.

monocytes: A phagocytic white blood cell that can live for years and has a role in immune regulation.

mucosal-associated lymphoid tissue (MALT): Mucus-producing cells essential to immune health that reside in the gut, nose, and upper respiratory tract. The mucosal immune system protects the surfaces bathed by external secretions. Also known as GALT.

mutation: A change in the DNA sequence of a particular gene that may prevent the gene from providing correct instructions for making a protein, resulting in abnormal proteins or cells.

natural killer lymphocyte (NK cell): A lymphocyte that is the first responder against viral infections. NK cells are part of the innate immune response.

neuropeptides: Small, proteinlike molecules consisting of amino acids and used by neurons to communicate with one another and with other cells.

neutrophil: A quick-acting scavenger phagocyte and the first line of defense against bacterial or fungal infections. The most predominant white blood cell in human blood, a neutrophil only lives a few hours in the tissues.

oxidants: Another word for free radicals.

oxidative stress: The process by which oxidants or free radicals damage cells and molecules and "stress" our optimal function.

peptides: Molecules consisting of two or more amino acids. Smaller than proteins, they typically contain no more than 50 amino acids.

Peyer's patches: Groups of lymphocytes in the small intestine.

phagocytes: White blood cells that engulf and destroy microbes. These include neutrophils, monocytes, and macrophages.

phytochemicals: Chemicals in plants that protect the plants against bacteria, viruses, and fungi. Humans can benefit from many of these chemicals for their own health.

plasma cells: Matured from B cells to produce antibodies.

platelets: Tiny blood cells essential for blood clotting.

probiotics: Live microbes, mostly bacteria such as the lactobacilli species, that help balance the microbes in the gut. They also have a role in helping the immune cells develop.

prostaglandins: Molecules that regulate inflammation.

protease inhibitors: Molecules that block the activity of enzymes (proteases) that break down proteins, preventing proteins from being degraded.

receptor: A molecule on the surface of the cell that recognizes specific signaling molecules, such as a histamine receptor that recognizes histamine or an adrenergic receptor that recognizes adrenaline (epinephrine).

remission: The absence of symptoms of active disease.

salivary IgA or secretory IgA: An immunoglobulin found primarily in the secretions of the body such as saliva. One of its roles is to facilitate the removal of microbes in the mouth and gut.

serum: The fluid part of the blood.

stress: The body's response to anything threatening, whether real or imagined. The stress response prepares the body to fight or flee.

substance P: A neuropeptide, made of 11 amino acids, that plays important roles in inflammation and pain. A proinflammatory molecule, it's involved in signaling pain responses.

T helpers (Th): Cells that activate other immune cells. The two primary categories are Th1 and Th2 and are distinguished by the cytokines they produce. Th1 cells are sometimes considered the inflammatory T cells, since they activate macrophages, while Th2 cells stimulate B cells to produce antibodies. Th17 is another T cell recently discovered.

Th1 helpers: Cells that increase the number of infection-fighting cells.

Th2 helpers: Cells that tell the B cells to get to work, to produce protective antibody molecules. Th2 cells drive the allergic response.

T killer cell: A cytotoxic cell that can kill other cells. It is most important in defending against pathogens that live inside cells.

T lymphocytes (T cells): A subset of lymphocytes that develop in the thymus and can further mature into T helpers and T regulatory cells.

T regulator (Treg): Cells that slow down, turn off, or accelerate a variety of immune processes.

thymus: The primary immune organ where T cells are produced and mature.

tumor suppressor genes: Genes that slow down cell division or cause cells to die at the appropriate time. They are also the DNA repair genes and can trigger apoptosis.

vaccines: Composed of dead or nonpathogenic forms of a microbe, vaccines prevent deadly or crippling diseases such as smallpox and polio. In general, a vaccine contains antigenic material from a specific organism, and this leads to antibody protection for future exposure to that organism.

white blood cells (WBCs): Blood cells involved in the immune response and in the destruction of microbes that cause infection. Also called leukocytes.

NOTES

Chapter 1

1 JE Graham, LM Christian, and JK Kiecolt-Glaser, "Stress, age, and immune function: towards a lifespan approach," *Journal of Behavioral Medicine* 29 (2006): 389–400.

2 LS Berk et al., "Stress hormone changes during mirthful laughter," *American Journal of the Medical Sciences* 298 (1989): 390–96; MP Bennett et al., "The effect of mirthful laughter on stress and natural killer cell activity," *Alternative Therapies in Health and Medicine* 9 (2003): 38.

3 J Kiecolt-Glaser et al., "Slowing of wound healing by psychological stress," *Lancet* 346 (1995): 1194–96; JP Gouin and JK Kiecolt-Glaser, "The impact of psychological stress on wound healing: methods and mechanisms," *Immunology and Allergy Clinics of North America* 31 (2011): 81–93. doi: 10.1016/j.iac.2010.09.010.

4 JP Gouin et al., "Chronic stress, daily stressors, and circulating inflammatory markers," *Health Psychology* 31 (2012): 264–68. doi: 10.1037/a0025536.

5 JK Kiecolt-Glaser, "Stress, food, and inflammation: psychoneuroimmunology and nutrition at the cutting edge," *Psychosomatic Medicine* 72 (2010): 365–59. doi: 10.1097/PSY.0b013e3181dbf489.

6 MJ Adams et al., "Thyroid cancer risk 40+ years after irradiation for an enlarged thymus: an update of the Hempelmann cohort," *Radiation Research* 174 (2010): 753–62.

7 MJ Adams et al., "Breast cancer risk 55+ years after irradiation for an enlarged thymus and its implications for early childhood medical irradiation today," *Cancer Epidemiology, Biomarkers, and Prevention* 19 (2010): 48–58.

8 E. Brender et al., "The spleen," *Journal of the American Medical Association* 294 (2005): 2660.

9 F Purchiaroni et al., "The role of intestinal microbiota and the immune system," *European Review for Medical and Pharmacological Sciences* 17 (2013): 323–33.

10 E McAllister et al., "Ten putative contributors to the obesity epidemic," *Critical Reviews in Food Science and Nutrition,* 49 (2009): 868–913.

11 "Chapter 11—Cytokines." http://www2.hawaii.edu/~johnb/micro/micro161/cytokines_chap11/Cytokines.htm.

12 "Health and research topics: community immunity ('herd' immunity)," National Institute of Allergy and Infectious Diseases, 2010, http://www.niaid.nih.gov/topics/pages/communityimmunity.aspx.

13 Plaisance K et al. Effect of antipyretic therapy on the duration of illness in experimental influenza A, Shigella sonnei, and Rickettsia rickettsii infections. *Pharmacotherapy* 2000 20 (12): 1417–22.

14 A Abbas, A Lichtman, and J Pober, *Cellular and Molecular Immunology* (Philadelphia: WB Saunders, 2000).

Chapter 2

1 CP Fagundes et al., "Depressive symptoms enhance stress-induced inflammatory responses," *Brain, Behavior, and Immunity* 31 (2013): 172–76. doi:10.1016/j.bbi.2012.05.006.

2 C Wedekind et al., "MHC-Dependent mate preferences in humans," *Proceedings of the Royal Society of London* 260 (1995), 245–49.

3 C Brooks, N Pearce, and J Douwes, "The hygiene hypothesis in allergy and asthma: an update," *Current Opinion in Allergy and Clinical Immunology* 13, no. 1 (2013): 70–77.

4 H Szajewska, "Early nutritional strategies for preventing allergic disease," *Israeli Medical Association Journal* 14, no. 1 (2012): 58–62.

5 "Outgrowing food allergies," National Institute of Allergic and Infectious Diseases, http://www.niaid.nih.gov/topics/foodAllergy/understanding/Pages/quickFacts.aspx.

6 R Valet, "Ugly plants worse for allergy patients," *ScienceDaily*, May 28, 2013. http://www.sciencedaily.com/releases/2013/05/130528122246.htm.

7 P Kidd, "Th1/Th2 balance: the hypothesis, its limitations, and implications for health and disease," *Alternative Medicine Review* 8 (2003): 223–46.

8 H Okada et al., "The 'hygiene hypothesis' for autoimmune and allergic diseases: an update," *Clinical and Experimental Immunology* 160, no. 1 (2010): 1–9.

9 AM Croft et al., "Helminth therapy (worms) for allergic rhinitis," *Cochrane Database of Systematic Reviews* 4 (2012): 1–46.

10 NR Lynch et al., "Effect of antihelmintic treatment on the allergic reactivity in children in a tropical slum," *Journal of Allergy and Clinical Immunology* 92, no. 3 (1993): 404–11.

11 M Yazdanbakhsh et al., "Allergy, parasites, and the hygiene hypothesis," *Science* 296 (2002): 490–94.

12 MR Waggoner, "Parsing the peanut panic: the social life of a contested food allergy epidemic," *Social Science and Medicine* 90 (2013): 49. doi:10.1016/j.socscimed.2013.04.031.

13 R Kristensen et al., "Perceived stress and risk of adult-onset asthma and other atopic disorders: a longitudinal cohort study," *Allergy* 67 (2012):1408–14.

14 PJ Busse et al., "Characteristics of allergic sensitization among asthmatic adults older than 55 years: results from the National Health and Nutrition Examination Survey, 2005–2006," *Annals of Allergy, Asthma, and Immunology* 110 no. 4 (2013): 247–52.

15 A Sapone et al., "Divergence of gut permeability and mucosal immune gene expression in two gluten-associated conditions: celiac disease and gluten sensitivity," *BMC Medicine* 9:23 (2011), 1–11. doi:10.1186/1741-7015-9-23.

16 "Autoimmune diseases fact sheet," Womenshealth.gov, http://www.womenshealth.gov/publications/our-publications/fact-sheet/autoimmune-diseases.html.

17 A Rubio-Tapia et al., "The prevalence of celiac disease in the United States," *American Journal of Gastroenterology* 107 (2012): 1538–44.

18 "Gluten-free diet fad: are celiac disease rates actually rising?," CBSNews.com, July 31, 2012, http://www.cbsnews.com/news/gluten-free-diet-fad-are-celiac-disease-rates-actually-rising/.

19 A Vilppula et al., "Increasing prevalence and high incidence of celiac disease in elderly people: a population-based study," *BMC Gastroenterology* 9:49 (2009):1–5.

20 M. Beck, "Clues to gluten sensitivity," *Wall Street Journal*, March 15, 2011. http://online.wsj.com/news/articles/SB10001424052748704893604576200393522456636.

21 Sapone, "Divergence of gut permeability and mucosal immune gene expression in two gluten-associated conditions."

22 J Alegria-Torres, et al. Epigenetics and Lifestyle. *Epigenomics* 2011, 3(3): 267-277.

23 http://commonfund.nih.gov/epigenomics/figure.aspx

24 R Roychoudhuri et al., "BACH2 represses effector programs to stabilize Treg-mediated immune homeostasis," *Nature* 498 (2013): 506–10. doi:10.1038/nature12199.

25 J Cárdenas-Roldán, A Rojas-Villarraga, and J Anaya, "How do autoimmune diseases cluster in families? A systematic review and meta-analysis," *BMC Medicine* 11:73 (2013). doi:10.1186/1741-7015-11-73.

26 R Root-Bernstein and D Fairweather, "Complexities in the relationship between infection and autoimmunity," *Current Allergy and Asthma Reports* 14, no. 1 (2014): 407–15. doi:10.1007/s11882-013-0407-3.

27 MF Cusick, J Libbey, and R Fujinami, "Molecular mimicry as a mechanism of autoimmune disease," *Clinical Review of Allergy and Immunology* 42, no. 1 (2012): 102–11.

28 Y Tomer and TF Davies, "Infection, thyroid disease, and autoimmunity," *Endocrine Review* 14, no. 1 (1993): 107–20. http://dx.doi.org/10.1210/edrv-14-1-107.

29 D Verthelyi, "Sex hormones as immunomodulators in health and disease," *International Immunopharmacology* 1, no. 6 (2001): 983–93.

30 B Annechien, M Heineman, and M Faas, "Sex hormones and the immune response in humans," *Human Reproduction Update* 11, no. 4 (2005): 411–23.

31 "NIH progress in autoimmune diseases research," National Institutes of Health, http://www.niaid.nih.gov/topics/autoimmune/Documents/adccfinal.pdf.

32 M. Cutolo et al., "Sex hormones influence on the immune system: basic and clinical aspects in autoimmunity," *Lupus* 13 (2004): 635–38.

33 D Furmana et al., "Systems analysis of sex differences reveals an immunosuppressive role for testosterone in the response to influenza vaccination," *Proceedings of the National Academy of Sciences* 111, no. 2 (2014): 869–74.

34 K Belge et al., "Advances in treating psoriasis," *F1000 Prime Reports* 6:4 (2014). doi:10.12703/P6-4.

35 J Kelly, Medscape Medical News. May 13, 2014. Lupus Studies Point to Gut Microbes, Epigenetics. http://www.medscape.com/viewarticle/825045?src=wnl_edit_specol&uac=161036AV

36 CJ Edwards, Costenbader KH. Epigenetics and the microbiome: developing areas in the understanding of the aetiology of lupus. *Lupus* 2014, 23: 505–506

37 C. Edwards, Commensal Gut Bacteria and the Etiopathogenesis of Rheumatoid Arthritis. *J. Rheumatology* 2008, 35:1477–1479. www.jrheum.org/content/35/8/1477

38 SM Vieira, Pagovich OE, and Kriegel MA. Diet, microbiota and autoimmune diseases. *Lupus* 2014, 23 (6): 518–526.

39 M Rincon, "Interleukin-6: from an inflammatory marker to a target for inflammatory diseases." *Trends in Immunology* 33, no. 11 (2012): 1–7. doi:10.1016/j.it.2012.07.003.

40 "Community immunity ('herd' immunity)," National Institute of Allergy and Infectious Diseases.

41 "Immunization," MedlinePlus, http://www.nlm.nih.gov/medlineplus/immunization.html.

42 FR Mooi et al., "Pertussis resurgence: waning immunity and pathogen adaptation," *Epidemiology & Infection* 142 (2014): 685–94.

43 JE Atwell et al., "Nonmedical vaccine exemptions and pertussis in California, 2010," *Pediatrics* 132 (2013): 624-30. doi:10.1542/peds.2013-0878.

44 KL Minaker, "Common clinical sequelae of aging," in L Goldman and AI Schafer, eds., *Cecil Goldman's Medicine*, 24th ed. (Philadelphia: Elsevier Saunders, 2011).

45 S Elahi et al., "Immunosuppressive CD71+ erythroid cells compromise neonatal host defence against infection," *Nature* 504 (2013): 158–62. doi:10.1038/nature12675.

46 Szajewska, "Early nutritional strategies for preventing allergic disease."

47 Minaker, "Common clinical sequelae of aging."

48 B Vogelstein and K Kinzler, "Cancer genes and the pathways they control," *Nature Medicine* 10 (2004): 789–99. doi:10.1038/nm1087.

49 "Fact sheet: BRCA1 and BRCA2: cancer risk and genetic testing," National Cancer Institute, http://www.cancer.gov/cancertopics/factsheet/Risk/BRCA.

50 R Kim et al., "Cancer immunoediting from immune surveillance to immune escape," *Immunology* 121, no. 1 (2007): 1–14. doi:10.1111/j.1365-2567.2007.02587.x.

51 RD Wood et al., "Human DNA repair genes, 2005," *Mutation Research* 577, no. 1–2 (2005): 275–83. http://dx.doi.org/10.1016/j.mrfmmm.2005.03.007.

52 DW Meek, "The p53 response to DNA damage," *DNA Repair* 3 (2004): 1049–56.

53 T Soussi and G Lozano, "p53 mutation heterogeneity in cancer," *Biochemical and Biophysical Research Communications* 331, no. 3 (2005): 834–42.

54 TB Tomasi et al., "Epigenetic regulation of immune escape genes in cancer," *Cancer Immunology, Immunotherapy* 55, no. 10 (2006): 1159–84.

Chapter 3

1 R Neal, "World's wonder drug," CBSNews.com, February 10, 2004, http://www.cbsnews.com/news/worlds-wonder-drug/.

2 H Markel, "The real story behind penicillin," PBS NewsHour, September 27, 2013, http://www.pbs.org/newshour/rundown/the-real-story-behind-the-worlds-first-antibiotic/.

3 "Summary of NDA approvals & receipts, 1938 to the present," FDA, http://www.fda.gov/AboutFDA/WhatWeDo/History/ProductRegulation/SummaryofNDAApprovalsReceipts1938tothepresent/default.htm.

4 http://www.centerwatch.com/drug-information/fda-approved-drugs/year/2013.

5 Q Gu et al., "Prescription drug use continues to increase: US prescription drug data for 2007–2008," NCHS Data Brief 42 (2010). http://www.cdc.gov/nchs/data/databriefs/db42.pdf.

6 "National Health Expenditure data," CMS.gov, http://www.cms.hhs.gov/NationalHealthExpendData/.

7 M Cokol et al., "Large-scale identification and analysis of suppressive drug interactions," Chemistry & Biology 21 (2014): 541–51. doi:10.1016/j.chembiol.2014.02.012.

8 University of Michigan Health System, "Seniors should watch for drug interactions when taking multiple medications," ScienceDaily, May 12, 2009. www.sciencedaily.com/releases/2009/05/090504211341.htm.

9 DJ DeNoon, "The 10 most prescribed drugs: most-prescribed drug list differs from list of drugs with biggest market share," WebMD, April 20, 2011, http://www.webmd.com/news/20110420/the-10-most-prescribed-drugs.

10 "Total number of retail prescription drugs filled at pharmacies," KFF.org, http://kff.org/other/state-indicator/total-retail-rx-drugs/.

11 "Tamiflu: clinical pharmacology," RxList, http://www.rxlist.com/tamiflu-drug/clinical-pharmacology.htm.

12 S Sheps, "Are over-the-counter cold remedies safe for people who have high blood pressure?," MayoClinc.org, http://www.mayoclinic.org/diseases-conditions/high-blood-pressure/expert-answers/high-blood-pressure/faq-20058281.

13 "Pneumonia fact sheet," American Lung Association, http://www.lung.org/lung-disease/influenza/in-depth-resources/pneumonia-fact-sheet.html.

14 "Sexual health and genital herpes (continued)," WebMD, http://www.webmd.com/genital-herpes/guide/sexual-health-genital-herpes?page=2.

15 KP Egan et al., "Immunological control of herpes simplex virus infections," Journal of Neurovirology 19 (2013): 328–45. doi:10.1007/s13365-013-0189-3

16 "Famvir: drug description," RxList, http://www.rxlist.com/famvir-drug.htm.

17 M. Sinead et al., "Herpes zoster vaccine effectiveness against incident herpes aoster and post-herpetic neuralgia in an older US population: a cohort study," PLoS Medicine 10 (2013): e1001420. doi:10.1371/journal.pmed.1001420.

18 MR Irwin et al., "Augmenting immune responses to varicella zoster virus in older adults: a randomized clinical trial of tai chi," Journal of the American Geriatric Society 55, no. 4 (2007): 511–17.

19 "Hepatitis C FAQs for the public," CDC, http://www.cdc.gov/hepatitis/c/cfaq.htm.

20 O Ogbru, "Interferon," MedicineNet.com, http://www.medicinenet.com/interferon/article.htm.

21 "Intron A," RxList, http://www.rxlist.com/intron-a-drug.htm.

22 "FDA approves new treatment for hepatitis C virus," RxList, http://www.rxlist.com/script/main/art.asp?articlekey=175372.

23 "Types of HIV/AIDS antiretroviral drugs," National Institute of Allergy and Infectious Diseases, http://www.niaid.nih.gov/topics/HIVAIDS/Understanding/Treatment/pages/arvdrugclasses.aspx.

24 ME O'Brien et al., "Patterns and correlates of discontinuation of the initial HAART regimen in an urban outpatient cohort," *Journal of Acquired Immune Deficiency Syndromes* 34 (2003): 407–14.

25 "Side effects of HIV medicines," AIDSinfo, http://aidsinfo.nih.gov/education-materials/fact-sheets/22/63/hiv-medicines-and-side-effects.

26 NHS Choices, "How antihistamines work," National Health Service, http://www.nhs.uk/Conditions/Antihistamines/Pages/How-does-it-work.aspx.

27 Discovery Fit & Health, "How does aspirin work?," Curiosity.com, http://curiosity.discovery.com/question/how-does-aspirin-work.

28 "Tylenol: clinical pharmacology," RxList, http://www.rxlist.com/tylenol-drug/clinical-pharmacology.htm.

29 E McNicol, "Ask the professor," *Tufts Journal*, April 2008, http://tuftsjournal.tufts.edu/2008/04/professor/01/.

30 "Nasalcrom: Nasalcrom consumer (continued)," RxList, http://www.rxlist.com/nasalcrom-drug/consumer-side-effects-precautions.htm.

31 "Seasonal allergy symptoms nationwide," WebMD, http://symptoms.webmd.com/seasonal-allergy-map-tool/antihistamines-1.

32 National Institute of Arthritis and Musculoskeletal and Skin Diseases, *Handout on Health: Atopic Dermatitis (A Type of Eczema)*, NIH Publication No. 13-4272. http://www.niams.nih.gov/Health_Info/Atopic_Dermatitis/default.asp.

33 "Autoimmune diseases fact sheet," Womenshealth.gov.

34 S Chandrashekara, "The treatment strategies of autoimmune disease may need a different approach from conventional protocol: a review," *Indian Journal of Pharmacology* 44 (2012): 665–71. doi:10.4103/0253-7613.103235.

35 "Hydroxychloroquine (Plaquenil)," American College of Rheumatology, https://www.rheumatology.org/Practice/Clinical/Patients/Medications/Hydroxychloroquine_(Plaquenil)/.

36 Healthwise Staff, "Methrotrexate for rheumatoid arthritis," WebMD, http://www.webmd.com/rheumatoid-arthritis/methotrexate-for-rheumatoid-arthritis.

37 KE Donahue et al., "Systematic review: comparative effectiveness and harms of disease-modifying medications for rheumatoid arthritis," *Annals of Internal Medicine* 148 (2008): 124–34.

38 "Anti-TNF," American College of Rheumatology, https://www.rheumatology.org/Practice/Clinical/Patients/Medications/Anti-TNF/.

39 "How do drugs and biologics differ?," Biotechnology Industry Organization, November 10, 2010, http://www.bio.org/articles/how-do-drugs-and-biologics-differ.

40 "Idiopathic thrombocytopenic purpurea (ITP)," MayoClinic.com, http://www.mayoclinic.org/diseases-conditions/idiopathic-thrombocytopenic-purpura/basics/definition/con-20034239.

41 "Antioxidants and health: an introduction," National Center for Complementary and Alternative Medicine, http://nccam.nih.gov/health/antioxidants/introduction.htm.

42 L Stojanovich, "Stress and autoimmunity," *Autoimmunity Reviews* 9 (2010): A271–76. doi:10.1016/j.autrev.2009.11.014.

43 "Multiple sclerosis: definition," MayoClinic.org, December 13, 2012, http://www.mayoclinic.org/diseases-conditions/multiple-sclerosis/basics/definition/con-20026689.

44 Healthwise Staff, "Interferon beta for multiple sclerosis," WebMD, http://www.webmd.com/multiple-sclerosis/interferon-beta-for-multiple-sclerosis.

45 LP Rowland, "Multiple sclerosis," in LP Rowland and TA Pedley, eds., *Merritt's Neurology*, 12th ed., (Philadelphia: Lippincott Williams and Wilkins, 2010), 902–18.

46 Lupus Foundation of America, "What is lupus?," Lupus.org, http://www.lupus.org/answers/entry/what-is-lupus.

47 "Lupus: definition," MayoClinic.org, http://www.mayoclinic.org/diseases-conditions/lupus/basics/definition/con-20019676.

Chapter 4

1 L Galland, "Diet and inflammation," *Nutrition in Clinical Practice* 25, no. 6 (2010): 634–40.

2 JR Mora, M Iwata, and UH von Andrian, "Vitamin effects on the immune system: vitamins A and D take centre stage," *Nature Reviews Immunology* 8 (2008): 685–98. doi:10.1038/nri2378.

3 ES Wintergerst et al., "Immune-enhancing role of vitamin C and zinc and effect on clinical conditions," *Annals of Nutrition and Metabolism* 50 (2006): 85–94.

4 J Manning et al., "Vitamin C promotes maturation of T-cells," *Antioxidants and Redox Signaling* 19 (2013): 2054–67.

5 LD Thomas et al., "Ascorbic acid supplements and kidney stone incidence among men: a prospective study," *JAMA Internal Medicine* 173, no. 5 (2013): 386–88. doi:10.1001/jamainternmed.2013.2296.

6 SN Han and SN Meydani, "Impact of vitamin E on immune function and its clinical implications," *Expert Review of Clinical Immunology* 2, no. 4 (2006): 561–67.

7 "Vitamin E fact sheet for health professionals," NIH Office of Dietary Supplements, http://ods.od.nih.gov /factsheets/VitaminE-HealthProfessional/.

8 S Salinthone et al., "α-Tocopherol (vitamin E) stimulates cyclic AMP production in human peripheral mononuclear cells and alters immune function," *Molecular Immunology* 53 (2013): 173–78. doi:10.1016 /j.molimm.2012.08.005.

9 E Mocchegiani et al., "Vitamin E-gene interactions in aging and inflammatory age-related diseases: implications for treatment: a systematic review," *Ageing Research Reviews* 4C (2014): 81–101. doi:10.1016/j. arr.2014.01.001.

10 "Millions of US children low in vitamin D- (70%)," *Health Research Report* 62 (2009). http:// healthresearchreport.me/z-in-progress-health-research-report-62-aug-2009/.

11 A Bowling, "Complementary and alternative medicine and multiple sclerosis," *Neurologic Clinics of North America* 29 (2011): 465–80.

12 MR von Essen et al., "Vitamin D controls T cell antigen receptor signaling and activation of human T cells," *Nature Immunology* 11 (2010): 344–49; doi:10.1038/ni.1851 10.1038/ni.1851.

13 KL Gibson et al., "B-cell diversity decreases in old age and is correlated with poor health status," *Aging Cell* 8 (2009): 18–25. doi:10.1111/j.1474-9726.2008.00443.x.

14 "Zinc fact sheet for health professionals," NIH Office of Dietary Supplements. http://ods.od.nih.gov/ factsheets/Zinc-HealthProfessional/.

15 M Dardenne, "Zinc and immune function," *European Journal of Clinical Nutrition* 56, Suppl. 3 (2002): S20–S23.

16 R Doty, "Smell and the degenerating brain," *Scientist* 27 (2013): 33–37.

17 J Arthur et al., "Selenium in the immune system," *Journal of Nutrition* 133 (2003): 1457S–59S.

18 JL Beard, "Iron biology in immune function, muscle metabolism and neuronal functioning," *Journal of Nutrition* 131, no. 2 (2001): 568S–80S.

19 JH Brock and V Mulero, "Cellular and molecular aspects of iron and immune function," *Proceedings of the Nutrition Society* 59 (2005): 537–40.

20 M Nairz et al., "The struggle for iron—a metal at the host-pathogen interface," *Cell Microbiology* 12 (2010): 1691–1702.

21 JK Chow et al., "Increased serum iron levels and infectious complications after liver transplantation," *Clinical Infectious Diseases* 51 (2010): e16–23.

22 SA Chacko et al., "Relations of dietary magnesium intake to biomarkers of inflammation and endothelial dysfunction in an ethnically diverse cohort of postmenopausal women," *Diabetes Care* 33, no. 2 (2010): 304–10.

23 A Jennings et al., "Intakes of anthocyanins and flavones are associated with biomarkers of insulin resistance and inflammation in women," *Journal of Nutrition* 144 (2014): 202–8; "Ingredients in chocolate, tea, berries could guard against diabetes," *ScienceDaily*, January 20, 2014, http://www.sciencedaily.com/releases/2014 /01/140120090647.htm.

24 RL Prior, X Wu, and K Schaich, "Standardized methods for the determination of antioxidant capacity and phenolics in foods and dietary supplements," *Journal of Agricultural and Food Chemistry* 53 (2005): 4290–302.

25 I Paur et al., "Antioxidants in herbs and spices: roles in oxidative stress and redox signaling," in IFF Benzie and S Wachtel-Galor, eds, *Herbal Medicine: Biomolecular and Clinical Aspects*, 2nd ed. (Boca Raton FL: CRC Press, 2011).

26 DL Katz et al. Cocoa and chocolate in human health and disease. *Antioxid Redox Signal.* 2011 Nov 15;15(10):2779–811.

27 M Monagas et al. Effect of cocoa powder on the modulation of inflammatory biomarkers in patients at high risk of cardiovascular disease. *Am J Clin Nutr* November 2009 90 (5): 1144–50.

28 M. Esser, et al., "Dark chocolate consumption improves leukocyte adhesion factors and vascular function in overweight men," *FASEB Journal* 28, no. 3 (2014): 1464–73. doi:10.1096/fj.13-239384.

29 FP Martin et al., "Metabolic effects of dark chocolate consumption on energy, gut microbiota, and stress-related metabolism in free-living subjects," *Journal of Proteome Research* 8 (2009): 5568–79. doi:10.1021/pr900607v.

30 KM Tuohy et al., "Up-regulating the human intestinal microbiome using whole plant foods, polyphenols, and/or fiber," *Journal of Agricultural and Food Chemistry* 60 (2012): 8776–82. doi:10.1021/jf205395.

31 RJ Jariwalla et al., "Restoration of blood total glutathione status and lymphocyte function following alpha-lipoic acid supplementation in patients with HIV infection," *Journal of Alternative and Complementary Medicine* 14 (2008): 139–46. doi:10.1089/acm.2006.6397.

32 S Larsen et al., "Simvastatin effects on skeletal muscle; relation to decreased mitochondrial function and glucose intolerance," *Journal of the American College of Cardiology* 61, no. 1 (2013): 44–53. doi:10.1016/j.jacc.2012.09.036.

33 "Omega-3 fatty acids," University of Maryland Medical Center, 2013, http://umm.edu/health/medical/altmed/supplement/omega3-fatty-acids#ixzz2wAGrwGtM.

34 AP Simopoulos, "Omega-3 fatty acids in inflammation and autoimmune diseases," *Journal of the American College of Nutrition* 21, no. 6 (2002): 495–505. doi:10.1080/07315724.2002.10719248.

35 J Dalli et al., "The novel 13S,14S-epoxy-maresin is converted by human macrophages to maresin1 (MaR1), inhibits leukotriene A4 hydrolase (LTA4H), and shifts macrophage phenotype," *FASEB Journal* 27 (2013): 2573–583. doi:10.1096/fj.13-227728.

36 P Romero et al., "Computational prediction of human metabolic pathways from the complete human genome," *Genome Biology* 6, R2 (2004). doi:10.1186/gb-2004-6-1-r2.

37 JM Daly et al., "Effect of dietary protein and amino acids on immune function," *Critical Care Medicine* 18, no. 2 (1990): S86–S159.

38 B Lesourd, "Protein undernutrition as the major cause of decreased immune function in the elderly: clinical and functional implications," *Nutrition Reviews* 53, no. 4 (1995): S86–S94. doi:10.1111/j.1753-4887.1995.tb01523.x.

39 C Castenada et al., "Elderly women accommodate to a low-protein diet with losses of body cell mass, muscle function, and immune response," *American Journal of Clinical Nutrition* 62 (1995): 30–39.

40 H Grimm and A Kraus, "Immunonutrition—supplementary amino acids and fatty acids ameliorate immune deficiency in critically ill patients," *Langenbeck's Archives of Surgery* 386 (2001): 369–76.

41 P Newsholme, "Why is L-glutamine metabolism important to cells of the immune system in health, postinjury, surgery or infection?," *Journal of Nutrition* 131, no. 9 (2001): 2515S–22S.

42 P Popovic et al., "Arginine and immunity," *Journal of Nutrition* 137, 6 Suppl. 2 (2007): 1681S–86S.

43 P Li et al., "Amino acids and immune function," *British Journal of Nutrition* 98, no. 2 (2007): 237–52.

44 S Hempel et al., "Probiotics for the prevention and treatment of antibiotic-associated diarrhea: a systematic review and meta-analysis," *Journal of the American Medical Association* 307, no. 18 (2012): 1959–69.

45 S De Kivit et al., "Regulation of intestinal immune responses through TLR activation: implications for pro- and prebiotics," *Frontiers in Immunology* 5 (2014): 60–67. doi:10.3389/fimmu.2014.00060.

46 AT Borcher et al., "Probiotics and immunity," *Journal of Gastroenterology* 44 (2009): 26–46.

47 "The truth about probiotics and your gut," WebMD, http://www.webmd.com/digestive-disorders/probiotics-10/slideshow-probiotics.

48 De Kivit, "Regulation of intestinal immune responses through TLR activation."

49 K Jones, "Probiotics: preventing antibiotic-associated diarrhea," *Journal for Specialists in Pediatric Nursing* 15 (2010): 160–62.

50 RJ Boyle et al., "Probiotic use in clinical practice: what are the risks?," *American Journal of Clinical Nutrition* 83 (2006): 1256–64.

51 Reid et al., "Oral use of *Lactobacillus rhamnosus* GR-1 and *L. fermentum* RC-14 significantly alters vaginal flora: randomized, placebo-controlled trial in 64 healthy women," *FEMS Immunology and Medical Microbiology* 35 (2003): 131–34.

52 Nermes et al., "Is there a role for probiotics in the prevention or treatment of food allergy?," *Current Allergy and Asthma Reports* 13, no. 6 (2013): 622–30.

53 T Matsuzaki et al., "Intestinal microflora: probiotics and autoimmunity," *Journal of Nutrition* 137 (2007): 798S–802S.

54 M Sanchez et al., "Effect of *Lactobacillus rhamnosus* CGMCC1.3724 supplementation on weight loss and maintenance in obese men and women," *British Journal of Nutrition* 111 (2013): 1507–19. doi:10.1017/S0007114513003875.

55 SK Sharma et al., "Mechanisms and clinical uses of capsaicin," *European Journal of Pharmacology* 720 (2013): 55–62. doi:10.1016/j.ejphar.2013.10.053.

56 M Hernández-Ortega et al., "Antioxidant, antinociceptive, and anti-inflammatory effects of carotenoids extracted from dried pepper (*Capsicum annuum* L.)," *Journal of Biomedicine and Biotechnology* 2012 (2012):524019. doi:10.1155/2012/524019.

57 Y Hagenlocher et al., "Cinnamon extract inhibits degranulation and de novo synthesis of inflammatory mediators in mast cells," *Allergy* 68, no. 4 (2013): 490–97. doi:10.1111/all.12122.

58 A Khan et al., "Cinnamon improves glucose and lipids of people with type 2 diabetes," *Diabetes Care* 26, no. 12 (2003): 3215–18.

59 JN Dhuley, "Anti-oxidant effects of cinnamon (*Cinnamomum verum*) bark and greater cardamom (*Amomum subulatum*) seeds in rats fed high fat diet," *Indian Journal of Experimental Biology* 37 (1999): 238–42.

60 TG Rodrigues et al., "In vitro and in vivo effects of clove on pro-inflammatory cytokines production by macrophages," *Natural Product Research* 23, no. 4 (2009): 319–26. doi:10.1080/14786410802242679.

61 P Josling, "Preventing the common cold with a garlic supplement: a double blind, placebo-controlled survey," *Advanced Therapies* 18, no. 4 (2001): 189–93.

62 E Alma et al., "The effect of garlic powder on human urinary cytokine excretion," *Urology Journal* 11, no. 1 (2014): 1308–15.

63 A Simonne, *Herbs and Garlic-in-Oil Mixtures: Safe Handling Practices for Consumers*, EDIS, University of Florida IFAS Extension publication FCS8743. http://edis.ifas.ufl.edu/fy487.

64 Y Ozaki et al., "Anti-inflammatory effect of *Zingiber cassumunar* Roxb. and its active principles," *Chemical and Pharmceutical Bulletin* 39 (1991): 2353–56.

65 P Palatty et al., "Ginger in the prevention of nausea and vomiting: a review," *Critical Reviews in Food Science and Nutrition* 53 (2013): 659–69. doi:10.1080/10408398.2011.553751.

66 "Ginger," University of Maryland Medical Center, http://umm.edu/health/medical/altmed/herb/ginger#ixzz2zH4e9fw7.

67 LJ Ming and AC Yin, "Therapeutic effects of glycyrrhizic acid," *Natural Product Communications* 8, no. 3 (2013): 415–18.

68 R Hearst et al., "An examination of antibacterial and antifungal properties of constituents of shiitake (*Lentinula edodes*) and oyster (*Pleurotus ostreatus*) mushrooms," *Complementary Therapies in Clinical Practice* 15, no. 1 (2009): 5–7.

69 JE Ramberg et al., "Immunomodulatory dietary polysaccharides: a systematic review of the literature," *Nutrition Journal* 9, no. 54 (2010): 1–22.

70 GT McAnlis et al., "Absorption and antioxidant effects of quercetin from onions, in man," *European Journal of Clinical Nutrition* 53 (1999): 92–96.

71 YB Shaik et al., "Role of quercetin (a natural herbal compound) in allergy and inflammation," *Journal of Biological Regulators and Homeostatic Agents* 20, no. 3–4 (2006): 47–52.

72 M Force et al., "Inhibition of enteric parasites by emulsified oil of oregano in vivo," *Phytotherapy Research* 14 (2000): 213–14.

73 M Martinez-Tomé et al., "Antioxidant properties of Mediterranean spices compared with common food additives," *Journal of Food Protection* 64, no. 9 (2001): 1412–19.

74 MR al-Sereiti, "Pharmacology of rosemary (*Rosmarinus officinalis* Linn.) and its therapeutic potentials," *Indian Journal of Experimental Biology* 37 (1999): 124–30.

75 JS Da Rosa et al., "Systemic administration of *Rosmarinus officinalis* attenuates the inflammatory response induced by carrageenan in the mouse model of pleurisy," *Planta Medica* 79, no. 17 (2013): 1605–14. doi:10.1055/s-0033-1351018.

76 SS Percival et al., "Bioavailability of herbs and spices in humans as determined by ex vivo inflammatory suppression and DNA strand breaks," *Journal of the American College of Nutrition* 31, no. 4 (2012): 288–94.

77 S Aydin et al., "Modulating effects of thyme and its major ingredients on oxidative DNA damage in human lymphocytes," *Journal of Agricultural and Food Chemistry* 53 (2005): 1299–305.

78 LC Tapsell et al., "Health benefits of herbs and spices: the past, the present, the future," *Medical Journal of Australia* 185, Suppl. 4 (2006): S4–S24.

79 ML Neuhouser et al., "A low-glycemic load diet reduces serum C-reactive protein and modestly increases adiponectin in overweight and obese adults," *Journal of Nutrition* 142 (2012): 396–74. doi:10.3945/jn.111.149807.

80 C Miglio et al., "Antioxidant and inflammatory response following high-fat meal consumption in overweight subjects," *European Journal of Nutrition* 52 (2013): 1107–14.

81 S Ley et al., "Associations between red meat intake and biomarkers of inflammation and glucose metabolism in women," *American Journal of Clinical Nutrition* 99 (2014): 352–60.

82 D Freed, "Do dietary lectins cause disease?," *British Medical Journal* 318, no. 7190 (1999): 1023–24.

83 AH Lichtenstein et al., "Diet and lifestyle recommendations revision 2006: a scientific statement from the American Heart Association Nutrition Committee," *Circulation* 114, no. 1 (2006): 82–96.

84 C Thomas, *50 Best Plants on the Planet* (San Francisco: Chronicle Books, 2013).

85 "What's new," Monterey Bay Aquarium Seafood Watch, http://www.seafoodwatch.org/cr/cr _seafoodwatch/sfw_whatsnew.aspx.

86 C Daley et al., "A review of fatty acid profiles and antioxidant content in grass-fed and grain-fed beef," *Nutrition Journal* 9 (2010): 10–22.

87 MB Schulze et al., "Processed meat intake and incidence of type 2 diabetes in younger and middle-aged women," *Diabetologia* 46, no. 11 (2003): 1465–73.

88 E. Haas with Daniella Chace, *The Detox Diet*, 3rd ed. (Berkeley, CA: Ten Speed Press, 2012).

89 T Barringer et al., "Effect of a multivitamin and mineral supplement on infection and quality of life: a randomized, double-blind, placebo-controlled trial," *Annals of Internal Medicine* 138, no. 5 (2003): 365–71. doi:10.7326/0003-4819-138-5-200303040-00005.

90 S Larsen et al., "Simvastatin effects on skeletal muscle: relation to decreased mitochondrial function and glucose intolerance," *Journal of the American College of Cardiology* 61, no. 1 (2013): 44–53. doi:10.1016/j. jacc.2012.09.036.

91 MJ Bolland et al., "Calcium supplements with or without vitamin D and risk of cardiovascular events: reanalysis of the Women's Health Initiative limited access dataset and meta-analysis," *British Medical Journal* 342 (2011): d2040. doi:10.1136/bmj.d2040.

92 IR Reid, MJ Bolland, and A Grey, "Does calcium supplementation increase cardiovascular risk?," *Clinical Endocrinology* 73 (2010): 689 95. doi:10.1111/j.1365-2265.2010.03792.x.

93 M Guasch-Ferre et al., "Dietary magnesium intake is inversely associated with mortality in adults at high cardiovascular disease risk," *Journal of Nutrition* 144 (2014): 55–60. doi:10.3945/jn.113.183012.

Chapter 5

1 JA Whitworth et al., "Cardiovascular consequences of cortisol excess," *Vascular Health and Risk Management* 1, no. 4 (2005): 291–99.

2 JK Kiecolt-Glaser and R Glaser, "Depression and immune function: central pathways to morbidity and mortality," *Journal of Psychosomatic Research* 53 (2002): 873–76.

3 MR Irwin et al., "Varicella zoster virus–specific immune responses to a herpes zoster vaccine in elderly recipients with major depression and the impact of antidepressant medications," *Clinical Infectious Diseases* 56 (2013): 1085–93. doi:10.1093/cid/cis1208.

4 N Rod et al., "Perceived stress and risk of adult-onset asthma and other atopic disorders: a longitudinal cohort study," *Allergy* 67 (2012): 1408–14.

5 T Ziemssen and S Kern, "Psychoneuroimmunology, cross-talk between the immune and nervous systems," *Journal of Neurology* 254, Suppl. 2 (2007): II/8–II/11. doi:10.1007/s00415-007-2003-8.

6 N Turrin and S Rivest, "Unraveling the molecular details involved in the intimate link between the immune and neuroendocrine systems," *Experimental Biology and Medicine* 229 (2004): 996–1006.

7 J Amat et al., "Medial prefrontal cortex determines how stressor controllability affects behavior and dorsal raphe nucleus," *Nature Neuroscience* 8, no. 3 (2005): 365-71.

8 R Ader, D Felten, and N Cohen, *Psychoneuroimmunology*, 5th ed. (London: Elsevier Academic Press, 2006).

9 C Riether et al., "Behavioural conditioning of immune functions: how the central nervous system controls peripheral immune responses by evoking associative learning processes," *Reviews in the Neursciences* 19 (2008): 1–17.

10 MU Goebel et al., "Behavioral conditioning of immunosuppression is possible in humans," *FASEB Journal* 16 (2002): 1869–73.

11 R Ader and N Cohen, "Behaviorally conditioned immunosuppression," *Psychosomatic Medicine* 37 (1975): 333–40.

12 JK Kiecolt-Glaser et al., "Marital quality, marital disruption, and immune function," *Psychosomatic Medicine* 49 (1987): 13–34.

13 S Cohen et al., "Chronic stress, glucocorticoid receptor resistance, inflammation, and disease risk," *Proceedings of the National Academy of Sciences of the United States of America* 109 (2012): 5995–99. doi:10.1073/pnas.1118355109.

14 S Cohen et al., "Social ties and susceptibility to the common cold," *Journal of the American Medical Association* 277 (1997): 1940–44.

15 SC. Segerstrom and GE Miller, "Psychological stress and the human immune system: a meta-analytic study of 30 years of inquiry," *Psychological Bulletin* 130, no. 4 (2004): 601–63.

16 JH Gruzelier, "A review of the impact of hypnosis, relaxation, guided imagery and individual differences on aspects of immunity and health," *Stress* 5 (2002): 147–63.

17 RK Wallace, H Benson, and AF Wilson, "A wakeful hypometabolic physiologic state," *American Journal of Physiology* 221 (1971): 795–99.

18 JA Dusek and H Benson, "A model of the comparative clinical impact of the acute stress and relaxation responses," *Minnesota Medicine* 92 (2009): 47–50.

19 H Benson, "The relaxation response: techniques and clinical applications," in *Ways of Health: Holistic Approaches to Ancient and Contemporary Medicine*, D Sobel, ed. (New York: Harcourt Brace Jovanovich, 1979), 331–51.

20 MK Bhasin et al., "Relaxation response induces temporal transcriptome changes in energy metabolism, insulin secretion and inflammatory pathways," *PLoS One* 8 (2013): e62817. doi:10.1371/journal.pone.0062817.

21 P Kaliman et al., "Rapid changes in histone deacetylases and inflammatory gene expression in expert meditators," *Psychoneuroendocrinology* 40 (2014): 96–98.

22 A Conrad and WT Roth, "Muscle relaxation therapy for anxiety disorders: it works but how?," *Journal of Anxiety Disorders* 21 (2007): 243–64.

23 N Grover et al., "Cognitive behavioural intervention in bronchial asthma," *Journal of the Association of Physicians of India* 50 (2002): 896–900.

24 MR Isa et al., "Impact of applied progressive deep muscle relaxation training on the level of depression, anxiety and stress among prostate cancer patients: a quasi-experimental study," *Asian Pacific Journal of Cancer Prevention* 14 (2013): 2237–42.

25 J Kabat-Zinn, "An outpatient program in behavioral medicine for chronic pain patients based on mindfulness meditation," *General Hospital Psychiatry* 4 (1982): 33-47.

26 J Kabat-Zinn, *Full Catastrophe Living: Using the Wisdom of Your Body and Mind to Face Stress, Pain, and Illness* (New York: Bantam Dell, 1990).

27 A Capetta, "10 super easy meditations to help you chill the hell out," iVillage, July 10, 2013, http://www.ivillage.com/relax-these-meditations/4-a-541017.

28 PH Koulivand, GM Khaleghi, and A Gorij, "Lavender and the nervous system," *Evidence Based Complement Alternative Medicine*, 2013;2013:681304. doi:10.1155/2013/681304.

29 EM Sibinga et al., "Mindfulness-based stress reduction for urban youth," *Journal of Alternative and Complementary Medicine* 17 (2011): 213–18.

30 M Rossman, *The Worry Solution* (New York: Three Rivers Press, 2010).

31 J Schneider et al., "Imagery and immune system studies: a summary of findings," in R. Kutzendorpf, ed., *Proceedings of 12th Annual Review of Mental Imagery* (New Haven, CT, 1991); D Bartlett et al., "The effects of music listening and perceived sensory experiences on the immune system as measured by interleukin-1 (IL1) and cortisol," *Journal of Music Therapy* 30, no. 4 (1993): 194–209.

32 MO Frenkel et al., "Mental practice maintains range of motion despite forearm immobilization: a pilot study in healthy persons," *Journal of Rehabilitation Medicine* 46 (2014): 225–32. doi:10.2340/16501977-1263.

33 MJ Weigensberg et al., "Imagine HEALTH: results from a randomized pilot lifestyle intervention for obese Latino adolescents using Interactive Guided Imagery," *BMC Complementary Alternative Medicine* 14 (2014): 28. doi:10.1186/1472-6882-14-28.

34 D Childre, H Martin, and D Beech, *The HeartMath Solution: The Institute of HeartMath's Revolutionary Program for Engaging the Power of the Heart's Intelligence*, reprint ed. (New York: HarperOne, 2000).

35 R McCraty et al., "The impact of an emotional self-management skills course on psychosocial functioning and autonomic recovery to stress in middle school children," *Integrative Physiological and Behavioral Sciences* 34 (1991): 246–68.

36 D Childre, *Freeze-Frame: One Minute Stress Management: A Scientifically Proven Technique for Clear Decision Making and Improved Health* (HeartMath System), 2nd ed. (Boulder Creek, CA: Planetary Publications, 1998).

37 M Antoni et al., "Cognitive-behavioral stress management reverses anxiety-related leukocyte transcriptional dynamics," *Biological Psychiatry* 71 (2012): 366–372.

38 M Seligman, *Learned Optimism* (New York: Pocket Books, 1991).

39 DC McClelland and AD Cheriff, "The immunoenhancing effects of humor on secretory IgA and resistance to respiratory infections," *Psychology and Health* 12 (1997): 329–44.

40 H Wahbeh et al., "Mind-body medicine and immune system outcomes: a systematic review," *Open Complementary Medicine Journal* 1 (2009): 25–34.

41 MP Bennett et al., "The effect of mirthful laughter on stress and natural killer cell activity," *Alternative Therapies in Health and Medicine* 9 (2003): 38.

42 KR Lebowitz et al., "Effects of humor and laughter on psychological functioning, quality of life, health status, and pulmonary functioning among patients with chronic obstructive pulmonary disease: A preliminary investigation," *Heart & Lung* 40 (2011): 317.

43 "Stress management," Mayo Clinic, http://www.mayoclinic.org/healthy-living/stress-management/in-depth/stress-relief/art-20044456.

44 Cohen, "Social ties and susceptibility to the common cold."

45 S Taylor et al., "Biobehavioral responses to stress in females: tend-and-befriend, not fight-or-flight," *Psychological Review* 107 (2000): 411–29.

46 ML Chanda and DJ Levitin, "The neurochemistry of music," *Trends in Cognitive Sciences* 17 (2013): 179–93.

47 SM Wang et al., "Music and preoperative anxiety: a randomized, controlled study," *Anesthesia and Analgesia* 94 (2002): 1489–94.

48 JA Voss et al., "Sedative music reduces anxiety and pain during chair rest after open-heart surgery," *Pain* 112 (2004): 197–203.

49 M Seligman, *Flourish: A Visionary New Understanding of Happiness and Well-being* (New York: Free Press, 2011).

50 A Croom, "Music, neuroscience, and the psychology of well-being: a précis," *Frontiers in Psychology* 2:393 (2011): 1–16. doi:10.3389/fpsyg.2011.00393.

51 E Haroon et al., "Psychoneuroimmunology meets neuropsychopharmacology: translational implications of the impact of inflammation on behavior," *Neuropsychopharmacology* 37 (2012): 137–62. doi:10.1038/npp.2011.205.

52 H Lavretsky et al., "A pilot study of yogic meditation for family dementia caregivers with depressive symptoms: effects on mental health, cognition, and telomerase activity," *International Journal of Geriatric Psychiatry* 28 (2013): 57–65. doi:10.1002/gps.3790.

53 DS Black et al., "Yogic meditation reverses NF-κB and IRF-related transcriptome dynamics in leukocytes of family dementia caregivers in a randomized controlled trial," *Psychoneuroendocrinology* 38 (2013): 348–55. doi:10.1016/j.psyneuen.2012.06.011.

54 AB Newberg et al., "Meditation effects on cognitive function and cerebral blood flow in subjects with memory loss: a preliminary study," *Journal of Alzheimer's Disease* 20, no. 2 (2010): 517–26. doi:10.3233/JAD-2010-1391.

55 "Practice the 12-minute yoga meditation exercise," Alzheimer's Research and Prevention Foundation, http://www.alzheimersprevention.org/research/12-minute-memory-exercise.

56 J Pennebaker et al., "Disclosure of traumas and immune function: health implications," *Journal of Consulting and Clinical Psychology* 56 (1988): 239–45; M Francis and JW Pennebaker, "Putting stress into words: the impact of writing on physiological, absentee, and self-reported emotional well-being measures," *American Journal of Health Promotion* 6 (1992): 280–87.

57 G Dvorsky, "Why we need to sleep in total darkness," io9, http://io9.com/why-we-need-to-sleep-in-total-darkness-1497075228.

58 SH Onen et al., "Prevention and treatment of sleep disorders through regulation of sleeping habits," *Presse Médicale*, 23, no.10 (1994): 485–89; "The sleep environment," National Sleep Foundation, http://www.sleepfoundation.org/article/how-sleep-works/the-sleep-environment.

59 "How does exercise help those with chronic insomnia?," National Sleep Foundation, http://sleepfoundation.org/ask-the-expert/how-does-exercise-help-those-chronic-insomnia.

60 "The truth about tryptophan," WebMD, http://www.webmd.com/food-recipes/features/the-truth-about-tryptophan.

61 "Natural sleep aids," WebMD, http://www.webmd.com/sleep-disorders/excessive-sleepiness-10/sleep-supplements-herbs.

62 "Lavender," University of Maryland Medical Center, http://umm.edu/health/medical/altmed/herb/lavender.

63 J Lytle et al., "Effect of lavender aromatherapy on vital signs and perceived quality of sleep in the intermediate care unit: a pilot study," *American Journal of Critical Care* 23 (2014): 242-9. doi:10.4037/ajcc2014958.

64 M Moeini et al., "Effect of aromatherapy on the quality of sleep in ischemic heart disease patients hospitalized in intensive care units of heart hospitals of the Isfahan University of Medical Sciences," *Iran Journal of Nursing and Midwifery Research* 15 (2010): 234–39.

65 W Sayorwan et al., "The effects of lavender oil inhalation on emotional states, autonomic nervous system, and brain electrical activity," *Journal of the Medical Association of Thailand* 95 (2012): 598–606.

66 "Stress and anxiety interfere with sleep," Anxiety and Depression Association of America, http://www.adaa.org/understanding-anxiety/related-illnesses/other-related-conditions/stress/stress-and-anxiety-interfere.

67 JK Smyth et al., "Effects of writing about stressful experiences on symptom reduction in patients with asthma or rheumatoid arthritis," *Journal of the American Medical Association* 281 (1999): 1304–9.

68 E Tobaldini et al., "One night on-call: sleep deprivation affects cardiac autonomic control and inflammation in physicians," *European Journal of Internal Medicine* 24 (2013): 664–70. doi:10.1016/j.ejim.2013.03.011.

69 P Matzner et al., "Resilience of the immune system in healthy young students to 30-hour sleep deprivation with psychological stress," *Neuroimmunomodulation* 20 (2013): 194–204. doi:10.1159/000348698.

70 M Ferrara and L Gennaro, "How much sleep do we need?," *Sleep Medicine Reviews* 5 (2001): 155–79.

71 "Melatonin," MedlinePlus, http://www.nlm.nih.gov/medlineplus/druginfo/natural/940.html.

72 A Carillo-Vico et al., "Melatonin: buffering the immune system," *Internal Journal of Molecular Science* 14 (2013): 8638–83. doi:10.3390/ijms14048638.

73 A Carillo-Vico et al., "A review of the multiple actions of melatonin on the immune system," *Endocrine* 7 (2005): 189–200.

74 SM Rajaratnam et al., "Sleep loss and circadian disruption in shift work: health burden and management," *Medical Journal of Australia* 199 (2013): S11–S15.

Chapter 6

1 RR Rosenkranz et al., "Active lifestyles related to excellent self-rated health and quality of life: cross sectional findings from 194,545 participants in the 45 and Up Study," *BMC Public Health* 13, no. 1 (2013): 1071–10.

2 Y Youm et al., "Inflammasome links systemic low-grade inflammation to functional decline in aging," *Cell Metabolism* 18 (2013): 519–32. doi:10.1016/j.cmet.2013.09.010.

3 DM Bhammar et al., "Effects of fractionized and continuous exercise on 24-h ambulatory blood pressure," *Medicine and Science in Sports and Exercise* 44, no. 12 (2012): 2270–76. doi:10.1249/MSS.0b013e3182663117.

4 M Holmstrug et al., "Multiple short bouts of exercise over 12-h period reduce glucose excursions more than an energy-matched single bout of exercise," *Metabolism* 63, no. 4 (2014): 510–19. doi:10.1016/j.metabol.2013.12.006.

5 RS Metcalfe et al., "Towards the minimal amount of exercise for improving metabolic health: beneficial effects of reduced-exertion high-intensity interval training," *European Journal of Applied Physiology* 112 (2012): 2767–75. doi:10.1007/s00421-011-2254-z.

6 NP Walsh et al., "Position statement. Part two: maintaining immune health," *Exercise Immunology Review* 17 (2011): 64–103.

7 LH Colbert et al., "Physical activity, exercise, and inflammatory markers in older adults: findings from the health, aging, and body composition study," *Journal of the American Geriatrics Society* 52, no. 7 (2004): 1098–104.

8 NA Mischel et al., "Physical (in)activity-dependent structural plasticity in bulbospinal catecholaminergic neurons of rat rostral ventrolateral medulla, *Journal of Comparative Neurology* 522, no. 3 (2014): 499–513. doi:10.1002/cne.23464.

9 C Cotman and N Berchtold, "Exercise: a behavioral intervention to enhance brain health and plasticity," *Trends in Neurosciences* 25, no. 6 (2002): 295–301. doi:http://dx.doi.org/10.1016/S0166-2236(02)02143-4.

10 S Behrman and KP Ebmeier, "Can exercise prevent cognitive decline?," *Practitioner* 258 (2014): 17–21, 2–3.

11 N Shoham et al., "Adipocyte stiffness increases with accumulation of lipid droplets," *Biophysical Journal* 106, no. 6 (2014): 1421–31. doi:10.1016/j.bpj.2014.01.045.

12 DB Reuben et al., "The associations between physical activity and inflammatory markers in high-functioning older persons: MacArthur studies of successful aging," *Journal of the American Geriatrics Society* 51 (2003): 1125–30.

13 KJ Stewart, "Role of exercise training on cardiovascular disease in persons who have type 2 diabetes and hypertension," *Cardiology Clinics* 22, no. 4 (2004): 569–86.

14 E Ford, "Does exercise reduce inflammation? Physical activity and C-reactive protein among US adults," *Epidemiology* 13, no. 5 (2002): 561–68; K Ogawa et al., "Resistance exercise training-induced muscle hypertrophy was associated with reduction of inflammatory markers in elderly women," *Mediators of Inflammation* 2010:171023 (2010): 1–7. doi:http://dx.doi.org/10.1155/2010/171023.

15 M Gleeson et al., "The antiinflammatory effects of exercise: mechanisms and implications for the prevention and treatment of disease," *Nature Reviews: Immunology* 11 (2011): 607–15.

16 Walsh, "Position statement"; H Bruunsgaard and B Pedersen, "Effects of exercise on the immune system in the elderly population," *Immunology and Cell Biology* 78 (2000): 523–31. doi:10.1111/j.1440-1711.2000.t01-14-.x.

17 PY Yang et al., "Exercise training improves sleep quality in middle-aged and older adults with sleep problems: a systematic review," *Journal of Physiotherapy* 58 (2012): 157–63.

18 F Li et al., "Tai chi and self-rated quality of sleep and daytime sleepiness in older adults: a randomized controlled trial." *Journal of the American Geriatric Society* 52 (2004): 892–900.

19 HS Driver and SR Taylor, "Exercise and sleep," *Sleep Medicine Reviews* 4, no. 4 (2000): 387–402. doi:http://dx.doi.org/10.1053/smrv.2000.0110.

20 Ogawa, "Resistance exercise training-induced muscle hypertrophy."

21 KJ Stewart, "Role of exercise training on cardiovascular disease in persons who have type 2 diabetes and hypertension," *Cardiology Clinics* 22, no. 4 (2004): 569–86.

22 Ford, "Does exercise reduce inflammation?"

23 U Das, "Exercise and inflammation." *European Heart Journal* 27 (2006): 1385.

24 P Jordan, *The Fitness Instinct: The Revolutionary New Approach to Healthy Exercise That Is Fun, Natural, and No Sweat* (Emmaus, PA: Rodale Press, 1999); M Jordan, *How to Be a Health Coach* (San Rafael, CA: Global Medicine Enterprises, 2013).

25 ME Nelson et al., "Physical activity and public health in older adults: recommendation from the American College of Sports Medicine and the American Heart Association," Medicine and Science in Sports and Exercise, 39 (2007): 1435–45. http://www.acsm-msse.org.

26 A Ross and S Thomas, "The health benefits of yoga and exercise: a review of comparison studies," *Journal of Alternative and Complementary Medicine* 16 (2010): 3–12. doi:10.1089/acm.2009.0044.

27 LA Gordon et al., "Effect of exercise therapy on lipid profile and oxidative stress indicators in patients with type 2 diabetes," *BMC Complementary and Alternative Medicine* 8 (2008): 21–31. doi:10.1186/1472-6882-8-21.

28 S Arora and J Bhattacharjee, "Modulation of immune responses in stress by Yoga," *International Journal of Yoga* 1 (2008): 45–55. doi:10.4103/0973-6131.43541.

29 T Kamei et al., "Decrease in serum cortisol during yoga exercise is correlated with alpha wave activation," *Perceptual and Motor Skills* 90 (2000): 1027–32.

30 A Ross et al., "Frequency of yoga practice predicts health: results of a national survey of yoga practitioners," *Evidence-Based Complementary and Alternative Medicine* 2012:983258 (2012). doi:10.1155/2012/983258.

31 PT Pullen et al., "Effects of yoga on inflammation and exercise capacity in patients with chronic heart failure," *Journal of Cardiac Failure* 14 (2008): 407-13. doi:10.1016/j.cardfail.2007.12.007.

32 CE Rogers, et al., "A review of clinical trials of tai chi and qigong in older adults," *Western J Nursing Research* 31 (2009):245-79. doi: 10.1177/0193945908327529.

33 SK Gatts and WH Woollacott, "How tai chi improves balance: biomechanics of recovery to a walking slip in impaired seniors," *Gait Posture* 25 (2007): 205–14.

34 MR Irwin et al., "Augmenting immune responses to varicella zoster virus in older adults: a randomized clinical trial of tai chi," *Journal of the American Geriatric Society* 55, no. 4 (2007): 511–17.

35 CW Wang et al., "Managing stress and anxiety through qigong exercise in healthy adults: a systematic review and meta-analysis of randomized controlled trials," *BMC Complementary and Alternative Medicine* 14 (2014): 8–17.

36 Y Yang et al., "Effects of a traditional Taiji/Qigong curriculum on older adults' immune response to influenza vaccine," *Medicine and Sport Science* 52 (2008): 64-76. doi:10.1159/000134285.

37 SH Yeh et al., "Regular tai chi chuan exercise enhances functional mobility and CD4CD25 regulatory T cells," *British Journal of Sports Medicine* 40, no. 3 (2006): 239–43.

38 LA Gonzalez et al., "Qigong improves balance in young women: a pilot study," *Journal of Integrative Medicine* 11 (2013): 241–45. doi:10.3736/jintegrmed2013038.

39 Y Ming et al., "Stress-reducing practice of qigong improved DNA repair in cancer patients," *Shanghai Qigong Institute, Second World Conference on Academic Exchange of Medical Qigong* (1993).

40 B Oh et al., "Medical qigong for cancer patients: pilot study of impact on quality of life, side effects of treatment and inflammation," *American Journal of Chinese Medicine* 36, no. 3 (2008): 459–72.

41 J Hanley et al., "Randomised controlled trial of therapeutic massage in the management of stress," *British Journal of General Practice* 53 (2003): 20–25.

42 D Atkins and D Eichler, "The effects of self-massage on osteoarthritis of the knee: a randomized, controlled trial," *International Journal of Therapeutic Massage and Bodywork*.6 (2013): 4–14.

43 S Jain and PJ Mills, "Biofield therapies: helpful or full of hype? A best evidence synthesis," *International Journal of Behavioral Medicine* 17 (2010):1–16. doi:10.1007/s12529-009-9062-4.

44 J Diamond, *Life Energy: Using the Meridians to Unlock the Hidden Power of Your Emotions* (New York: Dodd, Mead, 1985).

45 E Margulis, *On Repeat: How Music Plays the Mind* (New York: Oxford University Press, 2013).

Chapter 7

1   SC Kobasa et al., "Effectiveness of hardiness, exercise and social support as resources against illness," *Journal of Psychosomatic Research* 29, no. 5 (1985): 525–33.

2   SR Maddi, "The story of hardiness: twenty years of theorizing, research and practice," *Consulting Psychology Journal*, 54 (2002): 173–85.

3   JP Gouin et al., "Chronic stress, daily stressors, and circulating inflammatory markers," *Health Psychology* 31 (2012): 264–68. doi:10.1037/a0025536.

4   JK Kiecolt-Glaser, "Stress, food, and inflammation: psychoneuroimmunology and nutrition at the cutting edge" *Psychosomatic Medicine* 72 (2010): 365–69. doi:10.1097/PSY.0b013e3181dbf489.

5   A Halaris, "Inflammation, heart disease, and depression," *Current Psychiatry Reports* 15, no. 10 (2013): 400. doi:10.1007/s11920-013-0400-5.

6   T Bahorun et al., "Black tea reduces uric acid and C-reactive protein levels in humans susceptible to cardiovascular diseases," *Toxicology* 278, no. 1 (2010): 68–74.

7   R Glaser and JK Kiecolt-Glaser, "Stress-induced immune dysfunction: implications for health," *Nature Reviews Immunology* 5 (2005): 243–51.

8   "Practice the 12-minute yoga meditation exercise," Alzheimer's Research and Prevention Foundation, http://www.alzheimersprevention.org/research/12-minute-memory-exercise.

9   Black, "Yogic meditation."

10 JK Kiecolt-Glaser et al., "Yoga's impact on inflammation, mood, and fatigue in breast cancer survivors: a randomized controlled trial," *Journal of Clinical Oncology*, 32, no. 10 (2014):1040–49. doi:10.1200/JCO.2013.51.8860.

11 JD Creswell et al., "Mindfulness-based stress reduction training reduces loneliness and pro-inflammatory gene expression in older adults: a small randomized controlled trial," *Brain, Behavior, and Immunity* 26, no. 7 (2012): 1095–101.

12 J Pennebaker et al., "Disclosure of traumas and immune function: health implications," *Journal of Consulting and Clinical Psychology* 56 (1988): 239–45.

13 PG Frisina et al., "A meta-analysis of the effects of written emotional disclosure on the health outcomes of clinical populations," *Journal of Nervous and Mental Disease* 192, no. 9 (2004): 629–34.

14 JK Kiecolt-Glaser et al., "Omega-3 fatty acids, oxidative stress, and leukocyte telomere length: A randomized controlled trial." *Brain, Behavior, and Immunity* 28 (2013):16–24. doi:10.1016/j.bbi.2012.09.004.

15 YB Shaik et al., "Role of quercetin (a natural herbal compound) in allergy and inflammation," *Journal of Biological Regulators and Homeostatic Agents* 20, no. 3–4 (2006): 47–52.

16 HR Maurer, "Bromelain: biochemistry, pharmacology and medical use," *Cellular and Molecular Life Sciences* 58, no. 9 (2001): 1234–45.

17 KH Sturner et al., "Boswellic acids reduce Th17 differentiation via blockade of IL-1β-mediated IRAK1 signaling," *European Journal of Immunology* 44 (2014): 1200–12. doi:10.1002/eji.201343629.

18 Haas, *Detox Diet.*

19 KY Yeon et al., "Curcumin produces an anti-hyperalgesic effect via antagonism of TRPV1," *Journal of Dental Research* 89, no. 2 (2010): 170–74.

20 M Pirotta, "Arthritis disease—the use of complementary therapies," *Australian Family Physician* 39 (2010): 638–40.

21 NP Spanos et al., "Hypnosis, placebo, and suggestion in the treatment of warts," *Psychosomatic Medicine* 50, no. 3 (1988): 245–60.

22 C Clarey, "Olympians use imagery as mental training," *New York Times*, February 22, 2014.

23 K Crider et al., "Antibacterial medication use during pregnancy and risk of birth defects: National Birth Defects Prevention Study," *Archives of Pediatrics and Adolescent Medicine* 163, no. 11 (2009): 978–85. doi:10.1001/archpediatrics.2009.188.

24 M Pae et al., "The role of nutrition in enhancing immunity in aging," *Aging Disorders* 3, no. 1 (2012): 91–129.

25 "Key facts about influenza (flu) and flu vaccine," CDC, http://www.cdc.gov/flu/keyfacts.htm.

26 "Cold facts," McKinley Health Center, http://www.mckinley.illinois.edu/handouts/cold_facts.htm.

27 B Barrett et al., "Echinacea for treating the common cold," *Annals of Internal Medicine* 153 (2010): 769–77.

28 A Yamshchikov et al., "Vitamin D for treatment and prevention of infectious diseases: a systematic review of randomized controlled trials," *Endocrine Practice* 15, no. 5 (2009): 438–49.

29 JA Beard et al., "Vitamin D and the anti-viral state," *Journal of Clinical Virology* 50, no. 3 (2011): 194–200.

30 LK Mischley et al., "Safety survey of intranasal glutathione," *Journal of Alternative and Complementary Medicine* 19, no. 5 (2013): 459–63. doi:10.1089/acm.2011.0673.

31 KH Kyung, "Antimicrobial properties of allium species," *Current Opinion in Biotechnology* 23, no. 2 (2012):142–47. doi:10.1016/j.copbio.2011.08.004.

32 JP Anthony et al., "Plant active components—a resource for antiparasitic agents?," *Trends in Parasitology* 21 (2005): 462–68.

33 JP Heggers et al., "The effectiveness of processed grapefruit-seed extract as an antibacterial agent," *Journal of Alternative and Complementary Medicine* 8 (2002): 333–40.

34 X Su and DH D'Souza, "Grape seed extract for control of human enteric viruses," *Applied and Environmental Microbiology* 77, no. 12 (2011): 3982–87. doi:10.1128/AEM.00193-11.

35 A Altintas et al., "Characterization of volatile constituents from *Origanum onites* and their antifungal and antibacterial activity," *Journal of JAOAC International* 96, no. 6 (2013): 1200–8.

36 M Force et al., "Inhibition of enteric parasites by emulsified oil of oregano in vivo," *Phytotherapy Research* 14 (2000): 213–14.

37 "Goldenseal," Natural Medicines Comprehensive Database, www.naturaldatabase.com.

38 S Clement-Kruzei et al., "Immune modulation of macrophage pro-inflammatory response by goldenseal and astragalus extracts," *Journal of Medicinal Food* 11, no. 3 (2008): 493–98. doi:10.1089/jmf.2008.0044.

39 P Abidi et al., "The medicinal plant goldenseal is a natural LDL-lowering agent with multiple bioactive components and new action mechanisms," *Journal of Lipid Research* 47, no. 10 (2006): 2134-47.

40 "Licorice root," National Center for Complementary and Alternative Medicine, http://nccam.nih.gov/health/licoriceroot.

41 CM Bitler et al., "Olive extract supplement decreases pain and improves daily activities in adults with osteoarthritis and decreases plasma homocysteine in those with rheumatoid arthritis," *Nutrition Research* 27 (2007): 470–77.

42 Z Atai et al., "Efficacy of olive leaf extract in the treatment of minor oral aphthous ulcers," *American Journal of Infectious Diseases* 3, no. 1 (2007): 24–26.

43 KM Ahmed, "The effect of olive leaf extract in decreasing the expression of two pro-inflammatory cytokines in patients receiving chemotherapy for cancer. A randomized clinical trial," *Saudi Dental Journal* 25, no. 4 (2013): 141–47. doi:10.1016/j.sdentj.2013.09.001.

44 ME McNeil et al., "What are the risks associated with formula feeding? A re-analysis and review," *Breastfeeding Review* 18 (2010): 25–32.

45 J Barnett et al., "Low zinc status: a new risk factor for pneumonia in the elderly?" *Nutrition Reviews* 68, no. 1 (2010): 30–37.

46 WC Fischer and RE Black, "Zinc and the risk for infectious disease," *Annual Review of Nutrition* 24 (2004): 255–75.

47 http://www.advantagenutrition.us/nutricology-gastromycin-caps--150.htm.

48 "Cranberry juice fights urinary tract infections quickly," WebMD, http://www.webmd.com/women/news/20100823/cranberry-juice-fights-urinary-tract-infection-quickly.

49 S Altarac and D Papes, "Use of D-mannose in prophylaxis of recurrent urinary tract infections (UTIs) in women," *British Journal of Urology International* 113 (2014): 9–10. doi:10.1111/bju.12492.

50 KA Workowski and S Berman, "Sexually transmitted diseases treatment guidelines, 2010," *MMWR Recommendations and Reports* 59, RR-12 (2010): 1–110.

51 RS Griffith et al., "Success of L-lysine therapy in frequently recurrent herpes simplex infection: treatment and prophylaxis," *Dermatologica* 175 (1987): 183–90.

52 Loyola University Health System, "Shingles: a common and painful virus," *ScienceDaily*, February 26, 2014, www.sciencedaily.com/releases/2014/02/140226132752.htm.

53 AM Elvis and JS Ekta, "Ozone therapy: A clinical review," *Journal of Natural Science, Biology, and Medicine* 2 (2011): 66–70. doi:10.4103/0976-9668.82319.

54 S Zaky et al., "Preliminary results of ozone therapy as a possible treatment for patients with chronic hepatitis C," *Journal of Alternative and Complementary Medicine* 17, no. 3 (2011): 59–63. doi:10.1089/acm.2010.0016.

55 M Nermes et al., "Is there a role for probiotics in the prevention or treatment of food allergy?" *Current Allergy and Asthma Reports* 13, no. 6 (2013): 622–30.

56 AM Patterson et al., "Perceived stress predicts allergy flares," *Annals of Allergy, Asthma, and Immunology* 112, no. 4 (2014): 317–21. doi:10.1016/j.anai.2013.07.013.

57 ZQ Toh et al., "Probiotic therapy as a novel approach for allergic disease," *Frontiers in Pharmacology* 3 (2012). doi:10.3389/fphar.2012.00171.

58 RD Gray, "Effects of butterbur treatment in intermittent allergic rhinitis: a placebo-controlled evaluation," *Annals of Allergy, Asthma, and Immunology* 93, (2004): 56–60.

59 M Saeedi et al., "The treatment of atopic dermatitis with licorice gel," *Journal of Dermatological Treatment* 14, (2003): 153–57.

60 UC Danesch, "*Petasites hybridus* (Butterbur root) extract in the treatment of asthma—an open trial," *Alternative Medicine Review* 9, no. 1 (2004): 54–62.

61 L Mehl-Madrona, "Augmentation of conventional medical management of moderately severe or severe asthma with acupuncture and guided imagery/meditation, *Permanente Journal* 12, no. 4 (2008): 9–14.

62 Kiecolt-Glaser, "Stress, inflammation, and yoga practice."

63 Ö Özdemir, "Any role for probiotics in the therapy or prevention of autoimmune diseases? Up-to-date review," *Journal of Complementary and Integrative Medicine* 10, no. 1 (2013): 229–50. doi:10.1515/jcim-2012-0054.

64 E Laird et al., "Vitamin D deficiency is associated with inflammation in older Irish adults," *Journal of Clinical Endocrinology and Metabolism* 99, no. 5(2014): 1807–15. doi:10.1210/jc.2013-3507.

65 A Antico et al., "Can supplementation with vitamin D reduce the risk or modify the course of autoimmune diseases? A systematic review of the literature," *Autoimmune Reviews* 12, no. 2 (2012): 127–36. doi:10.1016/j.autrev.2012.07.007.

66 CS Zipitis and AK Akobeng, "Vitamin D supplementation in early childhood and risk of type 1 diabetes: a systematic review and meta-analysis," *Archives of Disease in Childhood* 93, no. 6 (2008): 512–17. doi:10.1136/adc.2007.128579.

67 AP Simopoulus, "Omega-3 fatty acids in inflammation and autoimmune diseases," *Journal of the American College of Nutrition* 21, no. 6 (2002): 495–505. doi:10.1080/07315724.2002.10719248.

68 RK Dissanayake and JV Bertouch, "Psychosocial interventions as adjunct therapy for patients with rheumatoid arthritis: a systematic review," *International Journal of Rheumatoid Disease* 13, no. 4 (2010): 324–34. doi:10.1111/j.1756-185X.2010.01563.x.

69 A Belluzzi et al., "Polyunsaturated fatty acids and inflammatory bowel disease," *American Journal of Clinical Nutrition* 71, suppl. (2000): 339S–42S.

70 B Chandran and A Goel, "A randomized, pilot study to assess the efficacy and safety of curcumin in patients with active rheumatoid arthritis," *Phytotherapy Research* 26(2012): 1719–25. doi:10.1002/ptr.4639.

71 NY Tang et al., "The anti-inflammatory effect of paeoniflorin on cerebral infarction induced by ischemia-reperfusion injury in Sprague-Dawley rats," *American Journal of Chinese Medicine* 38, no. 1 (2010): 51–64.

72 Z Rosman et al., "Biologic therapy for autoimmune diseases: an update," *BMC Medicine* 11 (2013): 88–92.

73 K White, "Safely manage autoimmune diseases," *Life Extension*, March/April 2014, 24–32.

74 W Zhang et al., "Mechanisms involved in the therapeutic effects of *Paeonia* in rheumatoid arthritis," *International Immunopharmacology* 14, no. 1 (2012): 27–31.

75 D Leverone and BJ Epstein, "Nonpharmacological interventions for the treatment of rheumatoid arthritis: a focus on mind-body medicine," *Journal of Pharmacy Practice* 23, no. 2 (2010): 101–9. doi:10.1177/0897190009360025; RK Dissanayake and JV Bertouch, "Psychosocial interventions as adjunct therapy for patients with rheumatoid arthritis: a systematic review," *International Journal of Rheumatic Disease* 13, no. 4 (2010): 324–34. doi:10.1111/j.1756-185X.2010.01563.x.

76 JK Smyth et al., "Effects of writing about stressful experiences on symptom reduction in patients with asthma or rheumatoid arthritis," *Journal of the American Medical Association* 281 (1999): 1304–9.

77 F Almutawa et al., "Systematic review of UV-based therapy for psoriasis," *American Journal of Clinical Dermatology* 14 (2013): 87–109. doi:10.1007/s40257-013-0015-y.

78 A Paradisi et al., "Effect of written emotional disclosure interventions in persons with psoriasis undergoing narrow band ultraviolet B phototherapy," *European Journal of Dermatology* 20 (2010): 599–605. doi:10.1684/ejd.2010.1018.

79 SA Gaylord et al., "Mindfulness training reduces the severity of irritable bowel syndrome in women: results of a randomized controlled trial," *American Journal of Gastroenterology* 106 (2011): 1678–88.

80 I Gupta et al., "Effects of gum resin of *Boswellia serrata* in patients with chronic colitis," *Planta Medica* 67 (2001): 391–95.

81 J Salazar et al., "Glucosamine for osteoarthritis: biological effects, clinical efficacy, and safety on glucose metabolism," *Arthritis* 2014:432463 (2014).

82 CK Kwoh et al., "Effect of oral glucosamine on joint structure in individuals with chronic knee pain: a randomized, placebo-controlled clinical trial," *Arthritis Rheumatology* 66, no. 4 (2014): 930–39. doi:10.1002/art.38314.

83 D Leverone and DB Epstein, "Nonpharmacological interventions for the treatment of rheumatoid arthritis: a focus on mind-body medicine," *Journal of Pharmacy Practice* 23, no. 2 (2010): 101–19. doi:10.1177/0897190009360025.

84 N Kimmatkar et al., "Efficacy and tolerability of *Boswellia serrata* extract in treatment of osteoarthritis of knee—a randomized double blind placebo controlled trial," *Phytomedicine* 10 (2003): 3–7.

85 JN Schad, "Stress caused adverse entanglement of the nervous and autoimmune systems: a case for MS," *Medical Hypotheses* 80 no. 2 (2013): 156–57. doi:10.1016/j.mehy.2012.11.016.

86 V Yadav et al., "Use and self-reported benefit of complementary and alternative medicine among multiple sclerosis patients," *International Journal of Multiple Sclerosis Care* 8 (2006): 5–10.

87 A Senders et al., "Mind-body medicine for multiple sclerosis: a systematic review," *Autoimmune Diseases* 2012:567324 (2012). doi:10.1155/2012/567324.

88 CM Greco et al., "Updated review of complementary and alternative medicine treatments for systemic lupus erythematosus," *Current Rheumatology Reports* 15, no. 11 (2013): 378. doi:10.1007/s11926-013-0378-3.

Chapter 8

1 S Agarwal, "Just add water: 3 delicious, totally-sippable metabolism boosters," IVillage, November 21, 2013, http://www.ivillage.com/boost-your-metabolism-and-burn-more-calories/4-a-546347.

INDEX

B

Bacterial infections, 22, 66, 70, 71
Barrett, Sondra, background of, viii–ix
B cells, **6**, 11, 12, <u>12</u>, **13**, 15
Be a Bird (Wing Waves), 192
Be a Wave (Core Wave), 192, **192**
Beef, grass-fed, 123
Belly Boost, 185, **185**
Benson, Herbert, 147, <u>148</u>
Beta-carotene, 98–99, <u>103</u>, <u>110</u>
Beverages, 294
  Beet-Orange Bliss, 295
  in I-PEP diet, <u>122</u>
  Mango-Strawberry Power-Up, 295
  Morning Energy Drink, 296
  Nut Milks—Almond, Cashew, Coconut, 294
  Tropical Fruit Smoothie, 296
  water variations, <u>297</u>
Biologics, drugs vs., <u>90</u>
Bladder infections, <u>65</u>. *See also* Urinary tract
      infections (UTIs)
Body scan exercise, <u>211</u>, 213
Bone loss, 135
Bone marrow, as immune organ, 3, 14, **14**
Boswellia, <u>203</u>, <u>204</u>, 235, 236
Brain, exercise improving, 168
Breakfasts, 239
  Hearty Oatmeal, 239
  Nice Rice, 240
  ProBowl, 240
  Scrambled Tofu with Turmeric, 241
  Toasted Oat Muesli, 243
  Veggie Frittata, 242
Bromelain, <u>203</u>, 212
Bronchitis
  causes of, 72, 197–98
  treatments for, 73–74, 220
Burst training, as exercise, 167–68
Butterbur, 227, 228
B vitamins, 133. *See also* Vitamin B$_5$; Vitamin B$_6$;
      Vitamin B$_{12}$
  absorption of, 134
  for immune support, 98, 101
  sources of, 101, 102, <u>103</u>

C

Caffeine, eliminating, 125
Calcium supplements, 135
Cancer, causes of, <u>58–59</u>
Cancer patients, qigong for, 180
Candida albicans, 22, <u>53</u>
Canker sores, 218, 222
Carbohydrates, improving sleep, <u>164</u>
Case studies, <u>64</u>, <u>65</u>
Cayenne pepper, 113
CBT, for stress management, 153–54
Celiac disease, 12, 13, 14, <u>44</u>, <u>51</u>, 87, 229–30

Change, hardiness principles for, <u>198</u>
Chemical exposure, reducing, <u>207</u>
Chicken pox, 177, 179, 222–23
Chi gung. *See* Qigong
Childre, Doc, 153
Chocolate, dark, as antioxidant, <u>104</u>
Chocolate allergy, <u>33</u>
Cholesterol reduction, <u>32</u>
Cinnamon, 113–14
Cleanse, 5-day juice, 124–25, <u>303</u>
Clove, 114
Coenzyme Q10 (CoQ10), 98, 105, 135, <u>203</u>, <u>204</u>
Coffee, eliminating, <u>124</u>
Cognitive behavioral therapy (CBT), 153–54
Cohen, Nicholas, 144
Colds, 60
  allergies vs., <u>39</u>
  exercise and, <u>171</u>
  preventing, 214–16
  treatments for, 66, 71–72, 219
Comfort foods, identifying, <u>119</u>
Cool Down Inflammation Prevention Program, xi,
      233
  components of
    gut healing, 205–6
    herbs and supplements, 202, <u>203</u>, 204, <u>204</u>
    mind-body techniques, 202
    nutrition, 201–2
  for infection protection, 214–18
  overview of, 206–7, <u>208–9</u>, <u>210–11</u>
  personalizing, 207, 210
  reducing chemical exposure in, <u>207</u>
  for specific conditions
    allergies, 224–30
    autoimmune diseases, 230–37
    chronic pain, 210–13
    diabetes, 235
    infections, 218–23
  success stories about, <u>32</u>, <u>75</u>, <u>106</u>
CoQ10. *See* Coenzyme Q10
Corticosteroids, <u>85</u>
Cortisol, as stress hormone, 139–40
Cough medicines, 71, 72
Cranberry juice and extracts, for urinary tract
      infections, 221
C-reactive protein (CRP), <u>52</u>, 174
Crohn's disease, 49, <u>50</u>, 234–35
Cultured foods, in I-PEP diet, <u>122</u>
Curcumin, <u>203</u>, 204, 232, 236. *See also* Turmeric
Cystitis. *See* Urinary tract infections (UTIs)
Cytokines, 3, 13, 20–21, <u>21</u>, 64, 140, 161, 174, 232

D

Dendritic cells, **6**, 10, 11
Depression, 141
Desserts
  Baked Apples, 287
  Blackberry-Ginger-Apple Crisp, 291

G

GALT, 20
Garlic, 95, 114, 217
Garlic/mullein flower ear oil, 220
Garlic oil, making, 114
Gastrointestinal tract, 19–20, 205–6, 230
Gastromycin, for digestive health, 221
Gender
    autoimmune disease and, 47–48
    unbalanced immune system and, 26
Gene expression, ix, 45, 53
Gene mutations, 7, 58, 59
Genes, immune imbalance and, 27–28, 27
Genetics, autoimmune disease and, 46
Ginger, 115, 203
Glaser, Ronald, 141
Glucosamine, 201, 235–36
Glutathione, 102, 105, 203, 216, 220
Gluten, 42–43, 44, 120
Gluten-free products, 44, 87, 120, 230
Gluten sensitivity, 44, 87, 119–20
Goals, writing about, 199
Goldenseal, 218
Grains, in I-PEP diet, 122
Grapefruit seed extract (GSE), 218
Grass-fed beef, 123
Gratitude, journaling about, 207
Graves' disease, 49, 50, 89
GSE, 218
Guided imagery, for stress management, 150, 152, 206, 213, 229
Gut-associated lymphoid tissue (GALT), 20

H

Haas, Elson, background of, viii, ix
Hardiness principles, 198
Hashimoto's thyroiditis, 49, 50, 53, 88
    treatments for, 68, 88–89, 233–34
Hay fever, natural treatments for, 226–28
Head Tap, 183, **183**
Health concerns, identifying, 196–99
Hepatitis
    treatments for, 80–81, 223
    types of, 79–80
Herbal medicine, 62. See also Herbs
Herbal teas, for improving sleep, 165
Herbs
    for cooking, 96
    in Cool Down Program, 203, 204, 204, 210
    immune-boosting, 95, 112–14, 116–17, 116
    in I-PEP diet, 122
Herpes infections, 61, 77–78
    treatments for, 78, 222, 223
Histamine, 8, 36, 117–18
HIV/AIDS, 81–82
HLAs, 28
Holmes, Thomas, 142, 143

Holmes and Rahe Stress Scale, 142, 143
Honey treatment, for allergies, 225
Human leukocyte antigens (HLAs), 28
Hygiene, for preventing infection, 215
Hygiene hypothesis, 39, 47
Hyperactive immune states, 5, 26, 28, 29, 33, 230.
    See also specific conditions

I

IBD. *See* Inflammatory bowel disease
IBS, 235
IgA, 15, 155, 156
IgE, 15
IgE antibodies, 35, **35**, 36, 43
IgG, 15
IgG antibodies, 43
IgM, 15
Illness, immune imbalance from, 27, 30
Imagery
    guided, 150, 152, 206, 213, 229
    uses for, xi, 212, 213, 227, 233
Immune cells, **6**. *See also* Lymphocytes;
    Phagocytes
    functions of, 14, 64
    in gut, 19–20
    influences on, 3
    interactions of, 11–13
    T and B lymphocytes, 11
Immune communications system, 20–22
Immune Diaries subjects
    asthma attacks, 42
    chocolate allergy, 33
    cold and sore throat treatment, 217
    conditioning by physical senses, 145
    diarrhea from stress, 142
    exercise, 175
    exercise breaks, 169
    Gastromycin for digestive protection, 221
    imagery for managing allergies, 152
    inflammation from a splinter, 10
    meditative toning, 159
    qigong, 182, 188
    seven key foods, 96
    sleep quality, 162, 163
Immune network, **4**, 5–11
Immune-Power Eating Plan. *See* I-PEP program
Immune Power 5-Day Cleanse, 124–25, 303
Immune system
    aging of, 56–57
    cancer and, 59
    effect of stress on, 143–46, 171–72
    environmental effects on, xi–xii
    healthy, protection from, xii, 2, 62
    organs of, 14–20
    overview of, 2–5
    quick guide to, 12, **13**
    stress weakening, 1

Vitamin E
    caution with, 91
    choosing supplement form of, 134–35
    correct dose of, 204
    immune functions of, 99–100
    selenium and, 102
    sources of, 103
    zinc and, 101
Vitiligo, 50
Vollaard, Niels, 167

W

Walking, 168, 181
Wash Your Face with Qi, 183, **183**
Water
    flavoring, 297
    for hydration, 122
Weight loss
    I-PEP program for, 125, 132
    success story about, 32
What's Your Outlook on Life? questionnaire, 154, 155
Wheat allergies, 42–45, 44, 229–30
White blood cells, 3, 71. *See also* Lymphocytes; Phagocytes
Whole Body Wake-Up Tap, 187

Whooping cough, 56
Worm infections, preventing allergies, 39–40
Writing
    emotional disclosure, 202, 207, 210, 229, 232–33, 234
    about goals, 199
    for stress management, 159–60

Y

Yeasts, infections from, 22–23, 74
Yoga, 176–77, 202
Yogurt, probiotics in, 110

Z

Zinc
    excessive, 97
    for immune function, 97, 98, 101, 110
    as natural treatment for
        colds and flu, 219
        Hashimoto's thyroiditis, 233
        pneumonia, 220
    for preventing infections, 215
    sources of, 101, 103, 110
    as supplement, 126, 133, 134, 135, 203, 204, 204
Zinc deficiency, 27, 101, 101, 220